T0337465

THE WASHINGTON MANUAL®
OF DERMATOLOGY
DIAGNOSTICS

M. Laurin Council, MD

Assistant Professor of Medicine
Division of Dermatology
Department of Internal Medicine
Washington University School of Medicine
St. Louis, Missouri

David M. Sheinbein, MD

Associate Professor of Medicine
Division of Dermatology
Department of Internal Medicine
Washington University School of Medicine
St. Louis, Missouri

Lynn A. Cornelius, MD

The Winifred and Emma Showman
Professor of Dermatology in Medicine
Division of Dermatology
Department of Internal Medicine
Washington University School of Medicine
St. Louis, Missouri

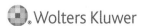

Philadelphia • Baltimore • New York • London
Buenos Aires • Hong Kong • Sydney • Tokyo

Executive Editor: Kel McGowan
Senior Product Development Editor: Kristina Oberle
Production Project Manager: Bridgett Dougherty
Design Coordinator: Teresa Mallon
Senior Manufacturing Coordinator: Beth Welsh
Prepress Vendor: SPi Global

9 8 7 6 5 4 3 2 1

Printed in China

Library of Congress Cataloging-in-Publication Data
The Washington manual of dermatology diagnostics / [edited by] M. Laurin Council, David M. Sheinbein, Lynn A. Cornelius.
    p. ; cm.
  Manual of dermatology diagnostics
  Includes bibliographical references.
  ISBN 978-1-4963-2317-0
 I. Council, M. Laurin, editor. II. Sheinbein, David M., editor. III. Cornelius, Lynn A., editor. IV. Washington University (Saint Louis, Mo.). School of Medicine, sponsoring body. V. Title: Manual of dermatology diagnostics.
  [DNLM: 1. Skin Diseases—diagnosis. 2. Integumentary System—pathology. WR 141]
  RL74
  616.5—dc23

                                             2015028761

To Arthur Eisen, MD, our mentor and friend.

Contributors

Milan J. Anadkat, MD
Associate Professor of Medicine
Division of Dermatology
Department of Internal Medicine
Washington University School of Medicine
St. Louis, Missouri

Susan J. Bayliss, MD
Professor of Medicine
Division of Dermatology
Department of Internal Medicine
Washington University School of Medicine
St. Louis, Missouri

Emily M. Beck, MD
Division of Dermatology
Department of Internal Medicine
Washington University School of Medicine
St. Louis, Missouri

Rachel L. Braden, MD
Division of Dermatology
Department of Internal Medicine
Washington University School of Medicine
St. Louis, Missouri

Kimberly L. Brady, MD
Division of Dermatology
Department of Internal Medicine
Washington University School of Medicine
St. Louis, Missouri

David Y. Chen, MD, PhD
Division of Dermatology
Department of Internal Medicine
Washington University School of Medicine
St. Louis, Missouri

Rebecca Chibnall, MD
Division of Dermatology
Department of Internal Medicine
Washington University School of Medicine
St. Louis, Missouri

Lynn A. Cornelius, MD
The Winifred and Emma Showman
  Professor of Dermatology in Medicine
Division of Dermatology
Department of Internal Medicine
Washington University School of Medicine
St. Louis, Missouri

M. Laurin Council, MD
Assistant Professor of Medicine
Division of Dermatology
Department of Internal Medicine
Washington University School of Medicine
St. Louis, Missouri

Shadmehr Demehri, MD, PhD
Division of Dermatology
Department of Internal Medicine
Washington University School of Medicine
St. Louis, Missouri

Kyle Eash, MD, PhD
Division of Dermatology
Department of Internal Medicine
Washington University School of Medicine
St. Louis, Missouri

Arthur Eisen, MD
Professor of Medicine
Division of Dermatology
Department of Internal Medicine
Washington University School of Medicine
St. Louis, Missouri

Shayna Gordon, MD
Division of Dermatology
Department of Internal Medicine
Washington University School of Medicine
St. Louis, Missouri

Ian Hornstra, MD, PhD
Assistant Professor of Medicine
Division of Dermatology
Department of Internal Medicine
Washington University School of Medicine
St. Louis, Missouri

Eva A. Hurst, MD
Associate Professor of Medicine
Division of Dermatology
Department of Internal Medicine
Washington University School of Medicine
St. Louis, Missouri

Heather Jones, MD
Division of Dermatology
Department of Internal Medicine
Washington University School of Medicine
St. Louis, Missouri

Monique Gupta Kumar, MD, MPhil
Assistant Professor
Departments of Dermatology and Pediatrics
Emory University School of Medicine
Atlanta, Georgia

Sena J. Lee, MD, PhD
Assistant Professor of Medicine
Division of Dermatology
Department of Internal Medicine
Washington University School of Medicine
St. Louis, Missouri

Caroline Mann, MD
Assistant Professor of Medicine
Division of Dermatology
Department of Internal Medicine
Washington University School of Medicine
St. Louis, Missouri

Ann G. Martin, MD
Associate Professor of Medicine
Division of Dermatology
Department of Internal Medicine
Washington University School of Medicine
St. Louis, Missouri

Katherine M. Moritz, MD
Division of Dermatology
Department of Internal Medicine
Washington University School of Medicine
St. Louis, Missouri

Jamie L. Mull, MD
Division of Dermatology
Department of Internal Medicine
Washington University School of Medicine
St. Louis, Missouri

Amy Musiek, MD
Assistant Professor of Medicine
Division of Dermatology
Department of Internal Medicine
Washington University School of Medicine
St. Louis, Missouri

Kathleen Nemer, MD
Division of Dermatology
Department of Internal Medicine
Washington University School of Medicine
St. Louis, Missouri

Urvi Patel, MD
Assistant Professor of Medicine
Division of Dermatology
Department of Internal Medicine
Washington University School of Medicine
St. Louis, Missouri

David M. Sheinbein, MD
Associate Professor of Medicine
Division of Dermatology
Department of Internal Medicine
Washington University School of Medicine
St. Louis, Missouri

Shaanan Shetty, MD
Division of Dermatology
Department of Internal Medicine
Washington University School of Medicine
St. Louis, Missouri

Karl Staser, MD, PhD
Division of Dermatology
Department of Internal Medicine
Washington University School of Medicine
St. Louis, Missouri

Kara Sternhell-Blackwell, MD
Assistant Professor of Medicine
Division of Dermatology
Department of Internal Medicine
Washington University School of Medicine
St. Louis, Missouri

Shivani V. Tripathi, MD
Division of Dermatology
Department of Internal Medicine
Washington University School of Medicine
St. Louis, Missouri

Christopher R. Urban, MD
Division of Dermatology
Department of Internal Medicine
Washington University School of Medicine
St. Louis, Missouri

Jason P. Burnham, MD
Department of Internal Medicine
Division of Infectious Diseases
Washington University School of Medicine
St. Louis, Missouri

Preface

Now is an exciting time to study the skin. New targeted therapies are emerging for severe forms of common conditions, such as psoriasis and urticaria. More advances have been made in the treatment of the most deadly skin cancer, melanoma, in the past 5 years than in the previous decades. On the cosmetic side, laser technology and the use of botulinum toxin have evolved to reverse the signs of aging. Now, more than ever, we are gaining greater insight into the science behind skin conditions and therefore developing novel therapeutic modalities.

Whether you are a medical student aspiring to become a dermatologist, an intern rotating through hospital wards, a primary care physician treating patients with skin concerns, or a specialist aiming to garner a greater understanding of dermatology, we hope that you will find this book to be a valuable resource. The *Washington Manual of Dermatology Diagnostics* covers the fundamentals of the study of the skin, hair, and nails. Basics, such as terminology used when describing skin lesion morphology and important steps of the skin exam, are covered in the first chapter. The structural importance of the skin and normal skin function are described in Chapter 2.

Chapters 3 to 10 describe the most common skin conditions, which one will encounter in medicine. Chapters 11 to 13 each elaborate on subspecialties of dermatology: dermatologic surgery, pediatric dermatology, and geriatric dermatology, respectively. This book also covers the importance of skin cancer prevention with sun protection (Chapter 14), common therapies used in dermatology (Chapter 15), and ends with a useful differential diagnosis reference (Chapter 16). We trust that you will find the information contained in the ensuing pages helpful in the care of your patients.

This manual would not be possible without the dedicated medical students, residents, and faculty of Washington University. We thank you for the countless hours of reviewing the literature and succinctly summarizing the most pertinent facts for this text, and we thank you for contributing classic examples of conditions from your image collections. Finally, and most importantly, we would like to thank the patients of our clinics and hospitals, for allowing us the opportunity to learn from you and allowing us to share what we have learned with others.

M. Laurin Council, MD

Contents

5 Reactive Disorders and Drug Eruptions 89

Shivani V. Tripathi, MD and Milan J. Anadkat, MD

6 Disorders of Pigmentation 117

Shaanan Shetty, MD and Caroline Mann, MD

7 Benign Skin Lesions 126
Shayna Gordon, MD and M. Laurin Council, MD

- Nevi
- Seborrheic Keratoses
- Acrochordons
- Angiomas
- Dermatofibroma
- Lentigines
- Sebaceous Hyperplasia
- Keloids
- Cysts
- Lipomas

8 Malignant Skin Lesions 137
David Y. Chen, MD, PhD, Amy Musiek, MD, and Lynn A. Cornelius, MD

- Basal Cell Carcinoma
- Squamous Cell Carcinoma and Actinic Keratoses
- Melanoma
- Cutaneous T-Cell Lymphoma

9 Disorders of the Hair and Nails 152
Katherine M. Moritz, MD and Ann G. Martin, MD

- Androgenetic Alopecia
- Alopecia Areata
- Telogen Effluvium
- Anagen Effluvium
- Trichotillomania
- Central Centrifugal Cicatricial Alopecia
- Discoid Lupus Erythematosus (see Chapter 10)
- Lichen Planopilaris
- Dissecting Cellulitis
- Folliculitis Decalvans
- Secondary Scarring Alopecias
- Hypertrichosis
- Hirsutism
- Nail Disorders

10 Cutaneous Manifestations of Systemic Disease 169

Urvi Patel, MD and Amy Musiek, MD

- **Lupus**
- **Dermatomyositis**
- **Sarcoidosis**
- **Scleroderma and Related Disorders**
- **Bullous Disorders**
- **Nutritional Deficiencies**

11 Dermatologic Surgery 183

Christopher R. Urban, MD and Eva A. Hurst, MD

- **Preoperative Assessment**
- **Procedural Techniques**
- **Wound Dressings**
- **Wound Healing**
- **Surgical Complications**

12 Pediatric Dermatology 199

Monique Gupta Kumar, MD, MPhil, Kara Sternhell-Blackwell, MD, and Susan J. Bayliss, MD

- **Neonatal and Infantile Dermatology**
- **Neonatal Acne (Cephalic Pustulosis)**
- **Aplasia Cutis Congenita**
- **Erythema Toxicum Neonatorum**
- **Milia**
- **Miliaria**
- **Nevus Sebaceus**
- **Subcutaneous Fat Necrosis**
- **Transient Neonatal Pustular Melanosis**
- **Pigmented Lesions**
- **Café Au Lait Macules**
- **Congenital Dermal Melanocytosis (Mongolian Spot)**
- **Congenital Melanocytic Nevi**
- **Spitz Nevus**
- **Vascular Lesions**
- **Capillary Malformation (Port-Wine Stain)**

- Cutis Marmorata Telangiectatica Congenita
- Infantile Hemangioma
- Nevus Simplex
- Dermatitis
- Atopic Dermatitis
- Contact Dermatitis (Allergic)
- Diaper Dermatitis
- Seborrheic Dermatitis
- Infectious Diseases
- Tinea
- Verrucae
- Molluscum Contagiosum
- Miscellaneous
- Acne Vulgaris
- Erythema Multiforme

13 Geriatric Dermatology 222
Kathleen Nemer, MD and David M. Sheinbein, MD

- Actinic Purpura
- Erythema Ab Igne
- Leg Ulcers
- Skin Maceration
- Xerosis/Pruritus

14 Sun Safety 239
Rachel L. Braden, MD and Kimberly L. Brady, MD

- Sunscreens

15 Dermatologic Therapies 246
Kyle Eash, MD, PhD and Ian Hornstra, MD, PhD

- Topical Therapy Overview
- Glucocorticosteroids
- Retinoids
- Phototherapy
- Selected Antimicrobials
- Topical Immunomodulators and Chemotherapeutics
- Systemic Immunosuppressive and Immunomodulatory Agents

The Skin Exam

Rebecca Chibnall, MD, Susan J. Bayliss, MD, and
Arthur Eisen, MD

Unlike other medical disciples, dermatology is a predominantly visual field. By directly observing and palpating the skin, one can obtain vital information, which can lead to the correct diagnosis and treatment. Pointed questions and, occasionally, ancillary tests, are also useful to this regard. This chapter covers the nuances of examination of the skin.

1. DERMATOLOGIC HISTORY

- History of present illness
  - In most medical specialties, a thorough history is obtained first from the patient followed by a physical exam. In dermatology, the physical exam is essential to achieving a diagnosis, so it is best to obtain the medical history before, during, and after physical examination. Key questions to ask include the following:
    - "How long?"
    - "Does it hurt or itch?"
    - "What treatments have you tried?"
    - "Have you had any other symptoms?"
- Past medical history
  - Obtaining a focused past medical history is also essential to the dermatologic exam. Questions that are helpful to ask include, "Have you had similar rashes before?" This may assist in the diagnosis, and if previous treatments have been employed, they may assist in treatment as well. Prior to prescribing any systemic medications, other illnesses should be documented.

2. INDICATIONS FOR TOTAL-BODY SKIN EXAM

- In 2009, the U.S. Preventive Services Task Force (USPSTF) reported insufficient evidence for or against screening for skin cancer at any age. These recommendations are currently under review, and a new statement is anticipated in the near future.[1] The 2009 report did, however, suggest risk assessing for the following:
  - Patients with history of extensive sun exposure or sunburn
  - Patients with fair skin over age 65
  - Patients with clinically atypical nevi
  - Patients with more than 50 nevi
- In 2012, the USPSTF gave a grade "B" recommendation to the practice of counseling fair-skinned children, adolescents, and young adults ages 10 to 24 about reducing their risk of skin cancer. They concluded that "insufficient" evidence existed for similar counseling for adults.[2]

- Our recommendations are that any fair-skinned individual who has had considerable sun exposure during the early periods of his or her life needs to be examined at least yearly. Individuals who have numerous nevi should also be examined annually. Additionally, patients with a family history of melanoma in a first-degree relative also warrant an annual skin exam. Patients should be instructed in the ABCDEs of melanoma, which are as follows:
  - A—Asymmetry
  - B—Border irregularity
  - C—Color variation
  - D—Diameter > 6 mm (the size of a pencil eraser)
  - E—Evolution

3. EXAMINATION TOOLS

- Potassium hydroxide mount (Fig. 1-1)
  - This technique is useful for diagnosing dermatophyte infections and can be easily employed in any clinic equipped with a microscope. The following steps will ensure an adequate and clinically helpful sample:
    - Hold a microscope slide perpendicular to the skin just inferior to the area identified for scraping. Using a 15-blade scalpel, vigorously scrape the scale from the edge of the lesion onto the slide.
    - Apply a cover slip to the portion of the slide with scale pieces. Place 1 to 2 drops of 20% KOH with dimethylsulfoxide (DMSO) beneath the coverslip so that the entire field is covered.
    - Blot excess KOH with a paper towel. This allows the scale to be evenly distributed and prevents KOH from coming into contact with the microscope objective
    - Scan the slide at low power (10×) searching for fungal elements, which appear as refractile, large, branching hyphae that cross cell membranes.
    - Higher-power examination of a suspicious area (40×) confirms the diagnosis.
  - This technique may also be used for diagnosis of scabies. Vigorous scraping of suspected burrows or papules should be performed in order to maximize the ability to find the mite.
- Culture
  - Occasionally, lesions will present with crust, purulent drainage, or ulceration. If infection is suspected, a culture swab may be taken in an attempt to identify the causative organism. If crust is present, it should be removed and the exudate below swabbed for aerobic culture. Fungal cultures may also be performed in this way; however, if a deeper tissue infection is suspected, a tissue biopsy and culture will have greater yield.
  - Cultures or PCR may also be performed for viruses such as herpes simplex and varicella-zoster. Viral transport medium must be used, and vesicles should be deroofed or crust removed. The serum at the base should be vigorously swabbed to give the highest possible yield. PCR results can be available relatively quickly, whereas culture results generally take 7 to 10 days.
- Biopsy
  - The gold standard for precise diagnosis of many skin conditions remains tissue biopsy. The two most commonly employed techniques are shave biopsy (Fig. 1-2)

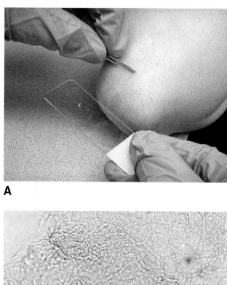

A

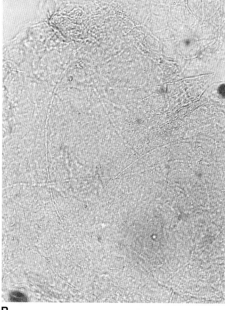

B

Figure 1-1. A: Skin scraping for a potassium hydroxide preparation. **B:** Positive prep for hyphae and yeast forms. (Courtesy of David Sheinbein.)

and punch biopsy (Fig. 1-3). Both are relatively simple and noninvasive procedures that can be quickly performed in an outpatient setting. Shave biopsies are best utilized for lesions concerning for neoplasms such as nonmelanoma skin cancers or atypical moles. Care should be taken to entirely remove pigmented lesions through shave biopsy so as to not encounter sampling error. Punch biopsies are

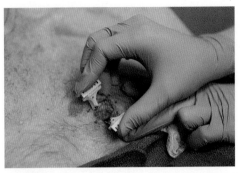

Figure 1-2. The shave biopsy technique. (Courtesy of
M. Laurin Council, MD.)

best employed for rashes or other inflammatory skin processes. The best site for
a punch biopsy depends on the patient's rash. For ulcerated or necrotic lesions,
the leading edge of the rash, especially if there is erythema, will give the highest
yield. For primary blistering disorders, biopsy should be performed at the edge
of the blister to include some intact skin as well. Steps taken for biopsy should
be as follows:

o Identify and mark the site of biopsy. Obtain informed consent from the patient.
Set up all supplies including properly labeled specimen cups.

o Cleanse the area, and then using a small-gauge (we recommend 30-gauge)
needle, infiltrate the area with 1% lidocaine with epinephrine 1:100,000 so
that a wheal is formed.

o For shave biopsy, a scalpel is used parallel to the skin or in a "scooping" fashion
to remove the suspicious lesion. For punch biopsy, a firm twisting motion is
employed perpendicular to the skin until the desired depth is achieved. The
portion of tissue removed with the punch tool can then be gently lifted with
forceps and snipped with scissors at the base.

o Tissue specimens should then be handled with care with forceps and placed in
appropriately labeled specimen cups containing formalin.

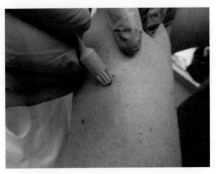

Figure 1-3. The punch biopsy technique.
(Courtesy of M. Laurin Council, MD.)

○ Hemostasis in shave biopsy can be achieved with electrocautery, firm pressure, or a 20% aluminum chloride solution. Hemostasis in punch biopsy can be achieved with the means above, but more commonly one or two simple interrupted sutures are placed using 4-0 nylon suture material.

4. MORPHOLOGY OF SKIN LESIONS

• In dermatology, terms using to describe specific lesions or patterns of lesions are standardized. Primary lesions are covered in Table 1-1. Secondary lesions, or lesions that appear as a result of an underlying or exogenous process, are demonstrated in Table 1-2. Table 1-3 describes various patterns of dermatologic lesions.

Table 1-1	Primary Lesions	
Macule	• Nonpalpable • <1 cm in diameter	
Patch	• Nonpalpable • >1 cm in diameter	
Papule	• Palpable • <1 cm in diameter	
Plaque	• Palpable • >1 cm in diameter	

continued on following page

Nodule	• Palpable, but deeper than a papule • Often >1 cm in diameter	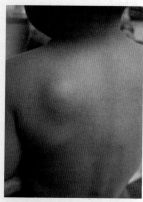
Vesicle	• Palpable and filled with fluid • <1 cm in diameter	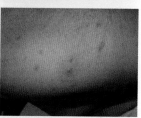
Pustule	• Palpable and filled with purulent fluid • <1 cm in diameter	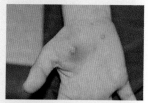
Bullae	• Palpable and filled with fluid • >1 cm in diameter	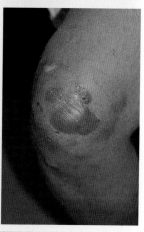

Table 1-2	Secondary Lesions	
Scale	• Keratin accumulation from the stratum corneum (outermost layer of skin)	
Crust	• Dried exudate or transudate. Can be hemorrhagic (blood), purulent (pus), or serous (serum)	
Fissure	• Linear crack in the skin often from excessive dryness	
Excoriation	• Traumatic injury to the skin	
Erosion	• Partial loss of the epidermis	
Ulcer	• Full-thickness loss of the epidermis. Can extend even deeper	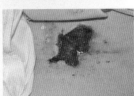

Table 1-3	Patterns of Dermatologic Lesions
Linear	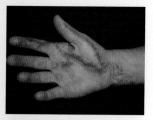
Annular	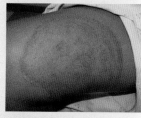
Arcuate	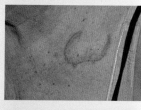
Serpiginous	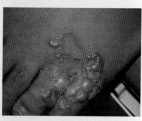
Livedoid	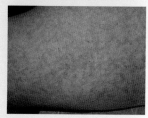

REFERENCES

1. U.S. Preventive Services Task Force. Screening for skin cancer: U.S. Preventive Services Task Force Recommendation Statement. *Ann Intern Med* 2009;150:188–193.
2. U.S. Preventive Services Task Force. Counseling for skin cancer: U.S. Preventive Services Task Force Recommendation Statement. *Ann Intern Med* 2012;157:1–8.

2 Basic Science of the Skin

Karl Staser, MD, PhD and Shadmehr Demehri, MD, PhD

Skin, the largest organ in the human body, regulates immunity, circulation, body temperature, sun protection, barrier function, physical sensation, and appearance.[1] The skin also hosts diverse and site-specific microbes: commensal bacteria, which mediate skin development, infection resistance, and tumorigenesis.[2] Here, we discuss the structure and function of normal skin highlighting each aspect in the context of disease processes.

1. BASIC ANATOMY

- **Epidermis**, the outermost layer of the skin, consists principally of keratinocytes, averages 50 μm in thickness, and completely turns over approximately every 50 days. Histologically, the epidermis contains five strata, each representing a different stage of keratinocyte migration and maturation.[3]
  - **Stratum basale** (innermost): Typically a one- to three-cell layer, the stratum basale contains the basal keratinoctyes, the stem cell reserve pool for skin regeneration. The basal keratinocytes attach to the extracellular matrix of the basement membrane via **hemidesmosomes.** The stratum basale also contains pigment producing **melanocytes**, antigen-presenting **Langerhans cells**, and touch receptor–mediating **Merkel cells**.
  - **Stratum spinosum**: This layer of viable, outward migrating keratinocytes histologically appears "spiny" due to contracted microfilaments in **desmosomes**, structures composed of desmogleins and other molecules critical to epidermal integrity.
  - **Stratum granulosum**: This layer contains maturing keratinocytes filled with lamellar and keratohyalin granules, structures that mediate keratin and lamellar membrane formation, respectively, in the stratum corneum.
  - **Stratum lucidum**: This thin "clear layer" of dead keratinocytes just below the corneum serves as an additional reinforcing layer, found almost exclusively in the thickest skin (e.g., palms, soles).
  - **Stratum corneum** (outermost): Composed of approximately 20 flattened anucleated corneocytes strengthened by corneodesmosomes within a network of hydrophobic lipid, including ceramides, cholesterol, and free fatty acids (e.g., the "lamellar membrane"). This layer serves as a physical and immunologic barrier, modulates drug penetrance, and provides the microenvironment for commensal microbiota.
- **Clinical correlations:** Pathologic processes occurring in the epidermis typically demonstrate scaling, blistering, and/or crusting. **Examples**:
  - **Psoriasis**, which, among other mechanisms, results from increased keratinocyte proliferation and maturation, classically presents with distinctive silver-scaled pink papules and plaques.
  - **HSV infection**, which results in keratinocyte necrosis, presents with blistering and crusting.

○ **Seborrheic keratosis,** a common benign epidermal neoplasm, presents as a "stuck on," well-demarcated lesion, commonly with a waxy, scaled character.

• **Dermis,** the layer located just below the epidermis (Fig. 2-1), provides structural support and facilitates nutrition and immune cell trafficking through its blood supply. Structural components include elastin, collagen, and the extrafibrillar matrix (i.e., "ground substance," composed of water, glycosaminoglycans such as hyaluronan, proteoglycans, and glycoproteins). Histologically, the dermis contains three distinct anatomical zones:

  • **Papillary dermis:** This uppermost, cellular layer of the dermis intercalates with the rete ridges of the epidermis, increasing the contact surface area between the epidermis and the vascular dermis, thus facilitating fine innervation and the exchange of nutrients, oxygen, and waste. The papillary dermis contains loosely arranged collagen types I, II, III, and VII.

  • **Reticular dermis:** Predominantly composed of densely packed collagen type I, this lower layer of the dermis reinforces the skin's structural integrity; contains hair follicles, sweat glands, and nerve fibers; and serves as a critical conduit for the blood and lymphatic supply. Horizontal vessels in the reticular dermis join the subpapillary plexus that give rise to papillary capillaries and lymphatics supplying the epidermis.

  • **Subcutaneous tissue:** Histologically, adipocytes and the presence of arteries and veins distinguish this dermal layer. This fatty tissue cushions the skin and provides a conduit for the large vessels that give rise to the horizontal vessels of the reticular dermis. This layer directly connects to the underlying deep fascia via fibrous bands.

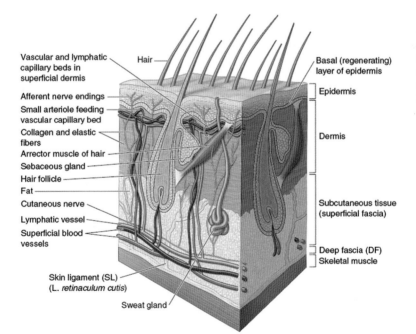

Figure 2-1. Anatomy of the skin. (From Moore KL, Agur AMR, Dalley AF. *Clinically Oriented Anatomy.* 7th ed. Baltimore, MD: Lippincott Williams & Wilkins; 2014.)

- **Clinical correlations:** Pathologic processes confined to the dermis typically present as deeper papules or nodules lacking prominent changes on the skin surface. **Examples**:
  - **Neurofibromas,** a dermal neoplasm, present as prominent papules or nodules but lack discernible scaling, crusting, or blistering.
  - **Panniculitis,** such as **erythema nodosum,** may present as very thin, tender, red-brown nodules or plaques with no overlying epidermal changes.
- **Hair** functions in thermoregulation, hygiene, and social-sexual communication. Individual hairs cycle between anagen (active growth, ~85% of hairs), telogen (resting, ~15%), and catagen (cessation of growth, ~1%). Histologically, the **hair follicle** is composed of the **hair bulb** (deep portion), **isthmus** (middle portion), and the **infundibulum** (superficial portion).
  - The **hair bulb,** the site from which the entire follicle originates in the deep dermis, centers on the hair **papilla**, a nonregenerating structure comprised of connective tissue and capillaries. The papilla reinforces and feeds the **hair matrix**, a collection of epithelial cells and melanocytes giving rise to the **hair shaft**.
  - The **hair shaft** contains a medulla, cortex, and cuticle, which, combined with the cuticle and root sheaths, contain at least 54 different keratin proteins. Compared to epidermal keratins, hair keratins contain increased sulfur in head and tail domains, allowing cross-links, which strengthen hair fibers.
  - The **hair bulge** rests at the insertion site of the arrector pili muscle. Multipotent stem cells localized within the hair bulb mediate epidermal regeneration, wound healing, and, possibly, neural regeneration.
  - The **arrector pili** muscles cause hair erection (i.e., "goose bumps") and can serve as a source of neoplastic leiomyosarcoma.
  - **Hair follicles** escape immune detection (i.e., "immunologically privileged"), similar to the anterior chamber of the eye, testis, brain, and placenta.
  - **Clinical correlations:** The presence and style of hair remain fundamental attributes to self-identity and social communication. As such, disorders related to hair growth can psychosocially devastate patients. **Examples**:
    - **Androgenic alopecia,** or "male pattern baldness," results from dihydrotestosterone (DHT) stimulation, which promotes facial hair growth but inhibits scalp hair growth.
    - **Scarring alopecia** processes such as **lichen planopilaris** and **discoid lupus** destroy the upper hair follicle and its stem cells, resulting in permanent loss of the follicle.
    - **Nonscarring alopecia** processes such as **alopecia areata**, which results from pathologic T-cell attack on hair matrix cells, do not destroy the stem cell pool, permitting complete regrowth.
    - **Neoplasms** such as **trichodiscoma** or **fibrofolliculoma** may arise from cells of the hair follicle.
    - **Fungus** (tinea capitis), **lice**, and **crabs** (pediculosis pubis) commonly infest hair-bearing areas. Depending on severity, fungal infections can cause either scarring or nonscarring alopecia.
- **The pilosebaceous unit** describes the anatomical structure comprised of the hair follicle, sebaceous glands, and apocrine or eccrine sweat glands.
  - **Eccrine sweat glands,** which are found on every cutaneous surface except the vermilion lip, clitoris, labia minora, and the external auditory canal, originate in perifollicular secretory coils located at the junction of the dermis and subcutaneous tissue. These coils attach to the eccrine duct, which extends upward through

the dermis to extrude sweat via the acrosyringium (i.e., "sweat pore"). Sweat is a sterile, hypotonic solution consisting of NaCl, K^+, HCO_3^-, and antimicrobial peptides (AMPs) such as dermcidin. Eccrine sweat glands receive innervation from muscarinic, α_1, β_2, β_3, and purinergic receptors. Histologically, the eccrine sweat gland consists of three cell types: **large clear cells** secrete electrolytes and water, interspersed **dark cells** contain basophilic granules likely composed of sialomucin, and surrounding **myoepithelial cells** promote the outward movement of fluid.

- **Apocrine sweat glands** are found on the external auditory canal (ceruminous glands), eyelid margins (glands of Moll), portions of the nostril, vermilion border of the lip, axilla, areola, nipple, and anogenital region. Like the eccrine sweat gland, apocrine sweat glands originate at the junction of the dermis and the sub-cutaneous tissue. In contrast to the eccrine sweat gland, the apocrine duct extends through the middermis to directly connect to the hair follicle, where it extrudes its contents. Apocrine sweat contains sterile, odorless, and acidic fluid rich in lipids including cholesterol, cholesterol esters, triglycerides, fatty acids, and squalene. This lipid, when processed by the skin's microbiota, produces bromhidrosis, that is, "body odor." Apocrine sweat glands receive innervation from β_2, β_3, purinergic, and, to a lesser degree, muscarinic receptors.

- **Sebaceous glands** produce sebum, an oily substance composed of triglycerides, wax esters, squalene, and free fatty acids. Sebum lubricates the skin and reinforces its barrier function. Sebaceous glands also extrude diverse proteins important to endocrinologic and immunologic function. In most body sites, sebaceous glands associate with and directly connect to the hair follicle. Exceptions include sebaceous glands in the labia (Tyson glands), eyelids (meibomian glands), areolae (Montgomery tubercles), and vermilion lips/oral mucosa (Fordyce granules).

- **Clinical correlations:**
  - **Hyperthermia** can result from impaired sweating and cooling.
  - **Hyperhidrosis,** or excessive sweating, can significantly impair quality of life. Commonly affected areas included the axilla, palms, soles, back, buttocks, and groin.
  - **Acne vulgaris** correlates with androgen-mediated sebaceous gland activity. Increased sebum production creates the milieu for pustule formation.
  - **Sebaceous hyperplasia,** which presents as a pink-yellow crateriform papule typically on the face, can be mistaken for basal and squamous cell carcinoma.
  - **Neoplasms,** including **sebaceous carcinoma, eccrine hidradenoma,** and **apocrine gland carcinoma,** arise from adnexal structures.
  - **Muir-Torre syndrome,** a heritable variant of hereditary nonpolyposis colorectal carcinoma (HNPCC) syndrome that results from mutations in DNA mismatch repair genes, may present as multiple sebaceous gland tumors in the context of a family history of gastrointestinal malignancy.

- **Cutaneous innervation** depends on specialized microanatomical structures with high sensitivity for specific types of sensation. Cutaneous sensation facilitates critical human activities, including feeding, sexuality/mating, and avoiding harm (i.e., pain).[4]

- **Merkel cells,** oval receptor cells located in the epidermal stratum basale, synapse with somatosensory afferents and mediate light touch discrimination. Merkel cells are found in the highest concentration in the fingertips, lips, and external genitalia.

- **Free nerve endings,** branching, nonencapsulated nerve fibers terminating in the stratum granulosum, detect pain, temperature, and mechanical stimuli including stretch, pressure, and touch.

- **Tactile (Meissner) corpuscle,** an unmyelinated nerve encapsulated by connective tissue and lamellated Schwann cells, localizes to the papillary dermis and mediates low-frequency (30- to 50-Hz) vibratory sensation. Tactile corpuscles are found in highest concentrations in the fingers, palms, and soles (i.e., glabrous or non–hair-bearing skin).

- **Lamellar (pacinian) corpuscle,** a single afferent nerve encapsulated in lamellated Schwann cells and fibroblasts, has a distinctive "onion-like" appearance, localizes to the deep dermis, and mediates high-frequency (250- to 350-Hz) vibration of the skin. Lamellar corpuscles are found in the highest concentrations in the hand, where they compose 10% to 15% of cutaneous receptors.
- **Bulbous (Ruffini) corpuscle,** a spindle-shaped encapsulated receptor with enlarged dendritic endings, localizes to the deep dermis and likely mediates cutaneous stretch sensations. Bulbous corpuscles are found in the highest concentrations in the fingertips, lips, and external genitalia. They compose approximately 25% of cutaneous receptors in the hand.
- **Clinical correlations:**
  - **Erythromelalgia,** a disorder characterized by burning and erythema of the extremities, results from gain-of-function mutations in *SCN9A*, a gene that encodes a voltage-gated sodium channel subunit.
  - **Autosomal recessive insensitivity to pain** results from loss-of-function mutations of *SCN9A*. This disorder leads to unintentional self-mutilation and, potentially, accidental death.[5]
  - **Schwannomas, neuromas, neurofibromas**, and related tumors arise from Schwann cells (and their precursor cells) encapsulating axons in the cutaneous tissue.
  - **Merkel cell carcinoma,** a highly anaplastic neuroendocrine tumor, classically presents as a rapidly growing red-purple papule or nodule on the head or neck of an older male. However, pathologists now prefer to call these tumors **primary neuroendocrine carcinoma of the skin**, as they do not appear to arise directly from a clonogenic Merkel cell population.
- **Specialized skin sites** include the scalp, nails, palms and soles, and mucous membranes.
  - **Scalp** skin contains a high concentration of hair follicles, sebaceous glands, and blood vessels, explaining hair oiliness and the brisk bleeding of head lacerations.
  - **Volar** skin (palms and soles) contains a prominent keratinized stratum corneum and an increased concentration of eccrine sweat glands.
  - **The mucous membranes** lack a stratum corneum and thus are nonkeratinized.
  - **Finger and toenail** skin contains a **nail plate** composed of a thick layer of clear keratin (corresponding to the stratum corneum) overlying the **nail bed**, a thin layer of viable epidermal cells. Other distinctive structures include the **eponychium** (corresponding to the cuticle) and the **hyponychium**, thickened epidermis at the distal aspect of the nail bed reinforcing the nail against exterior insult.

2. CELLULAR AND MOLECULAR BIOLOGY

- **Epidermal cells** include keratinocytes, melanocytes, Merkel cells, and Langerhans cells.
  - **Keratinocytes** form the substance of the epidermis. These ectoderm-derived cells proliferate and migrate outward from their reserve pool along the stratum basale and, in wound healing, from the bulge of the hair follicle. Keratinocytes produce keratin, the key epidermal structural protein, and rely on specialized adherens junctions for epidermal integrity.

- **Keratin** intermediate filaments underpin the structural integrity of the epidermis and participate in cellular signaling. Keratins 5 and 14 predominate in the stratum basale, while keratins 1, 2, and 10 predominate in upper epidermal layers. Keratin gene mutations underpin **epidermolysis bullosa** and **epidermolytic ichthyosis** diseases, many of which lead to severe debility or fatality at an early age.[6]
- **Keratohyalin granules** contain loricrin and profilaggrin, proteins critical to the barrier and water retention functions of the stratum corneum. Filaggrin mutations underlie **ichthyosis vulgaris** and some cases of **atopic dermatitis/eczema**. Hypothetically, in atopic dermatitis, filaggrin dysfunction permits increased antigen penetration, leading to immune hypersensitivity and inflammation.
- **Hemidesmosomes** connect keratinocytes along the stratum basale to the basement membrane. Autoantibodies directed against hemidesmosome-localized transmembrane collagen XVII (i.e., BPAG2) and cytoskeletal linker BP230 (i.e., BPAG1) underpin **bullous pemphigoid**, a disease characterized by tense blistering.
- **Desmosomes,** a specialized adherens junction composed of desmoglein, desmocollin, and plakins, connect keratinocytes to each other within the epidermis. Autoantibodies directed against desmoglein-1 and desmoglein-3 underpin **pemphigus** group (e.g., vulgaris, foliaceous), diseases characterized by flaccid blistering. Desmoglein proteins reinforce hair follicle integrity, just as in the epidermis. Genetic mutations in desmoglein and other desmosome-related proteins underpin some **palmoplantar keratosis, ectodermal dysplasia,** and hair follicle malformation syndromes.
- **E6** and **E7**, viral peptides expressed by the human papillomavirus, inhibit keratinocyte **p53** and **Rb**, promoting malignant transformation in HPV-associated **squamous cell carcinoma**. HPV-associated squamous cell hyperplasia also results in verruca vulgaris (warts). Finally, keratinocytes, altered molecularly by UV damage or other insults, give rise to **actinic keratosis, basal cell,** and **squamous cell carcinoma**.

- **Melanocytes,** neural crest–derived pigmented cells located in the stratum basale, determine skin color through their synthesis of melanin, a product of tyrosine oxidation. Via dendritic processes, melanocytes transfer melanin-containing melanosomes to neighboring keratinocytes in the epidermis. Melanin refracts light and protects against UV damage. Accordingly, dark-skinned individuals, who have the highest concentrations of eumelanin, have the lowest risk of **melanoma**, a common and potentially fatal neoplasm of melanocytes. Fair-skinned red-haired individuals, who have high concentrations of pheomelanin, a relatively poor photoprotective molecule, have the highest risk of melanoma. Of note, melanin production indicates existing UV damage—therefore, one could argue that no tan is a "safe tan."
  - **α-MSH** (melanocyte-stimulating hormone) activates **MC1-R** (melanocortin-1 receptor), which ultimately transcribes **MITF** (microphthalmia-associated transcription factor). MITF regulates the expression of genes critical to melanin synthesis. Mutations in *MITF* underpin a subtype of **Waardenburg syndrome**, a disease characterized by heterochromia, white forelock, and hearing impairment.
  - **Tyrosinase** hydroxylates tyrosine to DOPA, the rate-limiting step in melanin synthesis. Mutations in tyrosinase and associated transporter proteins underlie **oculocutaneous albinism.**
  - **C-kit receptor tyrosine kinase** modulates melanocyte migration and survival. Inactivating *KIT* mutations result in **piebaldism** (white forelock, patchy

hypopigmentation), while activating mutations correlate with certain forms of **melanoma**.

- ○ **RAS-RAF-MEK-ERK** signaling pathway activating mutations, especially those in *BRAF,* are found in many melanomas.
- ○ **Neurofibromin,** the protein product of the *NF1* gene, negatively regulates RAS-RAF-MEK-ERK signaling. *NF1* mutations underpin **neurofibromatosis type 1**, a disease characterized by multiple neurofibromas and pigmented **café au lait macules**, which contain hyperactive melanocytes. *NF1* mutations also correlate with certain forms of **melanoma**.

• **Merkel cells** are specialized touch receptors (see **Cutaneous innervation**).
• **Langerhans cells** are specialized dendritic cells (DCs), antigen-presenting cells of the immune system (see **Adaptive immunity**).
• **Dermal cells** include fibroblasts, endothelial cells, smooth muscle cells, Schwann cells, adipocytes, specialized epithelial cells (e.g., eccrine cells, apocrine cells; sebocytes), and inflammatory cells.

- • **Fibroblasts** synthesize and extrude the major components of the extracellular matrix, including collagens, laminins, elastin, fibrillins, and the macromolecules of the extrafibrillary matrix.
  - ○ **Collagen,** a hydroxyproline-enriched α-helix trimer, exits the cell as procollagen before cross-linking with other structural proteins to create collagen fibrils, the backbone of the extracellular matrix. Many of the 28 known collagen types and their isoforms localize to the skin. Of note, collagen types I, III, and V compose much of the dermis, and collagen IV reinforces the basement membrane. **Deficiency in vitamin C**, a cofactor for lysyl and prolyl hydroxylases, results in defective collagen trimer formation and causes **scurvy**, a disease characterized by bleeding mucous membranes, spongy gums, and petechiae, all consequences of impaired wound healing. Genetic mutations in collagen and collagen-related genes result in **Ehlers-Danlos syndrome**, a disease characterized by hyperextensible skin and joints, easy bruising, and vascular anomalies. **Hypertrophic scars** and **keloids** result from increased numbers of fibroblasts and collagen density in the dermis.
  - ○ **Elastin**, a highly cross-linked hydrophobic protein, and **fibrillin**, the main protein constituent of microfibrils, form **elastic fibers**, extracellular matrix molecules that allow skin to reform its original shape following stretching. Elastic fibers maintain the structural integrity of many organ systems, a point demonstrated by the systemic consequences of **Marfan syndrome**, a disease resulting from autosomal dominant mutations in **fibrillin** and the resultant increase in TGFβ signaling. Marfan patients present with long slender limbs, arachnodactyly, scoliosis, pes planus, hyperextensible joints, unexplained stretch marks, eye pathology (e.g., subluxation or ectopia lentis, glaucoma, cataracts, retinal detachment), mitral valve prolapse, aortic aneurysm or dissection, and spontaneous pneumothorax.
  - ○ **Fibronectin** and **laminin** reinforce cell-to-collagen and cell-to-basement membrane connections, respectively.
  - ○ **Proteoglycans,** negatively charged molecules such as heparan sulfate, chondroitin sulfate, and keratin sulfate, capture nutrients, growth factors, and water by attracting cations such as Na^+, K^+, and Ca^{2+}.
  - ○ **Hyaluronic acid,** a nonproteoglycan polysaccharide, absorbs large amounts of water and resists compressive forces.

- **Endothelial cells** form veins, arteries, arterioles, venules, and capillaries. Endothelial cells regulate body temperature, nutrient and oxygen delivery, and waste disposal.
  - **CD31, CD34,** and **PAL-E** mark blood vessels histologically.
  - **FGFR** and **VEGFR** modulate vasculogenesis and angiogenesis. Bevacizumab, a monoclonal antibody against VEGF-A, carries FDA approval in the treatment of several cancers.
  - **Selectins, ICAMs,** and **VCAMs** on the endothelial lumen modulate leukocyte chemotaxis.
  - **Vascular neoplasms** include **infantile hemangiomas, Kaposi sarcoma,** and **angiosarcoma.**
  - **Vasculitides** result from either immune complex–mediated inflammation or anti-neutrophil cystoplasmic antibodies (ANCA), which incite neutrophil-endothelial adherence and inflammatory effector release. Prominent dermatologic vasculitides include small-vessel (e.g., **urticarial, Henoch-Schönlein, drug-** or **infection-induced**), small-to-medium (e.g., **cryoglobulinemia, Churg-Strauss, granulomatosis with polyangiitis**), and, less commonly, medium-vessel vasculitis (e.g., polyarteritis nodosa). Large-vessel vasculitides (e.g., temporal arteritis, Takayasu's) rarely have prominent skin findings, as these vessels localize to deeper tissue.
  - **Vasculopathies** result from microvascular occlusion (noninflammatory). The causes are numerous and include platelet plugging (e.g., **TTP**), agglutination (noninflammatory **cryoglobulinemia**), infection (e.g., **fungal, pseudomonas, strongyloidiasis, leprosy**), embolic (e.g., **cholesterol, oxalate**), coagulopathic (e.g., **warfarin necrosis**), occlusive (e.g., **lymphoma**), and toxic (e.g., **brown recluse spider**'s sphingomyelinase D)
- **Schwann cells,** the principal glial cells of the peripheral nervous system, encase nerve axons to provide growth factors and conductive myelination.
  - **S100** antibody detects for Schwann cells as well as melanocytes, adipocytes, Langerhans cells, DCs, myoepithelial cells, and macrophages.
  - **Myelin** insulates nerves and is comprised of cholesterol, other lipids, water, and proteins, including **myelin basic protein**. Antibodies against myelin basic protein may contribute to **multiple sclerosis**.
  - **Neoplasms** arising from Schwann cells and their precursors include **plexiform neurofibromas** and **Schwannoma**.
- **Adipocytes** contain lipid in the deep dermis. **Panniculitis**, or inflammation of the fat, results from many mechanisms, including autoimmune, infectious, and neoplastic.
- **Smooth muscle cells** in the skin localize to arterial walls and arrector pili muscle. These structures, as well as the dartos muscle in the scrotum, serve as potential cells of origin for **leiomyoma** and **leiomyosarcoma** arising in the skin.
- **Specialized epithelial cells** include apocrine cells, eccrine cells, and sebocytes (see **The pilosebaceous unit**).

3. IMMUNOLOGY

Cells of the **immune system** defend against pathogens, modulate tumorigenesis, and, in their dysregulation, effect inflammatory disorders such as psoriasis and lupus. Although convention has divided the immune system into the **innate** and **adaptive** systems, we increasingly appreciate the complex and inextricable interaction between all molecules, cells, and tissues of the immune system.[7]
- **Innate immunity** includes immune modalities activating in an antibody-independent fashion: complement, toll-like receptors (TLRs), AMPs, cytokines,

and myeloid cells such as macrophages, neutrophils, eosinophils, basophils, mast cells, and innate lymphoid cells (ILCs) (e.g., natural killer cells).

- **Innate antimicrobial molecules** include AMPs, TLRs, and complement.
  - **Antimicrobial peptides (AMPs),** low molecular weight (~5- to 15-kD) proteins synthesized in the skin by keratinocytes, eccrine/apocrine epithelial cells, and sebocytes, directly defend against bacteria, fungi, and, likely, viruses. Examples include **dermcidin**, **human β-defensin**, **lysozyme**, and **psoriasin**. Pathogens and secreted cytokines can induce AMP expression, and AMPs can attract DCs and memory T cells via CCR6.
  - **Toll-like receptors (TLRs)** expressed on DCs and keratinocytes recognize pathogen-derived molecules. Once activated, TLRs signal in a similar fashion as the IL-1 receptor, activating NF-κB and subsequent interferon production.
  - **Complement** is activated by microbial polysaccharide interactions (alternate pathway), by other microbial carbohydrate interactions (lectin pathway), or by immune complex interactions (classical pathway). All pathways increase C3, and C3's cleave products attract phagocytes. Moreover, complement C5b assembly with C6 to C9 forms the membrane attack complex, which directly lyses microbial cells.
- **Macrophages** phagocytize cells labeled with complement as well as cells expressing nonvertebrate carbohydrates. They additionally secrete colony factors (e.g., G-CSF), which promote neutrophil production and chemotaxis, present antigen to T and B cells, and critically modulate wound healing and angiogenesis.
- **Neutrophils,** which activated macrophages can recruit in large numbers from precursor cells in the bone marrow, serve as frontline defenders against microbes. Neutrophils kill via oxygen-dependent (e.g., the respiratory burst) and oxygen-independent (e.g., myeloperoxidase secretion) mechanisms.
- **Eosinophils** defend against parasites through IgE receptor (FcεR)–mediated degranulation of cytotoxic molecules and through the secretion of cytokines, leukotrienes, and prostaglandins. Eosinophil-mediated inflammation also underlies asthma and allergy.
- **Mast cells,** granular myeloid lineage cells, mediate wound healing, host defense, and response to toxic insult. IgE-sensitized mast cells promote inflammation of asthma and allergy, including **urticaria**, through the release of cytokines and vasoactive effectors such as histamine. Cutaneous **mastocytosis** may present as widely distributed red macules and patches.
- **Innate lymphoid cells** (ILCs), a recently devised nomenclature with newly discovered cell types, include natural killer (NK) cells and other lymphoid-derived cells that activate in an antibody-independent fashion. Our current understanding of ILCs is rapidly evolving.[8]
  - **Group 1 ILCs** (which includes NK cells) produce TNF and IFNγ and kill virus-infected and tumor cells.
  - **Group 2 ILCs** produce IL-4, IL-5, IL-9, and IL-13, mediate Th2 responses (see below), and help fight against parasite infection.
  - **Group 3 ILCs** produce IL-17 and IL-22 and likely modulate inflammatory disorders and tumorigenesis.
- **Adaptive immunity**, which regulates both cytotoxic and long-term antibody-dependent immunity (e.g., response to vaccination), includes DCs (a key antigen-presenting cell), T lymphocytes, B lymphocytes, and plasma cells or antibody-producing lymphocytes. Multiple subsets of T cells exist, including Th1, Th2, regulatory (or immunosuppressive) T cells, and the more recently described Th17 cells, which appear to critically modulate certain inflammatory disorders such as psoriasis.

- **Dendritic cells (DCs)** process and present antigen to adaptive immune cells, thus acting as intermediaries between the innate and adaptive immune systems. **Langerhans cells,** DCs located in the epidermis, express MHC class II and serve as powerful antigen-presenting cells that, following antigen capture, migrate to the lymphatic tissue to activate naive T cells.
- **T cells**
  - CD8⁺ T cells recognize MHC class I–presented intracellular antigens (e.g., virus, fungus, mycobacteria, tumor antigens). Cytotoxic CD8⁺ T cells affect killing through perforins, granzymes, granulysin, and FAS ligand interactions with Fas expressed on the target cell.
  - CD4⁺ T cells recognize MHC class II–presented antigens to modulate host defense against intracellular and extracellular antigens.
    - **CD4⁺IL-12R⁺ Th1** cells produce IFN-γ, TNF-β, and IL-2, which stimulate macrophages and cytotoxic lymphocytes to fight intracellular pathogens and tumor cells.
    - **CD4⁺IL-4R⁺ Th2** cells produce IL-5, IL-4, and IL-13, which stimulate macrophages, eosinophils, and B cells, promoting plasma cell differentiation and antibody production.
    - **CD4⁺IL-23⁺ Th17** cells, which have more recently been described, produce IL-17 and help fight *Candida* and *Staphylococcus* infections. Th17 cells also promote psoriasis and eczema, and monoclonal antibodies directed against the Th17 pathway may effectively treat these diseases.
  - **Tregs** suppress adaptive immune responses through secretion of IL-10, IL-35, and TGF-β, through conversion of ATP to adenosine (a cytotoxin), and through CTLA-4 interactions with MHC class II complex. **Ipilimumab,** a drug that carries FDA approval for the treatment of metastatic **melanoma**, inhibits CTLA-4 to promote antitumor cytotoxicity.
- **B cells** receive activating signals from T cells, which induce them to plasma cells that secrete antigen-specific immunoglobulin antibodies. **Plasma cells** produce IgM (primary responses), IgG (secondary immune responses, i.e., long-term immunity), IgA (mucosal surfaces), IgE (allergy and anaphylaxis), or IgD (function largely unknown).

REFERENCES

1. Bolognia J, Jorizzo JL, Schaffer JV. *Dermatology*. 3rd ed. Philadelphia, PA: Elsevier Saunders; 2012. http://hdl.library.upenn.edu/1017.12/1337728
2. Belkaid Y, Segre JA. Dialogue between skin microbiota and immunity. *Science* 2014;346(6212):954–959.
3. Elston DM, Ferringer T. Dermatopathology. In: *Requisites in dermatology*. 2nd ed. Philadelphia, PA: Elsevier Saunders; 2008. http://hdl.library.upenn.edu/1017.12/1338118
4. Purves D, Williams SM. *Neuroscience*. 2nd ed. Sunderland, MA: Sinauer Associates; 2001.
5. Hoeijmakers JG, Faber CG, Merkies IS, et al. Painful peripheral neuropathy and sodium channel mutations. *Neurosci Lett* 2015;596:51–59.
6. Toivola DM, Boor P, Alam C, et al. Keratins in health and disease. *Curr Opin Cell Biol* 2015;32C:73–81.
7. Parham P, Janeway C, Louis A. Duhring fund. In: *The immune system*. 3rd ed. New York: Garland Science; 2009.
8. Diefenbach A, Colonna M, Koyasu S. Development, differentiation, and diversity of innate lymphoid cells. *Immunity* 2014;41(3):354–365.

Inflammatory Disorders

Emily M. Beck, MD and Sena J. Lee, MD, PhD

Inflammatory disorders of the skin encompass several common dermatologic complaints. Some conditions, such as allergic contact dermatitis, may be clinically limited while others, such as acne and psoriasis, are chronic conditions that may span the course of years.

1. ACNE

1.1. Background
- Acne affects 85% of young adults ages 12 to 24 and may persist into adulthood.[1]
- This multifactorial disorder is driven by genetics, hormonal influences, sebum production, comedone formation, and the bacterium, *Propionibacterium acnes*.
  - Genetics largely determines number and activity of sebaceous glands.
  - Adrenarche heralds the onset of adrenal production of dehydroepiandrosterone sulfate (DHEAS), which leads to increased sebum production.
  - Increased cohesiveness of follicular-based keratinocytes leads to follicular plugging, accumulation of keratin, and proliferation of *P. acnes* at the base of the hair follicle.
  - *Propionobacterium acnes,* a gram-positive rod, triggers a robust inflammatory response.
  - Increasing pressure secondary to keratin accumulation can lead to comedone rupture, triggering a vigorous inflammatory reaction.

1.2. Clinical Presentation
One or more subtypes may be observed in any given patient (Fig. 3-1).
- Comedonal acne
  - Characterized by open and closed comedones
    - Closed comedones, commonly called whiteheads, are small, round, skin-colored papules.
    - Open comedones, commonly called blackheads, are small, round, skin-colored papules with a central black open core reflective of lipid oxidation of keratin.
  - Lesions are most commonly seen on the forehead, nose, cheeks, and chin. Eyelids are generally spared.
- Inflammatory acne
  - Characterized by erythematous papules, pustules, nodules, and cysts.
  - Inflammatory lesions frequently result in the development of postinflammatory hyperpigmentation and scarring.
  - The violaceous macules of postinflammatory hyperpigmentation may resolve over the course of months.
  - Resultant scarring is permanent and difficult to treat.

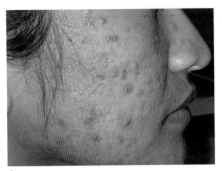

A

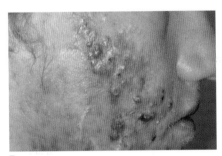

B

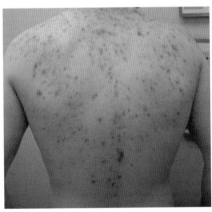

C

Figure 3-1. Forms of acne vulgaris. **A:** Inflammatory acne. **B:** Nodulocystic acne. **C:** Truncal acne. (Courtesy of David Sheinbein, MD.)

- Acne subtypes
  - Acne fulminans
    - Adolescent males are most commonly affected.
    - Symptoms include rapid development of fever, arthralgias, inflammatory papules, cysts, and hemorrhagic crusts.
    - Laboratory abnormalities include elevated erythrocyte sedimentation rate, leukocytosis, proteinuria, and osteolytic lesions.
    - SAPHO syndrome is a subset characterized by **s**ynovitis, **a**cne, **p**ustulosis, **h**yperostosis, and **o**steitis.
  - Acne conglobata
    - Adolescent males are most commonly affected.
    - Symptoms include severe nodulocystic, scarring inflammatory acne with possible sinus tract formation.
    - Acne conglobata, hidradenitis suppurativa, dissecting cellulitis of the scalp, and pilonidal cysts form the follicular occlusion tetrad.
    - PAPA syndrome is an autosomal dominant variant composed of **p**yogenic **a**rthritis, **p**yoderma gangrenosum, and **a**cne conglobata.
  - Postadolescent acne
    - Women with features of hyperandrogenism are most commonly affected.
    - Typical lesions are deep-set, erythematous papules on the lower cheeks and jawline.
    - Lesions tend to flare the week prior to menses.
  - Drug-induced acne
    - Typical lesions are monomorphic papules and pustules distributed on the chest and back.
    - The monomorphic morphology of drug-induced acne allows differentiation from the more heterogeneous appearance of acne vulgaris.
    - The most common drugs associated with acneiform eruptions include oral steroids, topical steroids, corticotropin, lithium, bromide, iodide, isoniazid, phenytoin, and epidermal growth factor receptor (EGFR) inhibitors.

1.3. Evaluation

- Acne is primarily a clinical diagnosis. Presence of comedones, red papules, pustules, and nodules on typically involved areas, such as face, chest, shoulders, and upper back, helps to make the diagnosis. If the pustular component is prominent and patient is unresponsive to typical acne treatment, bacterial culture and KOH prep should be done to rule out gram-negative folliculitis and Pityrosporum folliculitis, respectively.
- Careful review of contributing factors is recommended to optimize treatment.
- Check DHEAS and testosterone in the setting of obesity, hirsutism, irregular menses, and insulin resistance given concern for polycystic ovarian syndrome.
- Review the medication list for contributing drugs.

1.4. Treatment

Therapy is directed at normalizing keratinization, decreasing inflammation, and decreasing bacterial proliferation. Topical medications are first-line therapy for the management of mild comedonal and inflammatory acne. Oral antibiotics may be added for the control of moderate to severe inflammatory acne. In the event of severe,

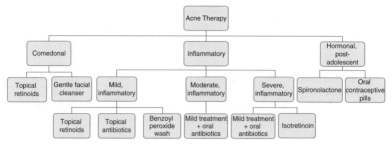

Figure 3-2. Overview of acne management based on clinical morphology and severity.

recalcitrant, nodulocystic, or scarring acne, isotretinoin may be used to prevent further scarring. In female patients with a predominantly hormone-induced cystic acne, oral contraceptive pills (OCPs) or spironolactone may be tried. See Figure 3-2 for an overview of acne management.

• Comedonal acne
  • Topical retinoids
    ○ Retinoids are vitamin A derivatives that promote normalization of keratinization and exhibit anti-inflammatory effects, which inhibit comedone formation making retinoids particularly effective at treating comedonal acne. Examples include adapalene, tretinoin, and tazarotene.
    ○ Retinoids are applied once daily at night given concern for inactivation by UV exposure. It may be applied 2 to 3 nights per week, and frequency may be increased, depending on tolerability.
    ○ Treatment is prophylactic and requires consistent application of affected areas, rather than spot treating active lesions. Initial flare is commonly observed in the first 4 weeks. Improvement is often observed in 8 to 12 weeks.
    ○ The most common side effects include xerosis, erythema, and photosensitivity. Drying or exfoliating agents should not be used in conjunction with topical retinoids. Daily use of moisturizer and broad-spectrum sunscreen is needed for increasing tolerability and successful treatment.
    ○ All topical retinoids (except for tazarotene, which is in category X) are in pregnancy category C. Topical retinoids are generally discontinued during pregnancy.
• Inflammatory acne
  • Combination of topical antibiotic and topical retinoid is generally effective in treating inflammatory acne. Oral antibiotic may be added for 3 to 6 months, if needed, to control cystic components. Isotretinoin is reserved for severe nodulocystic, scarring acne, or acne refractory to other therapies.
    ○ Clindamycin (gel, lotion, foam)
      – Binds bacterial ribosomal 50S subunit and inhibits protein synthesis.
      – An important side effect to be aware of is the development of gram-negative folliculitis.
    ○ Sodium sulfacetamide (lotion, wash, solution)
      – Inhibits dihydropteroate synthetase, which impairs folic acid synthesis.
      – The most common side effects are pruritus and xerosis.

- ○ Benzoyl peroxide (gel, wash)
  - Creates reactive oxygen species which directly damage bacterial proteins.
  - The most common side effect is skin irritation. Patients must take caution when using benzoyl peroxide as it is a bleaching agent.
- • Oral antibiotics
  - ○ Tetracyclines are the most commonly used class of oral antibiotics for acne treatment. Typically, this is given twice per day for 3 months at a time.
  - ○ Tetracyclines inhibit the bacterial 50S ribosomal subunit, which inhibits protein synthesis. Oral antibiotics exhibit both anti-inflammatory and antibacterial properties.
  - ○ Medication should be taken with a full glass of water to prevent the development of esophagitis.
  - ○ The most common class side effects include gastrointenstinal (GI) upset, esophagitis, and photosensitivity. Pseudotumor cerebri is a rare side effect.
    - Minocycline can cause blue-gray or muddy brown discoloration, autoimmune hepatitis, drug-induced lupus, or a drug hypersensitivity reaction.
    - Minocycline produces less photosensitivity than doxycycline, which may be advantageous in the summer.
- • Isotretinoin
  - ○ Isotretinoin is generally reserved for severe nodulocystic scarring acne due to its side effect profile. It is the only medication that offers a potential cure, meaning that other prescription acne medications would not be needed after treatment. It is given 0.5 to 1 mg/kg/d in divided doses twice daily. Cumulative dose of 150 mg/kg is generally needed to reduce the risk of relapse.
  - ○ Isotretinoin is a vitamin A derivative that normalizes epithelial keratinization, differentiation, and proliferation, decreases sebum production, and induces apoptosis of sebocytes.
  - ○ Side effects include xerosis, xerophthalmia, exacerbation of eczema, muscle and joint aches, mood changes, depression, anxiety, liver toxicity, and pseudotumor cerebri.
  - ○ Complete blood count (CBC), fasting lipid profile, and hepatic function panel should be checked before initiating therapy and monthly during therapy with dose changes. Lab abnormalities, such as elevated cholesterol, triglycerides, and transaminases, can be seen. Diet modification, omega-3 fatty acid supplementation, or dose modification may be help in hyperlipidemia, which generally self-resolves after completing therapy. Dose reduction or cessation of therapy may be required in cases of elevated transaminases.
  - ○ Isotretinoin is a potent teratogen and requires enrollment in the iPledge pregnancy prevention program to ensure appropriate administration.
    - Females of child-bearing potential are required to have two documented negative pregnancy tests 1 month apart prior to starting therapy. Two contraceptive measures must start 1 month prior to initial dose, and monthly negative pregnancy tests (serum beta-human chorionic gonadotropin) thereafter are required to continue therapy.
- • Postadolescent acne
  - • Oral contraceptive pills (OCPs)
    - ○ Most OCPs are comprised of both an estrogen and a progestin component. Older progestins have androgenic activity, but newer progestins have low or antiandrogenic activity.

- ◦ Several OCP formulations are food and drug administration approved for acne treatment: Ortho Tri-Cyclen, Estrostep, Yaz, Loryna, and Beyaz.
- ◦ Side effects include nausea, vomiting, breast tenderness, and weight gain. More serious side effects include hypertension and thromboembolism. Cardiovascular risk must be assessed to weigh risk versus benefit in each patient before starting OCP.
- • Spironolactone
  - ◦ Spironolactone blocks androgen receptors and inhibits the conversion of testosterone to dihydrotestosterone.
  - ◦ Dose of 50 to 200 mg a day divided in q12h doses for 3 to 6 months is generally needed to achieve improvement. Therapy may be continued for a few years, if needed.
  - ◦ Side effects include irregular menses, breast tenderness, hyperkalemia, headache, fatigue, and drug hypersensitivity reaction.
  - ◦ Given its antiandrogenic effects, spironolactone is a teratogen that may cause feminization of a male fetus. Contraceptive measures should be advised.

2. ROSACEA

2.1. Background
- • Rosacea is more common in women than men and in those with Fitzpatrick skin types I and II. The estimated prevalence in Caucasians is 14% in women and 5% in men.[2]
- • Rosacea is a multifactorial disorder modulated by UV exposure, innate immune system dysfunction, epidermal barrier dysfunction, and Demodex mite infestation.
- • Exacerbating factors include sunlight, strong wind, hot or spicy foods, alcohol, emotional distress, and topical skin irritants.

2.2. Clinical Presentation
- • Erythrotelangiectatic rosacea (Fig. 3-3A)
  - • Symptoms include persistent centrofacial erythema, flushing, telangiectasias, and increased skin sensitivity to irritants.
- • Papulopustular rosacea
  - • Symptoms include erythematous, dome-shaped papules and pustules in the centrofacial region.
  - • Papules last several weeks and fade to residual background erythema.
  - • Lack of comedones helps distinguish papulopustular rosacea from acne.
- • Phymatous rosacea
  - • Men are more commonly affected than women.
  - • Phymatous rosacea is characterized by nodular, soft tissue hypertrophy classically of the nose (rhinophyma, Fig. 3-3B).
  - • Patients may also develop phymatous changes of the chin (gnathophyma), ears (otophyma), glabella (glabellophyma), or forehead (metophyma).
- • Ocular rosacea
  - • Ocular manifestations of rosacea are common. Studies have shown a prevalence of ocular rosacea in 20.8% of patients with other features of rosacea.[3]
  - • Manifestations of ocular rosacea include xerosis, pruritus, stinging, burning, conjunctivitis, blepharitis, hordeola, chalazia, and rarely keratitis.

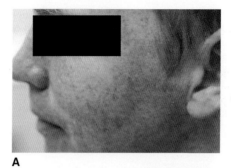

Figure 3-3. Rosacea. **A:** Erythrotelangiectatic rosacea. **B:** Rhinophymatous rosacea. (**A**, courtesy of M. Laurin Council, MD; **B**, courtesy of Eva Hurst, MD.)

2.3. Evaluation

- Rosacea is a clinical diagnosis that generally does not require laboratory evaluation. Patients exhibit erythema and telangiectases on the glabella, nose, cheeks, and chin in addition to erythematous papules in the papulopustular variant of rosacea.
- Differential diagnosis includes conditions that exhibit centrofacial erythema, such as seborrheic dermatitis or lupus erythematosus.
- If patients complain of photophobia, they should be evaluated by ophthalmology.

2.4. Treatment

Treatment focuses primarily on prevention. Patients should be advised to avoid common rosacea triggers and wear sunscreen daily. Centrofacial erythema and telangiectasia may be treated with topical antibiotics or vasoconstrictive agents or lasers. Papules and pustules may be prevented with the use of topical or oral antibiotics, or low-dose isotretinoin, if refractory to antibiotics. Phymatous rosacea treatment centers largely on surgical procedures for revision. Ocular rosacea treatment begins with warm compresses and gentle soap. If persistent, topical or oral antibiotics may be prescribed.

- Erythrotelangiectatic rosacea: This is the most difficult type to control. In addition to sun protection and trigger avoidance, topical antibiotics and vasoconstrictors are tried to varying degrees of success. Vascular lasers are often helpful.
  - Sunscreen with sun protection factor (SPF) 30+ daily
  - Trigger avoidance
  - Vasoconstrictors
  - Topical antibiotic/inflammatory (metronidazole, sulfacetamide-sulfur, azelaic acid)
  - Topical brimonidine tartrate (0.33% gel) daily
    - Alpha-2 adrenergic agonist.
    - Decreases centrofacial erythema for 12 or more hours when applied once daily. No rebound or worsening of disease was noted.[4]
  - Topical oxymetazoline (0.05% solution) daily
    - Imidazoline vasoconstrictor.
    - Case report demonstrates decreased centrofacial erythema in two patients when applied once daily. No rebound or sporadic flares were noted.[5]
  - Laser therapy
    - Pulsed dye laser (PDL), potassium titanyl phosphate laser, and intense pulsed light can be used to treat telangiectasias and persistent centrofacial erythema.
    - Multiple treatments are often required to produce good cosmetic outcomes.
    - Patients reported a statistically significant increased quality of life via the Dermatology Life Quality Index score after three PDL treatments.[6]
- Papulopustular rosacea
  Topical medications, one or a combination, should be tried first. Improvement is generally seen in 1 to 2 months. Oral antibiotic may be added for 2 to 3 months, if needed. A low-dose, submicrobial dose of doxycycline is also an option.
  - Topical treatments
    - Metronidazole gel or cream once or twice daily
    - Azelaic acid gel or cream twice daily
    - Sodium sulfacetamide—sulfur lotion, solution, or wash, once or twice daily
    - Clindamycin 1% gel, solution, or lotion once or twice daily
  - Systemic treatments
    - Oral antibiotics have been shown to decrease the appearance of papules and pustules. A short course of 4 to 12 weeks rapidly decreases inflammation.
    - Tetracycline antibiotics
      - Doxycycline 50 to 100 mg once or twice daily
      - Minocycline 50 to 100 mg once or twice daily
      - Tetracycline 250 to 500 mg once or twice daily
    - Macrolide antibiotics
      - Erythromycin 250 to 500 mg once or twice daily
      - Azithromycin 250 to 500 mg three times per week
    - Other antibiotics
      - Metronidazole 200 mg once or twice daily

- ○ Isotretinoin
  - – Lower doses of isotretinoin achieve acceptable therapeutic results (10 to 40 mg once daily), as compared to isotretinoin dose in acne.
  - – Requires strict counseling on avoidance of pregnancy, avoidance of blood donation, and possible side effects.
- Phymatous rosacea
  - Surgical revision debulks and recontours the nose. Revision options include partial-thickness excision, electrosurgery, and ablative laser.[7,8]
- Ocular rosacea
  - Artificial tears, warm compresses, and gentle lid washing
  - Metronidazole 0.75% gel
  - Cyclosporine 0.5% ophthalmic emulsion
  - Oral antibiotics as above if severe
  - Ophthalmologist evaluation if photophobia is present

3. ATOPIC DERMATITIS

3.1. Background

- Atopic dermatitis (AD) affects 19.3% of children 0 to 3 years old and gradually declines to 14.5% in children 10 to 13 years old.[9]
- Prior helminth infection has been associated with a decreased risk of atopic dermatitis.[10] Exposure to animals, endotoxin, and early daycare correlated with lower rates of AD.[11]
- Though the prevalence of AD declines with age, a substantial percentage continue to have symptoms into adulthood.[12]
- AD has a significant impact on quality of life in children secondary to chronic pruritus and sleep disturbance.[13]
- Children with AD are more prone to develop food allergies, asthma, and rhinitis.
- AD is a multifactorial disease based on genetics, epidermal barrier dysfunction, and environmental exposures as mentioned above.
  - Twins of affected individuals have a sevenfold increase risk of developing AD as compared to the general population.[14]
  - Epidermal skin barrier dysfunction promotes transepidermal water loss, which contributes to lesion development.[15]
  - Loss of filaggrin, a protein involved in skin barrier formation, has been described in the development of AD.[16]

3.2. Clinical Presentation

- Skin lesions (Fig. 3-4)
  - Acute
    - ○ More common in infants and young children
    - ○ Scaly, red papules and plaques with variable presence of vesicles, bullae, serosanguineous drainage, and excoriations
  - Subacute
    - ○ May be seen in any age group
    - ○ Scaly, red papules and plaques with variable crusting and excoriations
  - Chronic
    - ○ More commonly seen in adolescents and adults.
    - ○ Thickened, scaly, hyperpigmented plaques with accentuation of skin lines.
    - ○ Patients may also form prurigo nodules in response to chronic rubbing and scratching.

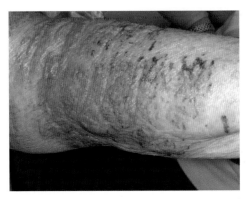

Figure 3-4. Severe atopic dermatitis. (Courtesy of David Sheinbein, MD.)

- Lesions by age
  - Infantile AD
    - ○ Characterized by acute and subacute lesions.
    - ○ Distributed on the cheeks, scalp, neck, trunk, and extensor surfaces of the extremities. The diaper area is usually spared given the retention of moisture.
  - Childhood AD
    - ○ Characterized primarily by acute and subacute lesions with some development of chronic lesions.
    - ○ Lesions assume a more classic AD pattern, affecting the flexural surfaces, neck, hands, feet, ankles, and wrists.
  - Adolescent and adult AD
    - ○ Characterized primarily by subacute and chronic lesions.
    - ○ Lesions are distributed in a classic AD pattern, with the hands and feet frequently being affected.
- Symptoms
  - Lesions are extremely pruritic and cause a significant disruption in quality of life.[17]
  - Given the child's distress and frustration of treating a chronic disease, parents of children with AD have a similarly decreased quality of life.[18]

3.3. Evaluation

- Atopic dermatitis is a clinical diagnosis, though patch testing, prick testing, and serology may be considered to identify contributing factors.

3.4. Treatment

Given the chronicity of atopic dermatitis, treatment requires dedication and patient compliance. Patients should be advised to avoid triggers and perform good dry skin care habits. Topical steroids are the first-line therapy for management of mild to moderate disease. Steroid potency should be chosen based on the age of the child, location, and severity of the lesion. If possible, steroid use should be avoided on the face. Instead, topical calcineurin inhibitors are recommended for facial lesions. Narrowband UVB phototherapy offers a low-risk treatment for persistent lesions unresponsive to steroids alone. Systemic medication such as cyclosporine is effective for achieving control of severe atopic dermatitis, but use should be limited given the concern for side effects.

- Avoidance of triggering factors
  - Decrease shower length and temperature
  - Decrease soap usage
  - Avoid products with fragrance
  - Avoid smoking
  - Avoid wool fabrics
- Emollients
  - Skin barrier dysfunction and increased transepidermal water loss require compensation in the form of ointment-based emollients.
  - Petroleum jelly should be applied, ideally to wet skin, multiple times daily.
- Topical steroids
  - Steroids are the mainstay of acute flare treatment. Steroids interact with nuclear receptors to decrease transcription of inflammatory mediators.
  - The potency should be based on the severity of the lesion. The steroid chosen should be able to quickly clear the lesion. Rapid clearance with an appropriately potent steroid helps prevent side effects of prolonged steroid application including atrophy, striae, skin fragility, and telangiectasias.
  - Steroids should be tapered as lesions resolve, though complete cessation may lead to rebound flares. Studies have shown that prophylactic maintenance application of steroids twice weekly in addition to emollients may prevent recurrence.[19]
  - Steroids should be avoided on the face given concern for side effects.
  - In infants and young children, low-potency, class V, VI, and VII steroids should be attempted before escalating therapy.
  - See Table 3-1 for a listing of corticosteroids by potency.
- Topical calcineurin inhibitors
  - Tacrolimus and pimecrolimus are unique anti-inflammatory agents most commonly used on the face. Topical calcineurin inhibitors allow control of

Table 3-1	Topical Corticosteroid Potency

Class I (superpotent)

Clobetasol propionate ointment, cream, gel, and foam 0.05%
Betamethasone dipropionate gel and ointment 0.05%
Fluocinonide cream 0.1%
Flurandrenolide tape 4 mcg/cm^2

Class II (high potency)

Clobetasol solution 0.05%
Betamethasone dipropionate cream 0.05%
Desoximetasone ointment and cream 0.25% and gel 0.05%
Fluocinonide gel, ointment, cream, and solution 0.05%
Mometasone furoate ointment 0.1%
Triamcinolone acetonide ointment 0.5%

Class III (high potency)

Triamcinolone acetonide ointment 0.1% and cream 0.5%
Betamethasone valerate ointment 0.1%
Fluticasone propionate ointment 0.005%

Class IV (medium potency)

Fluocinolone acetonide ointment 0.025%
Desoximetasone cream 0.05%
Fluocinolone acetonide ointment 0.025%
Hydrocortisone valerate ointment 0.2%
Mometasone furoate cream and lotion 0.1%

Class V (medium potency)

Fluocinolone acetonide cream 0.025% or oil and shampoo 0.01%
Fluticasone cream and lotion 0.05%
Hydrocortisone butyrate ointment, cream, and lotion 0.1%
Hydrocortisone valerate cream 0.2%

Class VI (low potency)

Alclometasone dipropionate ointment and cream 0.05%
Betamethasone valerate lotion 0.1%
Desonide gel, ointment, cream, lotion, and foam 0.05%
Fluocinolone cream and solution 0.01%

Class VII (low potency)

Hydrocortisone ointment 2.5%
Hydrocortisone ointment 1%

---

  inflammation while avoiding the side effects of steroids on the face including acneiform eruptions, perioral dermatitis, and skin thinning.
  - The most common side effects are transient stinging and burning. The sensation should fade with repeated application.
- Light therapy
  - Narrowband UVB (NB UVB) therapy may be used to treat severe or recalcitrant AD in older children; however, little is known of the long-term safety of light therapy in children. NB UVB therapy requires multiple visits to achieve a durable response.
  - A study of 25 AD patients demonstrated a 68% clearance rate after a mean of 24 NB UVB treatments. Side effects were generally mild and included erythema, HSV reactivation, and anxiety.[20]
  - Children receiving narrowband UVB therapy should have yearly skin screenings given the concern for increased risk of skin cancer.
- Cyclosporine
  - Cyclosporine rapidly clears severe, diffuse skin disease and may be considered an option to achieve short-term rapid control.
  - Long-term low-dose cyclosporine may also be used to control recalcitrant atopic dermatitis. Long-term courses have proven beneficial but are limited by side effects: hypertension, GI upset, hypertrichosis, and renal dysfunction.[21]
- Other immunomodulatory agents
  - Azathioprine and methotrexate may be considered as alternate systemic treatment options second to cyclosporine, producing similar results with a reported reduction in disease severity of 40%.[22]
  - Omalizumab, an anti-IgE antibody, has shown potential for the treatment of AD.[23]
  - Rituximab, an anti-CD20 antibody, has also shown potential for treatment-resistant AD.[24]

4. CONTACT DERMATITIS

4.1. Background

- Contact dermatitis is characterized by a pruritic, eczematous eruption in a body distribution correlated with the area of exposure. The acute phase manifests as vesicles on a well-defined erythematous patch or plaque with variable serosanguineous drainage and crusting. Chronic lesions present as well-demarcated, hyperpigmented, lichenified plaques with accentuation of skin lines.
- Lesions are most commonly found on the hands, feet, face, and arms and in a generalized eruptive pattern.[25]
- Contact dermatitis is divided into two broad categories: allergic contact dermatitis and irritant contact dermatitis.
  - Allergic contact dermatitis results from repeated exposure to a sensitizing agent. A rash is produced via a delayed type IV hypersensitivity reaction mediated primarily by T cells.
  - Irritant contact dermatitis does not require repeated exposures and is the result of local inflammation secondary to irritants such as soap, solvents, alkali, and acid.
- There is no age, gender, nor racial predilection for contact dermatitis, though different exposures predominate in different populations. For example, women have higher incidence of nickel allergy than men likely secondary to jewelry exposure.[26]
- The most common allergic contact allergens are nickel and poison ivy. Balsam of Peru is another important contact allergen.
  - Nickel allergic contact dermatitis
    - Nickel allergy was found in 34.4% of women and 8.9% of men in a European study by patch testing.[30] It is commonly found in costume jewelry, watches, denim snaps, and belt buckles. Lesions are commonly found on sites of nickel exposure such as the earlobes, around the umbilicus, wrists, and back of the neck.
    - Cell phones are a newer source of nickel exposure that may lead to development of lesions on the cheek and ear.
    - It is postulated that ear piercing in particular contributes to nickel allergy formation given the chronic exposure of nickel to a damaged cutaneous surface.[27]
    - Patients should be advised to wear nickel-free jewelry, snaps, and buckles. If unavoidable, they may try painting nickel-containing objects with clear nail polish to decrease the level of exposure. Sweating in the area of contact with nickel will aggravate the allergic dermatitis.
  - Poison ivy, poison oak, and poison sumac
    - These three plants are members of the family Anacardiaceae, genus *Toxicodendron*, and cause more allergic contact dermatitis than all other plants combined. In the United States, there are two varieties of poison ivy, two of poison oak, and one of poison sumac.
    - These plants contain urushiol and laccase, which oxidizes the urushiol to produce a black resin commonly observed as black spots on plants and areas of dermatitis.
    - Identification
      - Poison ivy and poison oak produce leaves with 3 green leaflets. "Leaves of three; let them be" is a common pneumonic used to remember avoidance.
      - Poison sumac has leaves with 5 or 7 leaflets that angle upward.
      - All three members of the *Toxicodendron* genus produce small green fruit that ripen to off-white to light tan fruit when mature.
    - Geographic distribution
      - Poison ivy is found across the United States. In the West, it is found as a low-growing shrub, whereas in the East, it is found as a climbing vine.

- Poison oak is found primarily in the Western United States.
  - Poison sumac is largely found in the Southeastern United States.
  o Lesions are characterized by weeping vesicles arranged in a linear fashion on an erythematous base. Shiny black dots may be present, reflecting the oxidation of urushiol. Lesions are very pruritic.
- Balsam of Peru
  o Balsam of Peru is complex resin comprised of over 400 chemicals derived from the tree *Myroxylon pereirae.* It is one of the most common allergens identified by the North American Contact Dermatitis Group.
  o Allergenic components of Balsam of Peru are found in fragrances, cosmetics, medicinal products, and food. Food sources may include vanilla, cinnamon, cloves, carbonated beverages, vermouth, and tomatoes.[28,29]
- Other common allergens include topical antibiotic (e.g., neomycin), fragrance, adhesives, rubber, latex, hair dye, nail polish, and metals (e.g., gold). See Table 3-2 for commonly patch tested substances.

Table 3-2	Components of the NACDG and True Test Patch Test Series
Compound	**Sources**
NACDG and True Test	
2-Mercaptobenzothiazole	Rubber, shoes
Colophony	Adhesives, chewing gum, violin bows
4-Phenylenediamine base	Hair dye, rubber
Neomycin sulfate	Topical antibiotics
Thiuram mix	Latex, rubber, adhesives
Formaldehyde	Preservatives, wrinkle-free clothing, cosmetics, shampoo, household cleaners
Epoxy resin	Uncured epoxy glue, adhesives, dental bonding agents, appliance finishes, varnish
Quarternium-15	Cosmetics, creams, lotions, shampoo, sunscreen
4-Tert-butylphenol formaldehyde resin	Adhesives, shoes
Mercapto mix	Rubber, gloves, boots, shoes, safety goggles
Potassium dichromate	Wet cement, welding fumes, chrome tanned leather, antirust paint
Balsam of Peru	Fragrances, pharmaceutical products, flavorings, sunscreen, shampoo
Nickel sulfate hexahydrate	Jewelry, snaps, zippers, buttons
Methylchloroisothiazolinone/ methylisothiazolinone	Cosmetics, shampoo, skin care products
Paraben mix	Cosmetics, skin care products
Fragrance mix I	Perfume, cologne, skin care products
Cobalt chloride	Nickel-plated objects, jewelry, cosmetics
Tixocortol-21-pivalate	Nasal spray
Budesonide	Asthma inhalers
Carba mix	Rubber, adhesives, gloves, safety goggles
Ethylenediamine dihydrochloride	Medicated skin creams
Imidazolidinyl urea	Cosmetics, shampoo, nail polish, deodorant
Diazolidinyl urea	Cosmetics, skin creams, pharmaceuticals

continued on following page

Compound	Sources
NACDG Only	
Benzocaine	Topical anesthetics
N-Isopropyl-N-phenyl-4-phenylenediamine	Black rubber
Sesquiterpene lactone mix	Cosmetics, creams, lotions, Asteraceae family plants (artichokes, chamomile, chrysanthemums, sunflowers, marigolds, and dandelions)
Methyldibromoglutaronitrile	Latex paint, adhesives, moist toilet wipes, cosmetics
Fragrance mix II	Perfume, cologne, skin care products
Cinnamic aldehyde	Perfume, cologne, flavoring agents
Amerchol L-101	Medicated ointments, furniture polish, cosmetics, textiles
DMDM hydantoin	Cosmetics, shampoos
Bacitracin	Topical antibiotics
Mixed dialkyl thioureas	Rubber, neoprene, shoes, wet suits
Glutaraldehyde	Disinfectants, leather and clothing tanners, dyes
2-Bromo-2-nitropropane-1,3-diol	Cosmetics, conditioner, shampoo, moisturizers, cleansing lotions
Propylene glycol	Cosmetics, personal lubricants, deodorant, hand sanitizers, food coloring
2-Hydroxy-4-methoxybenzophenone	Textiles, rubber, plastic, cosmetics, sunscreen
4-Chloro-3,5-xylenol	Creams, deodorants, disinfectants, conditioner
Ethyleneurea/melamine-formaldehyde mix	Textiles, draperies
Ethyl acrylate	Perfume, rubber, adhesives
Glyceryl monothioglycolate	Hair acid permanent wave solution
Tosylamide/formaldehyde resin	Nail polish
Methyl methacrylate	Dentures, fillings, fragrances
Disperse 106/124 mix	Blue linens, clothes
Iodopropynyl butyl carbamate	Cosmetics, water-based paint, wood preservatives
Compositae mix II	Cosmetics, shampoo, conditioner, oils, lotions
Hydrocortisone-17-butyrate	Topical steroids
Dimethylol dihydroxyethyleneurea	Draperies, permanent press clothing
Cocamidopropyl betaine	Shampoos, detergents, cleansing lotions
Triamcinolone acetonide	Topical steroids
True Test Only	
Caine mix	Topical anesthetics, cough syrup
Black rubber mix	Black rubber, boots, tires, scuba equipment, shoes, gloves
Thimerosal	Eye drops, ear drops, vaccines, cosmetics
Quinoline mix	Topical antibiotics

- Some are photocontact allergens and cause allergic dermatitis only when exposed to sunlight. Common ones include sunscreens (oxybenzone, octyl dimethyl para-aminobenzoic acid [PABA], and cinnamate), fragrance, and plants (lime, celery, parsnip).
- Airborne contact dermatitis is most commonly seen with plant allergens with diffuse involvement of exposed skin. It is most frequently seen with outdoor exposure to allergens carried by wind, but indoor exposure in the setting of a fireplace may also be seen.

4.2. Clinical Presentation

- Allergic contact dermatitis
  - Given the mechanism of delayed type IV hypersensitivity reaction, lesions develop days to weeks after exposure.
  - Characteristic features vary by chronicity.
    - Acute lesions are characterized by pruritic, erythematous, well-demarcated patches and plaques with variable vesicle formation and serosanguineous drainage (Fig. 3-5).
    - Chronic lesions are characterized by pruritic, hyperpigmented, thickened plaques with accentuation of skin lines.
  - Geometric or linear morphologic patterns are strongly suggestive of contact dermatitis; however, certain diffuse exposures such as shampoo may produce a widespread distribution pattern. In cases of severe localized contact dermatitis, id reaction, a diffuse nonspecific reactive dermatitis involving nonexposed areas, may be seen.
- Irritant contact dermatitis
  - Clinical presentation of irritant contact dermatitis may be subdivided into acute contact dermatitis, acute delayed irritant contact dermatitis, and cumulative irritant contact dermatitis.
    - Acute contact dermatitis
      - Characterized by rapid development of pain, burning, erythema, edema and variable vesiculation, bullae formation, and necrosis.
      - Potent acute irritants include acids, alkali solutions, and solvents.
    - Acute delayed irritant contact dermatitis
      - Characterized by the development of pain, burning, pruritus, xerosis, scaling, and fissuring on an erythematous background.
      - Results from exposure to moderate irritants such as benzalkonium chloride, which is a commonly used disinfectant.
      - Lesions may develop 8 to 24 hours after exposure.

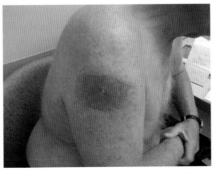

Figure 3-5. Allergic contact dermatitis, to adhesive in bandage. (Courtesy of David Sheinbein, MD.)

  ○ Cumulative irritant contact dermatitis
    – Characterized by the gradual development of burning, pruritus, erythema, xerosis, fissuring, hyperkeratosis, and accentuation of skin lines. Lesions tend to be less well defined than those of acute irritant dermatitis.
    – Results from repetitive exposure to mild irritants with insufficient time between exposures for restoration of skin barrier function.
    – Lesions develop days to weeks after chronic exposure.
    – Examples of mild irritants producing cumulative irritant contact dermatitis include soap and water.

4.3. Evaluation

- A careful history is critical in diagnosing either allergic or irritant contact dermatitis. Questions should be asked about all possible topical exposures. A history of exposure to known allergens versus irritants helps differentiate the two.
- The differential diagnosis includes atopic dermatitis, stasis dermatitis, seborrheic dermatitis, psoriasis, tinea, and rosacea. History and clinical exam are crucial in differentiating these diagnoses.
  - Atopic dermatitis is more frequently widespread, symmetric, and found in a classic distribution pattern on flexor surfaces.
  - Stasis dermatitis found on lower legs frequently has associated edema, varicosities, and hyperpigmentation. It is important to note that along with stasis dermatitis, one could also develop contact dermatitis, since chronicity and frequency of exposure to topical antibiotic, steroids, and emollients are increased.
  - Seborrheic dermatitis is more frequently symmetric and produces less well-defined erythematous patches with greasy, yellow scale.
  - Psoriasis is differentiated by the presence of erythematous plaques with adherent silvery scale.
  - A potassium hydroxide preparation may be performed to rule out tinea on the hands and feet.
  - Rosacea produces centrofacial erythema that may be confused with contact dermatitis, but the associated findings of telangiectasia, phymatous changes, and history of flushing help reach the correct diagnosis.
- Patch testing is the gold standard for identifying contact allergens (Fig. 3-6). The North American Contact Dermatitis Group's standard screening tray and True Test are most frequently used to screen for common allergens. See Table 3-2 for a list of included allergens.
  - Patch test trays are placed on the upper back, and the patient is instructed to return in 48 hours for removal. Patients should not get the patches wet or perform activities resulting in excessive sweating.
  - Patches are removed at 48 hours, allergens are marked, and any positive reactions are noted and scored. The patient is then asked to come back for a final read 72 hours to 1 week after initial patch placement.
  - Reactions are graded according to the international grading system for patch tests. See Table 3-3.

4.4. Treatment

The primary goal of treatment is to identify causative allergens and irritants and avoid exposure. Cessation of exposure will prevent further flares, though current episodes of dermatitis may take weeks to resolve. To hasten resolution of active lesions, clinicians may use topical steroids. If the reaction is particularly severe or diffuse, patients may take a short course of oral steroids to expedite clearance.

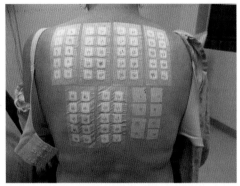

A

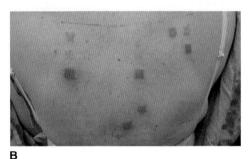

B

Figure 3-6. A: Patch test in place. **B:** Positive patch test results. (Courtesy of David Sheinbein, MD.)

- Topical steroids
  - Topical steroids are first-line therapy for mild to moderate, localized contact dermatitis. Generally, mid- to superpotent topical steroids are needed to resolve allergic contact dermatitis; for irritant contact dermatitis, high potency is rarely needed.
  - High-potency to superpotent topical steroids may be applied twice daily until lesions clear. Ointments are more effective than creams. One week of midpotency steroid is generally used on the face, if needed. Use of high potency on the face should be avoided.

Table 3-3	International Grading System for Patch Tests
Grade	**Reaction**
−	None
+/−	Unlikely reaction. Faint erythema
+	Weak reaction. Erythema, possible papules
++	Strong reaction. Erythema, infiltration, papules
+++	Very strong reaction. Erythema, bullae, ulcers, spreading
IR	Irritant reaction

- Side effects include atrophy, striae formation, telangiectasias, perioral dermatitis, purpura, acneiform, and rosacea-like lesions; however, given the transient nature of the disease, side effects are less common than when treating chronic conditions such as atopic dermatitis.
- Examples in order of increasing potency:
  o Triamcinolone 0.1% ointment BID
  o Desoximetasone 0.05% ointment BID
  o Clobetasol 0.05% ointment BID
- Oral steroids
  - A short course of oral steroids is effective in achieving rapid improvement of severe contact dermatitis. There is no difference in time to improvement, percentage with complete clearance, or recurrence between 5- and 15-day courses of prednisone observed in treatment of severe poison ivy.[30]
  - Side effects of oral steroids include hypertension, hyperglycemia, hyperlipidemia, cataracts, myopathy, striae formation, adrenal axis suppression, mood changes, insomnia, osteoporosis, and osteonecrosis; however, given the very short duration of therapy, side effects are limited.
  - Example
    o Prednisone 40 mg PO daily × 5 days

5. PITYRIASIS ROSEA

5.1. Background

- Pityriasis rosea (PR) is an acute, self-limited entity that commonly presents in young adults as a red, scaly rash. PR is slightly more common in females.
- The pathogenesis has not been definitively identified, but a viral etiology has been suggested based on the transient nature, case clustering, possible prodrome, and lack of recurrence suggesting immunity.
- Human herpesvirus (HHV) 6 and 7 have been extensively studied as the causative agents of PR; however, evidence is inconsistent.[31,32]

5.2. Clinical Presentation (Fig. 3-7)

- Onset typically begins with a solitary pink or salmon-colored, round to oval, patch or plaque with fine, trailing scale on the trunk. This is called the "herald patch."
- The herald patch slowly expands over the course of several days, after which, similar smaller lesions appear on the trunk and extremities. Lesions often follow Langer lines of cleavage and produce a "Christmas tree" pattern on the back.
- Patients may have a mild prodrome, but otherwise, lesions are typically asymptomatic and last 6 to 8 weeks. Lesions resolve completely without scarring.

5.3. Evaluation

- Diagnosis is largely clinical, though laboratory testing and biopsy may be helpful. Rapid plasma reagin (RPR) or the Venereal Disease Research Laboratory test (VDRL) is generally recommended for those who are sexually active to rule out secondary syphilis, which resembles PR. Follow up with confirmatory testing, if positive. If the eruption does not resolve within 3 months, a skin punch biopsy should be done to rule out other diagnoses on the differential.
- KOH preparation may be done to rule out tinea.

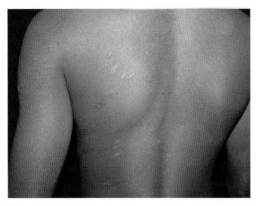

Figure 3-7. Pityriasis rosea. (Courtesy of Susan Bayliss, MD.)

• Drug reactions can produce a similar rash, so a careful review of the medication list is important.

5.4. Treatment

Since PR is a self-limited, generally asymptomatic disease, most cases require only education and reassurance. Patients suffering from pruritus may benefit from topical steroids, NB UVB, or oral antibiotics.
• Medium or high potency topical steroids applied twice daily may decrease pruritus. See Table 3-1 for a listing of corticosteroids by potency.
• NB UVB decreases extent of lesions and pruritus.[33]
• Erythromycin has been shown to speed resolution in some studies.[34]

6. PSORIASIS

6.1. Background

• Psoriasis is an immune-mediated disorder characterized by the development of thick, red plaques with adherent silvery scale commonly found on the scalp, extensor surfaces, hands, feet, and gluteal cleft.
• Worldwide prevalence in the adult population ranges from 0.91% to 8.5%.[35]
• Psoriasis can develop at any age; however, there are three peak ages of onset around puberty and fourth and sixth decades of life.[36]
• Systemic manifestations of psoriasis include psoriatic arthritis, increased risk of cardiovascular disease, and increased prevalence of metabolic syndrome.
    • Psoriatic arthritis can lead to crippling, erosive joint disease most commonly in the proximal interphalangeal (PIP) joints, and distal interphalangeal (DIP) joints of the fingers and toes.
    • Patients with psoriasis have a 2× increased risk of myocardial infarction (MI) and cardiovascular disease.[37]
    • Meta-analysis of over 1.4 million patients revealed an odds ratio of 2.1 in psoriatic patients for the development of metabolic syndrome, defined as a combination of three of five criteria including elevated fasting glucose, elevated

triglycerides, hypertension, decreased high-density lipoprotein, and elevated waist circumference.[38]
- Patients also suffer from psychosocial manifestations of their disease.
  - Patients with psoriasis report physical discomfort, impaired emotional functioning, negative body and self-image, and limitations in daily activities, social contacts, (skin-exposing) activities, and work.[39]
- Psoriasis results from a complex interplay between genetics, the innate and adaptive immunity, and triggering factors.
  - Twin association studies have demonstrated an increased prevalence of psoriasis in fraternal twins and an even higher prevalence in monozygotic twins, suggesting a strong genetic component.[40] Furthermore, a study of 5,197 families with psoriasis showed that 36% of the probands had one or more parents with psoriasis.[41]
  - HLA-Cw6 is the most commonly associated histocompatibility antigen. Its presence heralds an increased relative risk of development of psoriasis and earlier age of onset. Approximately 10% of HLA-Cw6–positive individuals will develop psoriasis.[42]
  - T lymphocytes drive inflammation in psoriasis. Supporting evidence includes association with specific HLA alleles, presence of oligoclonal lesional T cells, and response to T-cell–suppressive agents.[43–45]
  - Natural killer (NK) cells, part of the innate immune system, are increased in psoriatic lesions.[46] NK cells interact with CD1d receptors on keratinocytes. Activation of these receptors stimulates NK cells to produce IFN-gamma, which stimulates APCs.[47]
  - Innate and adaptive-derived cytokines and chemokines stimulate inflammation and keratinocyte proliferation.
    ○ Cytokines including IFN-gamma, IL-2, IL-12, IL-23, and IL-15 are increased in psoriatic skin. Anti-inflammatory cytokines such as IL-10 are decreased.
    ○ IL-12 and IL-23 are postulated to play a central role in lesion development, supported by the profound response to IL-12 and IL-23 inhibitors such as ustekinumab.
    ○ Proinflammatory innate cytokines including IL-1, IL-6, and TNF-alpha are also increased in lesional skin.
  - Triggering factors include infection, stress, drugs, trauma, and hypocalcemia.
    ○ Bacterial infections such as streptococcal pharyngitis are commonly implicated in the onset of guttate psoriasis.
    ○ High stress has been correlated with increased severity of skin lesions and joint symptoms.[48]
    ○ Medications such as ACE inhibitors, lithium, β-blockers, antimalarials, and NSAIDs have been shown to worsen psoriasis.
    ○ Psoriasis is well known to exhibit the Koebner phenomenon, meaning that cutaneous injury may trigger development of psoriatic lesions.
    ○ Hypocalemia is associated primarily with the development of pustular psoriasis.[49]

6.2. Clinical Presentation (Fig. 3-8)

There are several clinical variants of psoriasis. The main subtypes are chronic plaque psoriasis, guttate psoriasis, pustular psoriasis, and inverse psoriasis. Each of these variants may be associated with the development of psoriatic arthritis.

- Chronic plaque psoriasis
  - Characterized by erythematous, scaly, well-demarcated plaques.
  - Lesions are frequently found on the scalp, elbows, knees, hands, feet, and gluteal cleft.
  - Disease may be localized or widespread.
- Guttate psoriasis
  - Characterized by scattered small round to oval-shaped, erythematous, scaly, well-demarcated papules and plaques covering a widespread distribution.
  - Onset is frequently preceded by streptococcal pharyngitis, and lesions may spontaneously resolve. Neither penicillin nor erythromycin directed at streptococcal infection hastens resolution of lesions.[50]
  - This pattern is more frequently seen in children and young adults.
- Pustular psoriasis
  - Characterized by sterile, neutrophil-derived pustules in a generalized or localized pattern.

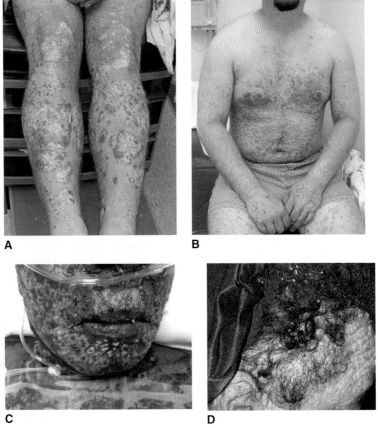

Figure 3-8. Variants of psoriasis. **A:** Psoriasis vulgaris. **B:** Moderate-severe plaque psoriasis. **C:** Pustular psoriasis. **D:** Scalp psoriasis. (Courtesy of David Sheinbein, MD.)

- Several variants exist, including palmoplantar pustulosis, acute generalized von Zumbusch, annular pattern, exanthematic type, and localized pattern.
  - Palmoplantar psoriasis is defined by the presence of sterile, pustules on the palms and soles on a background of erythematous, scaly plaques.
  - Von Zumbusch pattern is characterized by acute, generalized eruption of pustules on an erythematous background with pain and fever.
  - Annular pattern demonstrates pustules arranged in an annular fashion at the advancing edge of erythematous plaques.
  - Exanthematic type shows acute, widespread eruption of small pustules without background erythema, fever, or systemic symptoms.
  - Localized pattern is characterized by the development of pustules in pre-existing lesions of chronic plaque psoriasis.
- Inverse psoriasis
  - Lesions are typically located in the axillae, inguinal crease, inframammary folds, and gluteal cleft.
  - Characterized by well-demarcated thin red plaques with minimal scale.
  - Lesions may demonstrate fissures.
- Psoriatic arthritis
  - Characterized by progressive, erosive joint disease.
  - Estimates of the prevalence of psoriatic arthritis widely vary but is felt to be about 30%.[51]
  - Arthritis is more common in patients with more severe skin disease. However, it can also be seen in patients with none to minimal skin disease.
  - Several patterns exist including asymmetric mono- and oligoarthritis of the DIP and PIP joints, rheumatoid-like arthritis, arthritis mutilans, and spondylitis with sacroiliitis.
    - Asymmetric mono-/oligoarthritis of the DIP and PIP joints is the most common form of psoriatic arthritis. "Sausage digits" may result from vigorous inflammation of the distal digits.
    - Rheumatoid-like psoriatic arthritis produces symmetric polyarthritis of the MCPs, PIPs wrists, ankles, and elbows as in rheumatoid arthritis. Patients may have a positive or negative RF.
    - Arthritis mutilans is the most severe form of psoriatic arthritis characterized by progressive, destructive joint disease resulting in permanent deformity.
    - Spondylitis and sacroiliitis are more common in patients with HLA-B27 alleles. Prominent symptoms include axial joint pain with morning stiffness.

6.3. Evaluation

- Psoriasis is largely a clinical diagnosis, though careful review of contributing factors and screening for psoriatic arthritis is important. Psoriasis must be differentiated from other papulosquamous disorders including seborrheic dermatitis, cutaneous T-cell lymphoma (CTCL), and chronic eczema.
  - Sharp demarcation and thick, scaly, red plaques characteristic of psoriasis help to differentiate psoriatic lesions from those of seborrheic dermatitis, which are less well demarcated.
  - Epidermal atrophy and wrinkling followed by subsequent infiltration suggests CTCL. Biopsy would be warranted to rule out CTCL.

- Chronic eczema may produce scaly plaques, but they are frequently less well demarcated and less erythematous, allowing differentiation from psoriasis.
- Review the medication list for contributing factors.
- Check antistreptolysin O (ASO) titer in guttate psoriasis given possibility of streptococcal infection as an inciting factor.
- Check radiographs for erosion if psoriatic arthritis is suspected.
- Check rheumatoid factor and cyclic citrullinated peptide antibodies to help distinguish psoriatic arthritis from rheumatoid arthritis.
- Consider rheumatology referral if joint pain is not well controlled with standard therapies.

6.4. Treatment

Therapy is directed at effectively managing acute flares and maintaining a limited or disease-free maintenance phase. Both topical and systemic medications are enlisted. Topical medications comprise first-line therapy for limited disease. Steroids and calcineurin inhibitors reduce inflammation, while vitamin D analogues and retinoids help normalize epidermal differentiation. Topical therapies are often combined for treatment of mild to moderate psoriasis. Phototherapy is beneficial adjuvant therapy for treatment of plaques resistant to topical therapy or for more diffuse skin involvement. Systemic therapy should be utilized in those with recalcitrant, extensive disease and is mandated in patients with significant psoriatic arthritis.

- Topical therapy
  - Corticosteroids
    - Inhibit inflammation by interacting with nuclear receptors to decrease production of inflammatory cytokines.
    - Ointments have the highest efficacy, but creams may be better tolerated. Solutions and oils may be used on the scalp for increased ease of application.
    - Patients may wrap steroid ointment under plastic wrap to increase penetration and enhance efficacy.
    - Steroids should be applied twice daily until lesions resolve. Intermittent application thereafter several times per week helps maintain remission.[52]
    - Examples in order of increasing potency:
      - Fluocinolone 0.1% solution
      - Desonide 0.05% cream
      - Triamcinolone 0.1% cream
      - Triamcinolone 0.1% ointment
      - Fluocinonide 0.05% solution
      - Clobetasol 0.05% solution
      - Clobetasol 0.05% ointment
    - Side effects of topical steroid application include atrophy, striae formation, telangiectasia, perioral dermatitis, purpura, acneiform, and rosacea-like lesions. Application should be performed twice daily to areas of active inflammation. Maintenance therapy should be decreased to twice-weekly application to limit risks of cutaneous side effects.
  - Vitamin D analogues: calcipotriene
    - Inhibits epidermal proliferation, normalizes differentiation, and inhibits neutrophils.
    - Calcipotriene ointment applied twice daily resulted in a 70% reduction in lesion severity score after 8 weeks of treatment. Side effects were minimal, and

there was no significant difference in serum calcium levels between active and vehicle-only treatment groups.[53]
- Vitamin D analogues are frequently used in combination with topical steroids.
- Example
  - Calcipotriene 0.005% ointment or cream BID
• Topical retinoids: tazarotene
  - Inhibits epidermal proliferation and normalizes differentiation by binding to retinoic acid receptor (RAR)-beta and RAR-gamma.
  - Tazarotene gel application reduces erythema, plaque elevation, and pruritus as compared to vehicle.[54]
  - Tazarotene is less effective than topical steroids, though may be used in combination as a second-line therapy.
  - Side effects include burning, pruritus, and irritation.
  - Example
    - Tazarotene 0.1% or 0.05% gel once daily
• Calcineurin inhibitors
  - Inhibits production of proinflammatory cytokine IL-2.
  - Calcineurin inhibitors are particularly beneficial in the treatment of facial, genital, and intertriginous psoriasis given the absence of steroid-associated side effects in these sensitive areas.
  - Tacrolimus and pimecrolimus are both beneficial, though tacrolimus is somewhat more effective.[55]
  - Side effects including burning and irritation.
  - Examples
    - Tacrolimus 0.1% and 0.3% ointment BID
    - Pimecrolimus 1% cream BID
• Phototherapy
Narrowband UVB has become the phototherapy treatment of choice for diffuse cutaneous psoriasis, as its efficacy is nearly comparable to that of psoralen-UVA (PUVA) while demonstrating a superior safety profile. Phototherapy is administered two to three times per week, and the dose is gradually titrated to produce minimally perceptive erythema. Generally, 20 to 40 treatments over the course of a few months are required to achieve remission or significant improvement. Afterward, phototherapy can be tapered off or maintained at a less frequent schedule. For all wavelengths, eyes and genitalia are shielded in the light box, in addition to any unaffected areas.
• Narrowband UVB (NB UVB)
  - 311- to 313-nm light.
  - Absorbed by chromophores including nuclear DNA resulting in the formation of pyrimidine dimers and expression of p53. Both result in arrest of proliferation and p53 can lead to apoptosis. Narrowband UVB also reduces production of inflammatory cytokines.
  - NB UVB may be combined with calcipotriene or acitretin to increase efficacy.[56,57]
  - Side effects include erythema, xerosis, blistering, and reactivation of HSV.
  - Long-term side effects include photoaging and potential increased risk of skin cancer; however, a study of 3,867 patients did not show any increased risk of BCC, SCC, or melanoma in association with NB UVB treatment.[58]
• Psoralen with UVA (PUVA)
  - 320- to 400-nm light in combination with topical or oral psoralens.

- o Psoralens are photosensitizing agents that intercalate with DNA. UVA absorption stimulates DNA helix cross-linking, which inhibits DNA replication and leads to cell cycle arrest. Cells may then proceed through apoptosis.
- o Studies have shown PUVA with oral psoralens is more effective than NB UVB as monotherapy. NB UVB was more effective than PUVA with topical psoralens.[59]
- o PUVA may be combined with other medications to increase efficacy and reduce side effects.
    - – Methotrexate combined with PUVA resulted in faster clearing and decreased number of PUVA treatments compared to either monotherapy alone.[60]
    - – Oral retinoids combined with PUVA resulted in a 30% improvement in clearance rate as compared to PUVA alone.[61]
- o Cutaneous side effects include delayed erythema peaking at 72 to 96 hours posttreatment, persistent erythema, blistering, edema, pruritus, and stinging. Oral psoralen side effects include nausea and vomiting. PUVA induces cataract formation, so eye shielding during treatment as well as up to 24 hours posttreatment with UVA- and UVB-protective sunglasses is mandatory.
- o Long-term side effects include photoaging, actinic keratosis formation, lentigo formation, and increased risk of nonmelanoma skin cancers.
- • Systemic therapy
- • Methotrexate
    - o Inhibits dihydrofolate reductase, which impairs purine nucleotide synthesis, halting DNA and RNA synthesis.
    - o Generally, 15 to 20 mg weekly is needed to provide good control. Start at 7.5 mg weekly and titrate up by 2.5 mg every 2 weeks to achieve the required dose while checking CBC and LFT weekly. Administer the weekly dose in three divided doses every 12 hours (e.g., 15 mg per week dosing would give 5 mg every 12 hours for 3 doses per week).
    - o Folic acid 1 mg PO daily may be administered on off days to mitigate side effects.
    - o Side effects include hepatotoxicity, pancytopenia, nausea, mucositis, and photosensitivity. Potential for hepatotoxicity and pancytopenia requires laboratory monitoring with CBC and LFTs. Risk of hepatotoxicity is related to cumulative dose.
- • Cyclosporine
    - o Binds cyclophilin and inhibits production of IL-2.
    - o Results in rapid improvement of severe disease. Given its ability to produce rapid clearance, it is often used for short durations to achieve quick control of extensive, severe disease.
    - o Long-term, low-dose cyclosporine may be used for control of persistent psoriasis not cleared by other medicines, but is limited by side effects: nephrotoxicity, hypertension, increased risk of skin cancers, gastrointestinal disturbance, hypertrichosis, gingival hyperplasia, headache, and tremor.[62]
    - o Laboratory abnormalities include hyperkalemia, hyperuricemia, hypomagnesemia, and elevated lipid profile.
- • Systemic retinoids: acitretin
    - o Normalizes proliferation and differentiation via activation of RARs.
    - o Acitretin is indicated for use as first-line therapy for pustular or erythrodermic psoriasis or as second-line therapy for chronic plaque psoriasis.

- ○ May be combined with NB UVB as above to increase efficacy of both treatments.
- ○ Acitretin may be re-esterified to a related systemic retinoid called etretinate, particularly in the presence of alcohol. The half-life of etretinate is 120 days.
- ○ Side effects include xerosis, xerophthalmia, exacerbation of eczema, headaches, muscle and joint aches, mood changes, depression, and anxiety.
- ○ Laboratory abnormalities include increased cholesterol, triglycerides, and aminotransferases. Labs should be checked prior to, during, and after therapy.
- ○ Oral retinoids are potent teratogens. Pregnancy should be avoided for 3 years after stopping acitretin given re-esterification to etretinate as mentioned. For this reason, acitretin is generally avoided in women of child-bearing age.
- • Biologics
  - ○ Tumor necrosis factor (TNF) inhibitors
    - - Bind to TNF-alpha and impede its binding to TNF-alpha receptors.
    - - Excellent efficacy for treatment of skin lesions and psoriatic arthritis. Cost and side effects limit its use to those with moderate to severe psoriasis.
    - - Prior to treatment, patients should obtain a purified protein derivative (PPD), CBC, comprehensive metabolic panel (CMP), human immunodeficiency virus (HIV), and hepatitis B virus (HBV) and hepatitis C virus (HCV) serologic testing. While on treatment, patients should obtain a PPD annually and CBC and CMP every 3 to 12 months.
    - - Side effects include increased risk of infection, reactivation of latent tuberculosis, autoimmune antibodies, congestive heart failure, palmoplantar pustulosis, and hypersensitivity reactions.
    - - Examples
      - □ Etanercept 25 to 50 mg subcutaneously twice weekly
      - □ Infliximab 5 mg/kg IV infusion at 0, 2, and 6 weeks, and then every 8 weeks thereafter
      - □ Adalimumab 80 mg subcutaneously for the first dose, and then 40 mg subcutaneously at day 8 and every other week thereafter
  - ○ IL-12/IL-23 inhibitors: ustekinumab
    - - Binds to the p40 subunit of IL-12 and IL-23.
    - - Ustekinumab produces excellent clearance of skin lesions, but is not effective for psoriatic arthritis. 67.1% of patients receiving ustekinumab 45 mg achieved 75% improvement in their lesion severity by 12 weeks.[63]
    - - Side effects include increased risk of infections, reactivation of latent tuberculosis, and hypersensitivity reactions. Further studies are needed to evaluate the risks of cardiovascular disease and malignancy.
    - - Examples:
      - □ Ustekinumab 40 to 90 mg subcutaneously at 0 weeks, 4 weeks, and then every 12 weeks thereafter

7. SEBORRHEIC DERMATITIS

7.1. Background

- • Seborrheic dermatitis is a mild eczematous process characterized by greasy, flaky, yellow scales on an erythematous background. Pruritus is a common symptom. It predominates on areas of high sebum production, including the face, scalp, and upper trunk.

- There are two peak age distributions in infancy and later between the ages of 40 to 60 years old. Seborrheic dermatitis is more common in men than women.
- Seborrheic dermatitis in babies is often called "cradle cap." Cradle cap is very common, and studies have shown a prevalence of 71.7% in children < 3 months old with that number declining to 44.5% of children at 1 year of age.[64] The peak in infancy correlates with a transient period of sebaceous gland activity.
- The pathogenesis of seborrheic dermatitis is multifactorial and involves increased sebum production, *Malassezia globosa*, and an altered host immune response.[65–67]

7.2. Clinical Presentation

- Seborrheic dermatitis is characterized by greasy, flaky, yellow scales on poorly demarcated erythematous patches or thin plaques. Vesicles, crusting, and secondary infection are less frequently seen manifestations (Fig. 3-9).
- Lesions are most commonly found on areas of high sebum production including the face, scalp, and upper trunk. The eyebrows, nasal sidewalls, nasolabial folds, and glabella are classic areas of facial involvement.
- The rash is typically localized and follows a mild course; however, rarely, it may become generalized and produce erythroderma.
- Dandruff is a milder version with less inflammation. Pruritus is common.

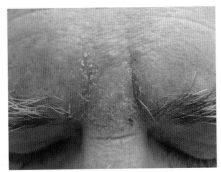

A

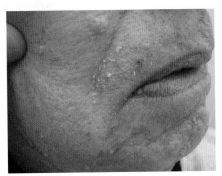

B

Figure 3-9. A,B: Seborrheic dermatitis. (Courtesy of David Sheinbein, MD.)

7.3. Evaluation

- Seborrheic dermatitis is primarily a clinical diagnosis with key features that distinguish it from other eczematous processes seen in a similar distribution.
- The differential diagnosis varies by age group.
  - The differential diagnosis of infantile and childhood seborrheic dermatitis includes atopic dermatitis, psoriasis, and tinea capitis.
    - Atopic dermatitis (AD) is associated with more intense inflammation, higher degree of pruritus, later age of onset, and more widespread distribution on the face, scalp, and extensor surfaces. AD also produces higher morbidity with greater disturbance in patient quality of life.
    - Psoriasis tends to have more well-demarcated, thick plaques with silvery, adherent scale as opposed to the greasy, flaky scale of seborrheic dermatitis.
    - Tinea capitis may produce a more robust inflammatory reaction and lead to hair loss. Fungal culture should be performed to rule out tinea capitis in high-risk populations.
  - The adult seborrheic dermatitis differential includes psoriasis, atopic dermatitis, contact dermatitis, rosacea, and acute lupus erythematosus.
    - Psoriasis is distinguishable as mentioned above by more well-demarcated thick, red plaques with adherent silvery scale. Distribution is often more widespread and includes the extensor surfaces. Nail findings and symptoms of inflammatory joint disease further distinguish psoriasis from SD.
    - Atopic dermatitis in the adult population is differentiated by its common distribution pattern on the flexor surfaces and hands.
    - Contact dermatitis typically follows a less symmetric pattern. Geometric or linear patterns in particular suggest contact dermatitis over SD. A history of exposure to potential allergens and irritants is key in differentiating contact dermatitis from seborrheic dermatitis.
    - Rosacea produces centrofacial erythema similar to SD, but the lack of scale differentiates rosacea from SD.
    - Similarly, acute lupus erythematosus produces centrofacial erythema as in SD, but it classically spares the nasolabial folds, allowing simple differentiation from SD.

7.4. Treatment

Seborrheic dermatitis is a chronic condition requiring routine application of therapeutic shampoos, solutions, and creams for continued control. Treatment is directed at minimizing erythema, scale, and pruritus. Topical products including antifungals and steroids are the mainstays of treatment. Topicals may be applied once or twice daily during acute flares and once or twice weekly thereafter for maintenance.

- Antifungal agents decrease the load of *Malassezia* yeast on affected skin.
  - Ketoconazole (KC) 2% shampoo or cream once or twice daily
  - Zinc pyrithione (ZPT) 1% shampoo once or twice daily
    - KC and ZPT have similar efficacy in SD management with a reported 73% and 67% reduction in total dandruff scores, respectively.[68]
  - Ciclopirox olamine (CPO) 1.5% shampoo once or twice daily
    - Comparison of CPO shampoo with KC shampoo demonstrated similar reductions in affected areas of 41.4 cm^2 and 48.2 cm^2, respectively. Patients reported higher levels of satisfaction in signs and symptoms with CPO shampoo.[69]

- Topical steroids decrease inflammation. Mild- and moderate-potency topical steroids were found to have a similar degree of efficacy.[70] Given their similar efficacy and decreased side effect profile, low-potency steroids should be tried first.
- Steroids may be applied once or twice daily during the acute phase.
- Maintenance should be attempted with antifungal agents. If unable to achieve disease-free maintenance state with antifungal agents alone, a topical steroid may be added with once- or twice-weekly application.
- Examples
  - Hydrocortisone 2.5% cream once or twice daily
  - Desonide 0.05% cream once or twice daily
  - Fluocinolone 0.01% solution once or twice daily

REFERENCES

1. Collier CN, Harper JC, Cafardi JA, et al. The prevalence of acne in adults 20 years and older. *J Am Acad Dermatol* 2008;58:56–59.
2. Berg M, Liden S. An epidemiological study of rosacea. *Acta Derm Venereol* 1989;69:419–423.
3. Spoendlin J, Voegel JJ, Jick SS, et al. A study on the epidemiology of rosacea in the UK. *Br J Dermatol* 2012;167:598–605.
4. Fowler J Jr, Jackson M, Moore A, et al. Efficacy and safety of once-daily topical brimonidine tartrate gel 0.5% for the treatment of moderate to severe facial erythema of rosacea: results of two randomized, double-blind, and vehicle-controlled pivotal studies. *J Drus Dermatol* 2013;12:650–656.
5. Shanler SD, Ondo AL. Successful treatment of the Erythema and flushing of Rosacea using a topically applied selective α1-adrenergic receptor agonist, Oxymetazoline. *Arch Dermatol* 2007;143:1369–1371.
6. Shim TN, Abdullah A. The effect of pulsed dye laser on the dermatology life quality index in erythematotelangiectatic rosacea patients: an assessment. *J Clin Aesthet Dermatol* 2013;6:30–32.
7. Bassi A, Campolmi P, Dindelli M, et al. *Laser surgery in rhinophyma. Giornale Italiano di dermatologia e venereologia*, 2014.
8. Prado R, Funke A, Brown M, et al. Treatment of severe rhinophyma using scalpel excision and wire loop tip electrosurgery. *Dermatol Surg* 2013;39:807–810.
9. Hong S, Son DK, Lim WR, et al. The prevalence of atopic dermatitis, asthma, and allergic rhinitis and the comorbidity of allergic diseases in children. *Environ Health Toxicol* 2012;27:e2012006.
10. Flohr C, Yeo L. Atopic dermatitis and the hygiene hypothesis revisited. *Curr Probl Dermatol* 2011;41:1–34.
11. Flohr C, Pascoe D, Williams HC. Atopic dermatitis and the 'hygiene hypothesis': too clean to be true? *Br J Dermatol* 2005;152:202–216.
12. Margolis JS, Abuabara K, Bilker W, et al. Persistence of mild to moderate atopic dermatitis. *JAMA Dermatol* 2014;150:593–600.
13. Chang YS, Chou YT, Lee JH, et al. Atopic dermatitis, melatonin, and sleep disturbance. *Pediatrics* 2014;134:e397–e405.
14. Thomsen SF, Ulrik CS, Kyvik KO, et al. Importance of genetic factors in the etiology of atopic dermatitis: a twin study. *Allergy Asthma Proc* 2007;28:535–539.
15. Elias PM, Schmuth M. Abnormal skin barrier in the etiopathogenesis of atopic dermatitis. *Curr Asthma Allergy Rep* 2009;9:265–272.
16. Palmer CN, Irvine AD, Terron-Kwiatkowski A, et al. Common loss-of-function variants of the epidermal barrier protein filaggrin are a major predisposing factor for atopic dermatitis. *Nat Genet* 2006;38:441–446.
17. Lewis-Jones S. Quality of life and childhood atopic dermatitis: the misery of living with childhood eczema. *Int J Clin Pract* 2006;60:984–992.

18. Gelmetti C, Boralevi F, Seité S, et al. Quality of life of parents living with a child suffering from atopic dermatitis before and after a 3-month treatment with an emollient. *Pediatr Dermatol* 2012;29:714–718.

19. Peserico A, Städtler G, Sebastian M, et al. Reduction of relapses of atopic dermatitis with methylprednisolone aceponate cream twice weekly in addition to maintenance treatment with emollient: a multicentre, randomized, double-blind, controlled study. *Br J Dermatol* 2008;158:801–807.

20. Jury CS, McHenry P, Burden AD, et al. Narrowband ultraviolet B (UVB) phototherapy in children. *Clin Exp Dermatol* 2006;31:196–199.

21. Haw S, Shin MK, Haw CR. The efficacy and safety of long-term oral cyclosporine treatment for patients with atopic dermatitis. *Ann Dermatol* 2010;22:9–15.

22. Thomsen SF, Karlsmark T, Clemmensen KK, et al. Outcome of treatment with azathioprine in severe atopic dermatitis: a five-year retrospective study of adult outpatients. *Br J Dermatol* 2015;172(4):1122–1124.

23. Sheinkopf LE, Rafi AW, Do LT, et al. Efficacy of omalizumab in the treatment of atopic dermatitis: a pilot study. *Allergy Asthma Proc* 2008;29:530–537.

24. Simon D, Hösli S, Kostylina G, et al. Anti-CD20 (rituximab) treatment improves atopic eczema. *J Allergy Clin Immunol* 2008;121:122–128.

25. Nethercott JR, Holness DL, Adams RM, et al. Patch testing with a routine screening tray in North America, 1985 through 1989: I. Frequency of response. *Dermatitis* 1991;2:122–129.

26. Teixeira V, Coutinho I, Gonçalo M. Allergic contact dermatitis to metals over a 20-year period in the Centre of Portugal: evaluation of the effects of the European directives. *Acta Med Port* 2014;27:295–303.

27. Larsson-Stymne B, Widström L. Ear piercing—a cause of nickel allergy in schoolgirls? *Contact Dermatitis* 1985;13:289–293.

28. Srivastava D, Cohen DE. Identification of the constituents of Balsam of Peru in tomatoes. *Dermatitis* 2009;20:99–105.

29. Cheman A, Rakowski EM, Chou V, et al. Balsam of Peru: past and future. *Dermatitis* 2013;24:153–160.

30. Curtis G, Lewis AC. Treatment of severe poison ivy: a randomized, controlled trial of long versus short course oral prednisone. *J Clin Med Res* 2014;6:429–434.

31. Yildirim M, Aridogan BC, Baysal V, et al. The role of human herpes virus 6 and 7 in the pathogenesis of pityriasis rosea. *Int J Clin Pract* 2004;58:119–121.

32. Chuh AA, Peiris JS. Lack of evidence of active human herpesvirus 7 (HHV-7) infection in three cases of pityriasis rosea in children. *Pediatr Dermatol* 2008;18:381–383.

33. Arndt KA, Paul BS, Stern RS, et al. Treatment of pityriasis rosea with UV radiation. *Arch Dermatol* 1983;119:381–382.

34. Bigby M. A remarkable result of a double-masked, placebo-controlled trial of erythromycin in the treatment of Pityriasis rosea. *Arch Dermatol* 2000;136:775–776.

35. Parisi R, Symmons DP, Griffiths CE, et al. Global epidemiology of psoriasis: a systematic review of incidence and prevalence. *J Investig Dermatol* 2013;133:377–385.

36. Swanbeck G, Inerot A, Martinsson T, et al. Age at onset and different types of psoriasis. *Br J Dermatol* 1995;133:768–773.

37. Lin HW, Wang KH, Lin HC, et al. Increased risk of acute myocardial infarction in patients with psoriasis: a 5-year population-based study in Taiwan. *J Am Acad Dermatol* 2011;64:495–501.

38. Armstrong AW, Harskamp CT, Armstrong EJ. Psoriasis and metabolic syndrome: a systematic review and meta-analysis of observational studies. *J Am Acad Dermatol* 2013;68:654–662.

39. de Korte J, Sprangers MA, Mombers FM, et al. Quality of life in patients with psoriasis: a systematic literature review. *J Invest Dermatol* 2004;9:140–147.

40. Grjibovski AM, Olsen AO, Magnus P, et al. Psoriasis in Norwegian twins: contribution of genetic and environmental effects. *J Eur Acad Dermatol Venereol* 2007;21:1337–1343.

41. Swanbeck G, Inerot A, Martinsson T, et al. A population genetic study of psoriasis. *Br J Dermatol* 1994;13:32–39.

42. Elder JT, Henseler T, Christophers E, et al. Of genes and antigens: the inheritance of psoriasis. *J Investig Dermatol* 1994;103:150S–153S.
43. Conrad C, Boyman O, Tonel G, et al. Alpha1beta1 integrin is crucial for accumulation of epidermal T cells and the development of psoriasis. *Nat Med* 2007;13:836–842.
44. Lin WJ, Norris DA, Achziger M, et al. Oligoclonal expansion of intraepidermal T cells in psoriasis skin lesions. *J Investig Dermatol* 2001;117:1546–1553.
45. Kryczek I, Bruce AT, Gudjonsson JE, et al. Induction of IL-17+ T cell trafficking and development by IFN-gamma: mechanism and pathological relevance in psoriasis. *J Immunol* 2008;18:4733–4741.
46. Cameron AL, Kirby B, Fei W, et al. Natural killer and natural killer-T cells in psoriasis. *Arch Dermatol Res* 2002;294:363–369.
47. Bonish B, Jullien D, Dutronc Y, et al. Overexpression of CD1d by keratinocytes in psoriasis and CD1d-dependent IFN-gamma production by NK-T cells. *J Immunol* 2000;165:4076–4085.
48. Harvima RJ, Viinamäki H, Harvima IT, et al. Association of psychic stress with clinical severity and symptoms of psoriatic patients. *Acta Derm Venereol* 1996;76:467–471.
49. Kawamura A, Kinoshita MT, Suzuki H. Generalized pustular psoriasis with hypoparathyroidism. *Eur J Dermatol* 1999;9:574–576.
50. Dogan B, Karabudak O, Harmanyeri Y. Antistreptococcal treatment of guttate psoriasis: a controlled study. *Int J Dermatol* 2008;47:950–952.
51. Mease PJ, Gladman DD, Papp KA, et al. Prevalence of rheumatologist-diagnosed psoriatic arthritis in patients with psoriasis in European/North American dermatology clinics. *J Am Acad Dermatol* 2013;69:729–735.
52. Katz HI, Hien NT, Prawer SE, et al. Betamethasone dipropionate in optimized vehicle. Intermittent pulse dosing for extended maintenance treatment of psoriasis. *Arch Dermatol* 1987;123:1308–1311.
53. Highton A, Quell J. Calcipotriene ointment 0.005% for psoriasis: a safety and efficacy study. *J Am Acad Dermatol* 1995;32:67–72.
54. Weinstein GD, Krueger GG, Lowe NJ, et al. Tazarotene gel, a new retinoid, for topical therapy of psoriasis: vehicle-controlled study of safety, efficacy, and duration of therapeutic effect. *J Am Acad Dermatol* 1997;37:85–92.
55. Wang C, Lin A. Efficacy of topical calcineurin inhibitors in psoriasis. *J Cutan Med Surg* 2014;18:8–14.
56. Takahashi H, Tsuji H, Ishida-Yamamoto A, et al. Comparison of clinical effects of psoriasis treatment regimens among calcipotriol alone, narrowband ultraviolet B phototherapy alone, combination of calcipotriol and narrowband ultraviolet B phototherapy once a week, and combination of calcipotriol and narrowband ultraviolet B phototherapy more than twice a week. *J Dermatol* 2013;40:424–427.
57. Spuls PI, Rozenblit M, Lebwohl M. Retrospective study of the efficacy of narrowband UVB and acitretin. *J Dermatol Treat* 2003;14:17–20.
58. Hearn RM, Kerr AC, Rahim KF, et al. Incidence of skin cancers in 3867 patients treated with narrow-band ultraviolet B phototherapy. *Br J Dermatol* 2008;159:931–935.
59. Almutawa F, Alnomair N, Wang Y, et al. Systematic review of UV-based therapy for psoriasis. *Am J Clin Dermatol* 2013;14:87–109.
60. Shehzad T, Dar NR, Zakria M. Efficacy of concomitant use of PUVA and methotrexate in disease clearance time in plaque type psoriasis. *J Pak Med Assoc* 2004;54:453–455.
61. Heidbreder G, Christophers E. Therapy of psoriasis with retinoid plus PUVA: clinical and histologic data. *Arch Dermatol Res* 1979;264:331–337.
62. Lowe NJ, Wieder JM, Rosenbach A, et al. Long-term low-dose cyclosporine therapy for severe psoriasis: effects on renal function and structure. *J Am Acad Dermatol* 1996;35:710–719.
63. Leonardi CL, Kimball AB, Papp KA, et al. Efficacy and safety of ustekinumab, a human interleukin-12/23 monoclonal antibody, in patients with psoriasis: 76-week results from a randomised, double-blind, placebo-controlled trial (PHOENIX 1). *Lancet* 2008;371:1665–1674.

64. Foley P, Zuo Y, Plunkett A, et al. The frequency of common skin conditions in preschool-aged children in Australia: seborrheic dermatitis and pityriasis capitis (cradle cap). *Arch Dermatol* 2003;139:318–322.

65. Ostlere LS, Taylor CR, Harris DW, et al. Skin surface lipids in HIV-positive patients with and without seborrheic dermatitis. *Int J Dermatol* 1996;35:276–279.

66. McGinley KJ, Leyden JJ, Marples RR, et al. Quantitative microbiology of the scalp in non-dandruff, dandruff, and seborrheic dermatitis. *J Investig Dermatol* 1975;64:401.

67. Sud N, Shanker V, Sharma A, et al. Mucocutaneous manifestations in 150 HIV-infected Indian patients and their relationship with CD4 lymphocyte counts. *Int J STD AIDS* 2009;20:771–774.

68. Piérard-Franchimont C, Goffin V, Decroix J, et al. A multicenter randomized trial of ketoconazole 2% and zinc pyrithione 1% shampoos in severe dandruff and seborrheic dermatitis. *Skin Pharmacol Appl Skin Physiol* 2002;15:434–441.

69. Ratnavel RC, Squire RA, Boorman GC. Clinical efficacies of shampoos containing ciclopirox olamine (1.5%) and ketoconazole (2.0%) in the treatment of seborrhoeic dermatitis. *J Dermatolog Treat* 2007;18:88–96.

70. Kastarinen H, Oksanen T, Okokon EO, et al. *Topical anti-inflammatory agents for seborrhoeic dermatitis of the face or scalp. Cochrane Database Syst Rev* 2014;(5):CD009446.

4 Infections and Infestations

Heather Jones, MD, Jason P. Burnham, MD,
and Kara Sternhell-Blackwell, MD

Infections and infestations are common dermatologic concerns. Some viral, bacterial, and fungal infections are limited to the skin, whereas others are systemic illnesses with more serious consequences. This chapter covers those conditions that affect patients of any age; additional information about childhood infections can be found in Chapters 5 and 12, Reactive Disorders and Pediatric Dermatology, respectively.

1. VERRUCAE

1.1. Background
- Papillomaviruses are nonenveloped, double-stranded DNA viruses that infect the skin and induce common warts, palmar and plantar warts, and flat warts.[1]

1.2. Clinical Features
- Common warts
  - Common warts are hyperkeratotic, exophytic, dome-shaped papules or plaques (Fig. 4-1).
  - Most frequently located on the fingers and dorsal surfaces of the hands but may occur anywhere on the skin.
  - Punctate black dots that represent thrombosed capillaries are characteristic. Shaving the surface results in bleeding.
  - HPV associations—HPV-1, HPV-2, HPV-4, HPV-27, and HPV-57.
- Palmar and plantar warts
  - Palmar and plantar warts appear as thick, endophytic papules with a central depression.
  - Plantar warts are often painful when walking due to deep inward growth.
  - HPV types 1, 2, 27, and 57 cause the majority of palmoplantar warts.[2]
- Flat warts
  - Flat warts are skin-colored to pinkish, smooth-surfaced, slightly elevated, flat-topped papules most commonly located on dorsal hands, arms, or face.
  - HPV associations—HPV types 3 and 10 and less commonly 28 and 29.
- Condyloma acuminata
  - Condylomata are discrete, sessile, smooth-surfaced exophytic papillomas, which may be skin colored, brown, or whitish.
  - Lesions are located on the external genitalia and perineum and may measure one to several millimeters in diameter.
  - HPV associations—HPV types 6 and 11.

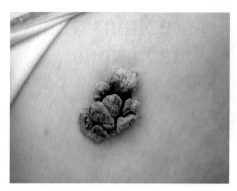

Figure 4-1. Common wart. (Courtesy of David Sheinbein, MD.)

1.3. Evaluation
- Warts are diagnosed based on morphology and anatomic location.
- Differential diagnosis
  - Seborrheic keratoses, squamous cell carcinomas, hypertrophic lichen planus, and corns.
  - Condyloma acuminata can be confused with condyloma lata of secondary syphilis.

1.4. Treatment
- There is no specific antiviral therapy to cure HPV. Current treatment modalities focus on destruction of visible lesions or induction of cytotoxicity against infected cells.
- Destruction is performed with cryotherapy or cantharidin.
  - Considerations include discomfort with cryotherapy and potential for formation of "doughnut" wart formation with cantharidin.
  - If lesions are many or recalcitrant to therapy, clinicians can combine therapy with salicylic acid preparations, imiquimod, or 5-fluorouracil.
- Genital HPV infection is typically widespread throughout the anogenital tract and recurrence rates are high.
  - Clinician-applied therapy includes cryotherapy, excision, and curettage.
  - Imiquimod, a topical immunomodulator approved for the treatment of genital HPV lesions, can be applied by patients.
  - HPV infection may cause cervical, vulvar, vaginal, penile, and anal malignancies. Patients with external HPV infection should be screened with Pap smears and physical exams for signs of dysplasia or malignancy.
  - Gardasil is a vaccine that protects against HPV types 6, 11, 16, and 18.

2. MOLLUSCUM CONTAGIOSUM

2.1. Background
- Family Poxviridae, double-stranded DNA virus.
- After the eradication of smallpox, molluscum contagiosum (MC) became the only remaining poxvirus to afflict humans.
- MC is a common, self-limited disease in children; however, in adults, it is usually considered a sexually transmitted disease.

2.2. Clinical Presentation

- MC lesions are firm, umbilicated, flesh-colored papules (see Fig. 12-20).
- Can occur anywhere on the skin. Widespread or large lesions may be seen in the setting of HIV or immunosuppression.

2.3. Evaluation

- MC is diagnosed clinically.
- Differential diagnosis: verrucae, condyloma acuminata, basal cell carcinoma, melanocytic nevi, and pyogenic granuloma. In immunocompromised patients, Cryptococcus or Histoplasma infections can mimic MC.

2.4. Treatment

- MC resolves spontaneously in immunocompetent children; however, the time interval between onset and clearance of infection can range from months to years.
- Therapeutic options include curettage, cryotherapy, or cantharidin (a blistering agent).
- Treatment of associated dermatitis with a topical corticosteroid can reduce itching and avoid autoinoculation.

3. SUPERFICIAL DERMATOPHYTES

3.1. Background

- Dermatophytoses are fungal infections caused by three genera of fungi—*Microsporum, Trichophyton*, and *Epidermophyton*[3]—that invade and multiply within keratinized tissue.

3.2. Clinical Features (Fig. 4-2)

- Tinea corporis
  - Dermatophyte infection of the skin of the trunk and extremities, excluding hair, nails, palms, soles, and groin.
  - Infection is generally restricted to the stratum corneum.
  - *Trichophyton rubrum* is the most common pathogen worldwide followed by *Trichophyton mentagrophytes.*
  - The typical incubation period is 1 to 3 weeks.
  - Characteristic lesions are sharply demarcated with a raised, erythematous, scaly, advancing border and central clearing. Scale may be diminished or absent if topical corticosteroids have been used (tinea "incognito").
  - Differential diagnosis: eczematous dermatitis, seborrheic dermatitis, pityriasis rosea, psoriasis, and contact dermatitis.
- Tinea cruris
  - Dermatophyte infection of the inguinal region.
  - The three most common causative agents are *Epidermophyton floccosum, T. rubrum*, and *T. mentagrophytes.*
  - Predisposing factors: obesity, excessive perspiration, and male sex.
  - Often coexistent with tinea pedis.
  - The first signs of infection are often erythema and pruritus in the perineal area.
  - Characteristic lesions are sharply demarcated erythematous plaques with peripheral scale. The scrotum is generally spared.
  - Differential diagnosis: cutaneous candidiasis, intertrigo, psoriasis, contact dermatitis, and mycosis fungoides.

- Tinea manuum
  - Dermatophyte infections of the palm and interdigital web spaces.
  - The typical causative organisms are the same as those for tinea pedis and cruris.
  - Infection is usually noninflammatory with hyperkeratosis on the palms, recalcitrant to treatment with emollients.
  - It is often unilateral and found in association with tinea pedis ("one-hand, two-foot disease").
  - Differential diagnosis: psoriasis, irritant or allergic contact dermatitis, and eczematous dermatitis.
- Tinea capitis
  - Dermatophyte infection of the scalp in children and adults.
  - The typical causative organisms are in two genera, *Trichophyton* and *Microsporum,* with *Trichophyton tonsurans* accounting for more than 90% of cases of tinea capitis in the United States.[4]

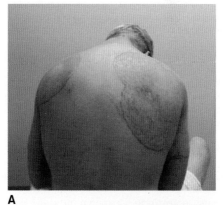

A

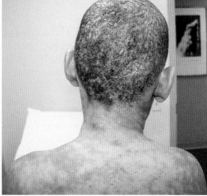

B

Figure 4-2. Tinea. **A:** Tinea corporis. **B:** Tinea capitis.

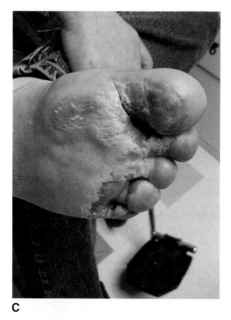

C

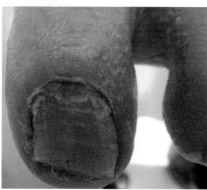

D

Figure 4-2. (*Continued*) **C:** Tinea pedis. **D:** Tinea unguium (onychomycosis). (Courtesy of David Sheinbein, MD.)

- Presentations of tinea capitis can range from noninflammatory scaling to a severe pustular eruption, with alopecia being the most common presentation.
- Advanced disease associated with an exaggerated host response to the organism can result in formation of boggy, purulent plaques with abscess formation and alopecia, known as a kerion.
- Occasionally, patients may become systemically ill with posterior cervical or postauricular lymphadenopathy.
- Differential diagnosis: seborrheic dermatitis, pustular psoriasis, and alopecia areata.

- Tinea pedis
  - Dermatophyte infection of the soles and interdigital web spaces on the feet.
  - The three most common organisms responsible for tinea pedis are *T. rubrum, T. mentagrophytes,* and *E. floccosum.*[5]
  - There are four major clinical types of tinea pedis—moccasin, interdigital, inflammatory, and ulcerative.
    - Moccasin—diffuse hyperkeratosis, erythema, and scaling on one or both plantar surfaces; may be associated with cell-mediated immunodeficiency
    - Interdigital—most common type with erythema, scaling, fissures, and maceration in web spaces
    - Inflammatory—vesicles and bullae on medial foot
    - Ulcerative—exacerbation of interdigital tinea pedis with ulcers and erosions in web spaces, seen in immunocompromised and diabetic patients
  - Differential diagnosis: eczematous dermatitis, tinea pedis caused by nondermatophytes including *Scytalidium dimidiatum.*
- Tinea unguium
  - Dermatophyte infection of the nail unit.
  - The most common causative pathogens are *T. rubrum, T. mentagrophytes,* and *E. floccosum.*
  - Toenail infections are more common than fingernail infections. With progression of infection, there is yellowing and thickening of the distal nail plate as well as onycholysis.
  - Differential diagnosis: candidiasis and onychodystrophy.

3.3. Diagnosis

- Potassium hydroxide prep (KOH) (Fig. 4-3)
  - Direct microscopy can be performed from a scraping of the scaly advancing border of a lesion (see Fig. 1-1).
  - In the case of tinea pedis, KOH preparation has a sensitivity of 77% and a specificity of 62%.[6] A negative test does not rule out the diagnosis, and a culture should follow the potassium hydroxide examination even if it is positive.

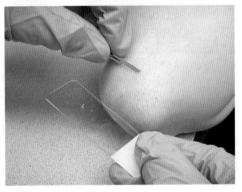

Figure 4-3. Potassium hydroxide preparation. (Courtesy of David Sheinbein, MD.)

3.4. Treatments

- Topical therapies—first line for uncomplicated, localized infections of tinea corporis, cruris, and pedis
  - These agents are generally applied twice daily until clinical signs and symptoms are improved, typically up to 4 weeks.
    ○ Clotrimazole—1% lotion, solution, or cream. Pregnancy category B. Over the counter (OTC) or by prescription (Rx)
    ○ Econazole—1% cream. Pregnancy category C. Rx
    ○ Miconazole—2% cream, lotion, powder. Pregnancy category C. OTC/Rx
    ○ Terbinafine—1% cream. Pregnancy category B. OTC
- Systemic agents
  - Terbinafine—indicated for onychomycosis and superficial fungal infections unresponsive to topical agents. Mycologic cure rates of 70% for toenails after 12 weeks and 80% for fingernails after 6 weeks. Pregnancy category B
  - Ketoconazole—indicated for superficial fungal infections unresponsive to topical therapy. Pregnancy category C
  - Griseofulvin—indicated for tinea capitis or onychomycosis. Drug of choice for treating dermatophyte infections resistant to topical agents in children with mycologic cure rates of 80% to 95%. Pregnancy category C

4. TINEA VERSICOLOR

4.1. Background

- Caused by *Malassezia furfur*, a microbe present in normal skin flora.
- *Malassezia* requires oil to grow, which accounts for its increased incidence in adolescents and preference for sebum-rich areas of the skin.

4.2. Clinical Features

- Usually presents with multiple oval to round patches or thin plaques with mild, fine scale. The lesions are often confluent centrally within areas of involvement, and seborrheic areas are the favored sites (Fig. 4-4).

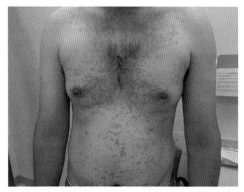

Figure 4-4. Tinea versicolor. (Courtesy of David Sheinbein, MD.)

- The most common colors are brown and whitish tan.
- Infection is generally asymptomatic.

4.3. Diagnosis
- KOH with visualization of both hyphal and yeast forms
- Differential diagnosis: pityriasis alba and postinflammatory hypopigmentation

4.4. Treatment
- Patients usually respond to topical antimycotic treatments including 2% ketoconazole or selenium sulfide shampoo, or topical azole cream.
- Systemic therapy is not generally indicated.

5. CANDIDIASIS

5.1. Background
- *Candida* species are responsible for mucocutaneous infections in immunocompetent hosts and disseminated infections in immunocompromised patients.
- Mucocutaneous candidiasis and disseminated infection are most commonly caused by *Candida albicans,* with *Candida tropicalis* being the second most common cause.
- Predisposing factors for mucocutaneous infection: diabetes mellitus, dry mouth, excessive sweat production, and use of corticosteroids or broad-spectrum antibiotics.
- Primary and secondary immunosuppression are the primary predisposing factors for disseminated candidiasis.
- *Candida glabrata* and *Candida krusei* have intrinsic fluconazole resistance that may be increasing in prevalence with the use of broad-spectrum antifungal agents.

5.2. Clinical Features
- Mucocutaneous *Candida* infection
  - Oral infection often presents with a white exudate resembling cottage cheese or thrush. Other presentations include adherent white plaques, denture stomatitis, angular cheilitis (perleche), and vulvovaginal infection.
  - Cutaneous infections present with markedly erythematous, occasionally erosive patches accompanied by satellite papules, most commonly involving the intertriginous areas (Fig. 4-5).
  - Infection can also occur in the periungual area and the diaper area in infants.
- Opportunistic *Candida* infection
  - Cutaneous lesions of disseminated candidiasis often present as firm pink papules or nodules on the trunk and extremities.
  - Other presentations include ecthyma gangrenosum–like lesions consisting of hemorrhagic bullae with necrotic eschar, pustules, and abscesses.

5.3. Diagnosis
- Mucocutaneous *Candida* infection—diagnosed with KOH examination demonstrating presence of budding yeast and pseudohyphae and by positive fungal culture.

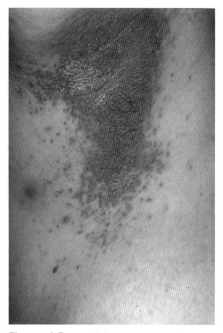

Figure 4-5. Candida. (Courtesy of Arthur Eisen, MD.)

- Opportunistic *Candida* infection—diagnosed with positive tissue or blood culture and demonstration of budding yeast and pseudohyphae in dermis.

5.4. Treatment

- Mucocutaneous *Candida* infection—removal of the predisposing factor is of primary importance. Topical nystatin and azole antifungals are generally effective. When oral therapy is required, systemic azoles are used.
- Opportunistic *Candida* infection—consultation with an infectious disease specialist is recommended.

6. HERPES SIMPLEX VIRUSES (HSV-1 AND HSV-2)

6.1. Background

- Herpes simplex virus type 1 (HSV-1) and type 2 (HSV-2) are large, double-stranded DNA viruses of the *Herpesviridae* family[7] with a worldwide distribution.
- HSV-2 is the cause of most genital herpes and is almost always sexually transmitted.[8]
- HSV-1 is usually transmitted during childhood nonsexually.
  - Recent studies have shown an increasing proportion of new genital herpes infections due to HSV-1 in the United States.[9]

- Genital HSV-2 infection increases the risk of human immunodeficiency virus (HIV) infection by at least twofold.[10]
- Host interaction—virus-host interaction includes three stages.
  - First stage: primary and nonprimary infections, which may be symptomatic or asymptomatic
    - Primary infections are first HSV infections in patients without pre-existing antibodies to HSV-1 or HSV-2.
    - Nonprimary infections are infections with one HSV type in patients with pre-existing antibodies to other HSV types.
  - Second stage: latency stage, in which the virus remains quiescent in the sensory ganglia
  - Third stage: reactivation resulting in recurrent infection with asymptomatic viral shedding or clinical manifestations

6.2. Clinical Features

- In primary genital infections, symptoms usually appear 4 to 7 days after sexual exposure.[7]
  - A prodrome of tender lymphadenopathy, malaise, anorexia, and fever followed by localized pain, tenderness, or burning often precedes mucocutaneous findings.
  - Painful grouped vesicles appear on an erythematous base and may become umbilicated. Vesicles progress to pustules, erosions, or ulcerations with a characteristic scalloped border before crusting and healing.
- Approximately 70% to 90% of people with symptomatic HSV-2 and 20% to 50% with symptomatic genital HSV-1 will have recurrence in the first year.[7]
  - A similar prodrome can precede recurrent lesions; however, the lesions are often fewer in number, with decreased severity and duration compared to the primary infection.
- HSV lesions can manifest in areas adjacent to the genitalia and should be considered in patients presenting with lesions on the abdomen, thighs, and buttocks (Fig. 4-6).

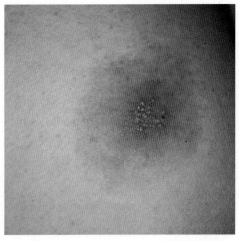

Figure 4-6. Primary HSV. (Courtesy of Arthur Eisen, MD.)

- The majority of primary orolabial infections are asymptomatic.
  - The most common sites of involvement are the mouth and lips, with recurrent lesions appearing on the vermillion border of the lip.
- Differential diagnosis
  - Orolabial herpes: aphthous ulcers, oral candidiasis, or erythema multiforme major or Stevens-Johnson syndrome
  - Genital herpes: trauma, syphilitic chancres, chancroid, and lymphogranuloma venereum

6.3. Diagnosis

- Viral culture, direct fluorescent antibody assays (DFA), molecular techniques, and serology can all be utilized for diagnosis. Identification of HSV by culture usually requires 2 to 5 days.
- Polymerase chain reaction (PCR) is increasingly being used as a rapid, sensitive, and specific method for detection of HSV in cerebrospinal fluid, skin, and other organs.

6.4. Treatment

- FDA-approved treatment of recurrent orolabial herpes in immunocompetent patients includes oral valacyclovir (2 g twice daily for 1 day), oral famciclovir (single dose of 1.5 g), and topical 1% penciclovir.
  - These treatments result in decreased duration of mucocutaneous lesions and decreased viral shedding, especially if taken at the first symptom or sign of recurrence.
- Intravenous acyclovir is used to treat severe infections in immunocompromised patients.
- Chronic suppressive therapy with oral antiviral agents is usually reserved for those with greater than six outbreaks per year. In addition to reducing outbreaks, chronic suppressive therapy reduces asymptomatic viral shedding and can prevent transmission of infection to susceptible partners.[11]

7. VARICELLA-ZOSTER VIRUS

7.1. Background

- Varicella-zoster virus (VZV) is a herpesvirus with a worldwide distribution that causes two distinct clinical syndromes.
- Since the introduction of the varicella vaccine in 1995, the overall incidence of varicella has decreased approximately 85%.
- Herpes zoster develops in approximately 30% of people over a lifetime,[12] with the risk of disease increasing with age.
- Transmission is usually via airborne droplets; however, direct contact with vesicular fluid represents another mode of spread.
- The incubation period ranges from 11 to 20 days.
- VZV travels to the epidermis via capillary endothelial cells and subsequently travels from mucocutaneous lesions to dorsal root ganglion cells where it remains latent.
- Herpes zoster represents reactivation of VZV, which may occur spontaneously or be triggered by stress, fever, illness, trauma, or immunosuppression.
  - During a zoster outbreak, the virus replicates in the dorsal root ganglion resulting in neuronal inflammation and painful ganglionitis.
  - Severe neuralgia worsens as the virus spreads down the sensory nerve.
  - Fluid from zoster vesicles can transmit VZV to seronegative individuals, leading to primary varicella infection.

7.2. Clinical Features

• Varicella
  • Begins with a prodrome of fever, malaise, and myalgia followed by an eruption of pruritic, erythematous macules, and papules (Fig. 4-7).
  • Lesions start on the head and spread downward to the trunk and extremities, rapidly evolving over 12 to 14 hours into clear vesicles surrounded by erythema.
  • The presence of lesions in all stages of development is a hallmark of varicella.
  • The disease is usually self-limited, and within 7 to 10 days, lesions crust over and heal.
  • Varicella in adolescents and adults is often more severe than in children, with increased number of skin lesions and more frequent complications.
  • Maternal varicella during the first 20 weeks of pregnancy is associated with a risk of congenital varicella syndrome with defects including low birth weight, cutaneous scarring, ocular abnormalities, psychomotor retardation, and hypoplastic limbs.
  • Severe neonatal varicella can occur when maternal infection develops between 5 days before and 2 days after delivery.

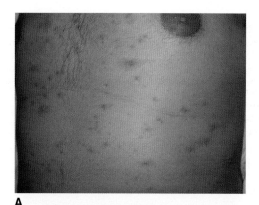

A

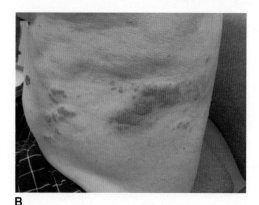

B

Figure 4-7. Varicella-zoster virus. **A:** Varicella. **B:** Zoster. (**A**, courtesy of Susan Bayliss, MD; **B**, courtesy of David Sheinbein, MD.)

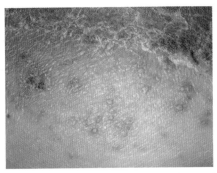

Figure 4-8. Impetigo. (Courtesy of David Sheinbein, MD.)

- Immunocompromised patients can have more extensive and atypical eruptions with higher morbidity and mortality.
- Herpes Zoster—reactivation of VZV may occur any time after primary varicella infection (Fig. 4-8).
  - Zoster outbreaks begin with a prodrome of pruritus, tingling, and pain.
  - While most patients develop a painful eruption of grouped vesicles on an erythematous base in a dermatomal distribution, a few patients have the prodrome without subsequent skin findings.
  - Lesions can involve more than one contiguous dermatome and occasionally cross midline.
  - Postherpetic neuralgia is the most common complication, characterized by dysesthetic pain that persists after cutaneous lesions have healed. More than 40% of people older than 50 years of age who have had zoster have postherpetic neuralgia.[13]
  - Additional complications from reactivation of VZV include involvement of the ophthalmic division of the trigeminal nerve with increased risk of ocular involvement.
    ○ When skin lesions are in the distribution of the nasociliary nerve, involving the nasal tip, dorsum, and root of the nose, ophthalmologic referral is necessary.
  - Involvement of the geniculate ganglion of the facial nerve with lesions affecting the external auditory canal, tympanic membrane, and anterior two-thirds of the tongue may result in partial facial paralysis, hearing loss, or vertigo.
- Differential Diagnosis
  - Varicella: viral exanthems, bullous arthropod reactions, and scabies
  - Herpes zoster: cellulitis, bullous impetigo, and localized contact dermatitis

7.3. Diagnosis
- Clinical diagnosis can usually be made with a thorough history and physical examination.
- Additional testing includes viral culture, serology, and PCR.

7.4. Treatment
- Varicella in immunocompetent patients can be treated symptomatically.
- Acyclovir can be used to decrease the duration and symptoms of disease if started within 24 to 72 hours of symptom onset.

- Oral acyclovir and valacyclovir are FDA approved for treatment of varicella in children (ages 2 to 17) while acyclovir is approved for adults.
  - In immunocompromised patients, intravenous acyclovir is indicated due to the increased risk of more severe disease and complications.
- Acyclovir, famciclovir, and valacyclovir are FDA approved for treatment of herpes zoster in immunocompetent patients to decrease duration and severity of skin findings and pain.
  - Antiviral therapy is best initiated within 72 hours of symptom onset; however, initiation up to 7 days after onset appears to be beneficial.

8. IMPETIGO

8.1. Background

- Impetigo is a common, contagious skin infection most commonly caused by *Staphylococcus aureus*. Infection can present in bullous and nonbullous forms.
- Group A beta-hemolytic *Streptococcus* (*Streptococcus pyogenes*) represents an important cause of nonbullous impetigo.

8.2. Clinical Features

- Nonbullous impetigo—early erythematous macules evolve into vesicles or pustules with late manifestations characterized by superficial erosions with "honey-colored" yellow crust (Fig. 4-6).
  - Local production of exfoliative toxins (ETA, ETB), which binds and cleaves desmosomal protein desmoglein-1. Less common.
  - Most commonly affected sites are the face and extremities.
  - Clinical course is usually self-limited, resolving without scarring.
- Bullous impetigo—early vesicles enlarge into flaccid bullae with little surrounding erythema. After blisters are broken, they develop a collarette of scale without yellow crusting.
  - *S. aureus* or *S. pyogenes* infection at sites of trauma with disruption of skin barrier. Represents 70% of cases.
  - The most commonly affected sites are the face, trunk, buttocks, axillae, and extremities.
  - Infection typically resolves in 3 to 6 weeks without treatment.
- Differential diagnosis
  - Nonbullous impetigo: insect bites, atopic dermatitis, inflamed dermatophytosis, and herpes simplex
  - Bullous impetigo: bullous insect bite reactions, thermal injury, and autoimmune bullous dermatoses

8.3. Diagnosis

- Impetigo is diagnosed clinically and with bacterial Gram stain and culture.

8.4. Treatment

- In otherwise healthy patients, topical mupirocin 2% ointment can be prescribed.
- Second-line treatment for uncomplicated disease includes oral first-generation cephalosporins, clindamycin, macrolides, or beta-lactamase–resistant penicillins. Topical agents are often equally effective for limited disease.
- For complicated infection, intravenous antibiotics may be required.

9. CELLULITIS

9.1. Cellulitis Background

- Cellulitis is a pyogenic infection of the deep dermis and subcutaneous tissue.
- The most commonly implicated organisms are *S. aureus* and group A *Streptococcus*. A mixture of gram-positive cocci and gram-negative anaerobes and aerobes is often found in cellulitis surrounding diabetic or decubitus wounds.
- Bacteria gain entry through breaks in the skin barrier.
- Predisposing factors: chronic lymphedema, diabetes, and peripheral neuropathy.

9.2. Clinical Features (Fig. 4-9)

- Cellulitis may be preceded by systemic signs or symptoms of infection including fever, chills, and malaise.
- Areas of infection present with inflammation, erythema, warmth, and pain. The borders are often ill defined.
- Severe infection can result in vesicles, pustules, or necrotic eschars.
- Occasionally ascending lymphangitis may be seen.
- Differential Diagnosis
  - Lower extremity cellulitis: deep venous thrombosis, lipodermatosclerosis, and stasis dermatitis

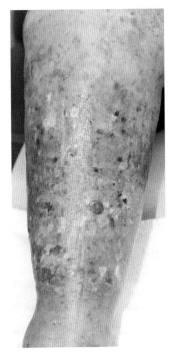

Figure 4-9. Cellulitis on severely actinic damaged skin. (Courtesy of M. Laurin Council, MD.)

9.3. Diagnosis

- Cultures of blood or cutaneous aspirates are not routinely recommended but should be considered in patients with malignancy on chemotherapy, neutropenia, severe cell-mediated immunodeficiency, or animal bites.[14]

9.4. Treatment

- For uncomplicated infection, a 5-day course of antimicrobials covering group A streptococci and *S. aureus* is recommended; however, treatment can be extended at clinician discretion.
  - If MRSA is not suspected, treatment with clindamycin, dicloxacillin, or cephalexin can be initiated.
- For patients with evidence of MRSA infection elsewhere, nasal colonization, history of intravenous drug abuse, or those fitting systemic inflammatory response syndrome criteria, MRSA coverage is recommended.
  - Vancomycin plus either piperacillin-tazobactam or meropenem is recommended for empiric treatment in severe infections.

10. ERYSIPELAS

10.1. Erysipelas Background

- Erysipelas is a superficial variant of cellulitis caused primarily by group A streptococci, affecting the dermis with prominent lymphatic involvement.
- Infection tends to occur in patients at the extremes of age, either very young or very old, and those severely debilitated or with chronic lymphedema or ulcers.

10.2. Clinical Features

- Infection classically involved the face; however, the most common location affected is the lower extremities.
- An abrupt onset of systemic symptoms occurs including fever, chills, and malaise.
- An erythematous plaque develops that is well-demarcated from uninvolved skin, unlike in cellulitis. The affected area is warm, tense, painful to palpation, and indurated.
- Regional lymphadenopathy may be present, and in severe disease, pustules, vesicles, and areas of hemorrhage and necrosis can develop.
- Differential diagnosis: cellulitis, inflammatory disorders, Sweet syndrome, and drug reactions.

10.3. Treatment

- Treatment is similar to that of cellulitis (see above).

11. FURUNCLES AND ABSCESSES

Abscesses and furuncles are collections of purulent material separated from the surrounding tissue. By definition, furuncles involve a hair follicle whereas abscesses can occur anywhere on the body.

11.1. Background

- Furuncles occur most often in adolescents and young adults.
- *S. aureus* is the most common causative organism.
- Predisposing factors: chronic colonization with *S. aureus*, diabetes mellitus, obesity, and certain immunodeficiency syndromes including chronic granulomatous disease.

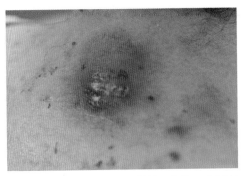

Figure 4-10. Abscess. (Courtesy of M. Laurin Council, MD.)

11.2. Clinical Features (Fig. 4-10)

- Abscesses present as inflamed, erythematous, and fluctuant collections of pus in a cutaneous site.
- Furuncles most commonly occur on the face, neck, axillae, buttocks, thighs, and perineum, presenting as firm, painful, erythematous nodules that progressively enlarge.
- Systemic symptoms are typically absent.
- Differential Diagnosis
  - Abscesses or furuncles presenting in the axillae and groin may be mistaken for hidradenitis suppurativa.

11.3. Diagnosis

- Can often be diagnosed by history and physical examination. Incision and drainage with culture can provide definitive diagnosis and guide antimicrobial therapy.

11.4. Treatment

- Uncomplicated furuncles may be treated with incision and drainage without additional systemic antimicrobials.
- The decision to administer antimicrobials directed against *S. aureus* in addition to incision and drainage should be based on presence of systemic inflammatory response criteria or a history of marked immunosuppression.[14]
- Given the prevalence of MRSA, empiric coverage with doxycycline, trimethoprim-sulfamethoxazole (TMP-SMX), or clindamycin is appropriate depending on local resistance patterns.
- For recurrent abscesses at sites of previous infection, Gram stain and culture of purulent material may be obtained to guide therapy and consideration given to decolonization with intranasal mupirocin or daily chlorhexidine washes.

12. METHICILLIN-RESISTANT *STAPHYLOCOCCUS AUREUS*

12.1. Background

- Methicillin-resistant *Staphylococcus aureus* (MRSA) refers to isolates that are resistant to all available beta-lactam antibiotics, including penicillins and cephalosporins.[15]

- First recognized in the early 1960s, MRSA was largely confined to health care facilities; however, since the mid-1990s, it has been increasing in prevalence in the community.[16]
- Skin and soft tissue infections (SSTIs) represent the majority of community-acquired MRSA (CA-MRSA) infections, with furunculosis being the most common manifestation.
- Methicillin resistance is caused by altered penicillin-binding protein (PBP2a) resulting in decreased affinity for beta-lactam antibiotics.

12.2. Diagnosis and Treatment

- When an *S. aureus* infection is suspected, culture and susceptibility testing should be performed.
- For uncomplicated, nonpurulent cellulitis, empiric treatment for beta-hemolytic streptococci is recommended as the role of CA-MRSA is unknown.
  - Empiric therapy for CA-MRSA is recommended for patients who do not respond to initial treatment or develop systemic toxicity.
- For purulent cellulitis, empiric therapy for CA-MRSA is recommended pending culture results.[17]
  - Empiric coverage of CA-MRSA in outpatients with SSTIs includes clindamycin, TMP-SMX, tetracyclines, and linezolid.
- For hospitalized patients with complicated SSTIs, MRSA should be considered pending culture results.
  - Treatment options include intravenous vancomycin, oral or intravenous linezolid, intravenous daptomycin, or intravenous ceftaroline.

13. NECROTIZING FASCIITIS

13.1. Background

- Necrotizing fasciitis is a severe infection of the subcutaneous tissue that results in rapidly progressive destruction of fat and fascia.
- There are two clinical types, both associated with high mortality, up to 70%.
  - Type I necrotizing fasciitis is a polymicrobial infection with aerobic and anaerobic bacteria.
  - Type II necrotizing fasciitis is due to group A streptococci.

13.2. Clinical Presentation

- Predisposing factors, type I: diabetes, surgery, trauma, immunosuppression, alcoholism, NSAIDs, peripheral vascular disease, chronic venous insufficiency, decubitus ulcers, Bartholin or vulvovaginal abscesses, and malignancy.[18]
  - Type I infections tend to occur on the lower extremities.
- Predisposing factors, type II: trauma, muscle strain, childbirth, varicella infection, intravenous drug use, and surgery.[18]
- Initially, necrotizing fasciitis may mimic cellulitis, muscle strain, or uncomplicated minor trauma.
- The site of initial bacterial invasion is often minor and is undetectable in 20% of cases.
- Inoculation can occur at the site of minor abrasions, insect bites, splinters, or injection drug sites.
- Pain out of proportion to physical examination findings is characteristic of necrotizing fasciitis. However, physical exam may reveal anesthesia of affected areas due to destruction of superficial nerves.

- Tissue destruction can progress at rates of 1 inch per hour.
- Systemic symptoms are common but nonspecific, including fever, chills, malaise, fatigue, myalgias, and anorexia.
- Erythema is the most common cutaneous manifestation, which can progress to a reddish-purple discoloration associated with blisters or bullae.
  - Development of bullae signifies extensive tissue destruction.
  - Lesions can have dusky blue central discoloration, weeping blisters or bullae, and border cellulitis.[19]
  - Subcutaneous tissue may have a wooden feel.
- *Aeromonas hydrophila* infections can occur in patients with trauma and exposure to a water source or rarely in patients who use leeches.
- *Vibrio vulnificus* is a cause of necrotizing fasciitis in patients exposed to warm salt water, typically from the Gulf of Mexico.
  - Infection is more likely to occur in immunosuppressed patients. Inoculation can occur via exposure of small abrasions and wounds to contaminated salt water. Puncture wounds from fish, crustaceans, or other sea creatures can also result in infection when they occur in colonized water sources.

13.3. Evaluation

- Necrotizing fasciitis is suggested by history, physical examination, and imaging findings.
- Gas (though not in type II infections) or subcutaneous edema may be seen on computed tomography, magnetic resonance imaging, or ultrasonography.
  - No imaging studies can definitively rule out necrotizing fasciitis. Therefore, when suspicion of the diagnosis is high, surgical exploration should occur. Surgical exploration provides definitive diagnosis.
- Laboratory findings suggestive of necrotizing fasciitis include elevated levels of creatinine, aspartate aminotransferase, creatine phosphokinase, and leukocytosis with a left shift.

13.4. Treatment

- The mainstay of treatment is surgical debridement.
- Empirically, broad-spectrum antibiotics should be initiated with vancomycin or linezolid plus piperacillin-tazobactam or a carbapenem, or plus ceftriaxone and metronidazole.[14]
  - Antibiotic treatment should be directed toward pathogens cultured intraoperatively.
  - Mixed infections should be treated with broad-spectrum antibiotics, as previously mentioned.
- In confirmed cases of group A streptococcal or *Clostridium* infections, penicillin plus clindamycin is the treatment of choice.[14]
  - For staphylococcal infections, vancomycin should be used in the presence of methicillin resistance, while nafcillin, oxacillin, cefazolin, and clindamycin are all reasonable in its absence.[14]
  - *Aeromonas hydrophila* infections are best treated with doxycycline plus ciprofloxacin or ceftriaxone.[14]
  - *Vibrio vulnificus* infection is best treated with doxycycline plus ceftriaxone or cefotaxime.[14]
- Family members and close contacts of patients with group A streptococcal infections should be considered for prophylactic administration of penicillin (or other

agent to which the index organism is susceptible) to prevent a serious infection as their risk is increased 50-fold compared to the general population.[20]
- Supportive care with intravenous fluids is often required due to copious fluid losses from wound sites. In severe or refractory cases of group A streptococcal infection, intravenous immunoglobulin may be of benefit.[21]

14. SCABIES

14.1. Background
- Scabies is caused by the mite *Sarcoptes scabiei* var. *hominis* and has a worldwide distribution.
- The entire life cycle of the host-specific mite is completed in the epidermis.
- Transmission occurs via direct contact with an infested person and less frequently by sexual contact or fomites.
- The number of mites living on an affected person is typically <15; however, individuals with crusted scabies may have thousands of mites on the skin surface.

14.2. Clinical Features
- The incubation period between exposure and symptom onset can range from days to months, with the immune system taking 2 to 6 weeks to become sensitized to the mite during a first infestation.
- Pruritus can develop before the onset of skin findings and can be severe.
- Skin findings consist of small erythematous papules symmetrically distributed and typically involve the web spaces of the hands, flexural aspects of the wrists, axillae, waist, ankles, feet, and buttocks.
  - Infants, elderly, and immunocompromised patients may have involvement of the scalp and face.
- The pathognomonic sign is the burrow, representing the tunnel through which the female mite traveled while laying eggs.
- Crusted scabies is found in patients with compromised immune systems, including the elderly, HIV positive or transplant recipients, and those with decreased sensory functions. Infestation in this population can exceed one thousand mites on the skin surface and presents with marked acral hyperkeratosis.
- Differential diagnosis: atopic dermatitis, arthropod bites, and allergic contact dermatitis.

14.3. Diagnosis
- Diagnosis is confirmed by light microscopy examination of skin scrapings from infested areas. Visualization of adult mites, eggs, or fecal pellets confirms diagnosis.

14.4. Treatment
- Two topical treatments, 1 week apart, with permethrin 5% cream is recommended. The topical agent is applied to entire body surface, excluding the face, and left on overnight.
  - At the time of treatment, all clothing and linens should be washed in hot water or stored in a sealed bag for 10 days.
- Skin lesions and pruritus may persist for 2 to 4 weeks or longer after successful treatment, referred to as "postscabietic" dermatitis.

15. LICE (PEDICULOSIS)

15.1. Background
- Body Lice—aka pediculosis corporis
  - Pediculosis corporis is caused by *Pediculus humanus* var. *corporis.*
  - Important human diseases are transmitted via the body louse including *Rickettsia prowazekii,* responsible for endemic typhus; *Borrelia* species, responsible for relapsing fever; and *Bartonella* species, the causative agent for trench fever, bacillary angiomatosis, and endocarditis.
  - Transmission of organisms occurs when lice fecal pellets cross the skin barrier due to excoriations.
- Head Lice—aka pediculosis capitis
  - Pediculosis capitis is caused by the head louse, *Pediculus capitis,* an obligate human parasite that lives only on the hairs of the scalp.
  - Head lice have a worldwide distribution. Children aged 3 to 11 years have the highest incidence. Infestation is more frequently seen in girls.
  - Transmission is via direct head-to-head contact or contact with fomites such as brushes and hair accessories.
  - The nits (eggs) are cemented to hair shafts.
  - Females may live up to 30 days, taking blood meals every 4 to 6 hours.

15.2. Clinical Features
- Body Lice
  - Body lice primarily reside on the clothing of their host, rather than the skin.
  - Infestation results in severe pruritus with the most commonly affected areas being the back, neck, shoulders, and waist.
  - Skin lesions present as erythematous macules or papules, crusts, or excoriations.
- Head Lice
  - During a first infestation, symptoms may not appear until 2 to 6 weeks after exposure as an immunologic response must develop to lice saliva and excreta.
  - Pruritus then develops and excoriations, erythema, and scaliness are common findings, limited in distribution to the scalp and neck.
  - In repeat infestations, symptoms appear within the first 24 to 48 hours after exposure.

15.3. Diagnosis
- Diagnosis is made by direct visualization of the louse or eggs.
  - Inspection of clothing and especially clothing seams is required for diagnosis of body lice.
  - For head lice, diagnosis is made by visual identification of lice or eggs on scalp hair.

15.4. Treatment
- Body Lice
  - First-line treatment is eliminating clothing and bedding of infested persons in tightly sealed bags. If this is not possible, topical treatment with permethrin 5% cream and fumigating or laundering clothes in hot water is recommended.
- Head Lice
  - Topical treatments include permethrin 1% rinse or lotion or permethrin 5% cream; however, resistance is common. No resistance in the United States has

been found against malathion 0.5% lotion or gel, and this remains a good option. Oral ivermectin and ivermectin lotion are alternative therapeutic options. With all topical preparations, two applications performed 1 week apart are advised.

16. SYPHILIS

16.1. Background

- Syphilis is a sexually transmitted infection caused by *Treponema pallidum* subspecies *pallidum* and is associated with various dermatologic manifestations depending on the stage of disease.
- Globally, syphilis is a leading cause of ulcerative genital disease, particularly in low-income countries.
- In the United States, syphilis is a male-predominant disease due to its high incidence in men who have sex with men (MSM).

16.2. Clinical Presentation

- Incubation period varies inversely with inoculum size (10 to 90 days), but on average, primary lesions appear 21 days after exposure.[18]
  - Three to ten weeks after the appearance of the primary chancre, hematogenous dissemination of bacteria results in secondary syphilis.
  - Untreated, the lesions of secondary syphilis will spontaneously disappear in 3 to 12 weeks.
  - Approximately 25% of patients will have a recurrence of secondary syphilis in the absence of treatment, 90% of which occur in the first year.[22]
  - Patients then enter the latent stage of syphilis. Over a period of years, patients have either spontaneous cure or progression to tertiary syphilis.
- Syphilis can be transmitted during the primary and secondary stages via direct contact with infective tissue.
- Syphilis facilitates the transmission of HIV.[23–25]
- Primary syphilis (Fig. 4-11A)
  - The initial lesion of primary syphilis can be papular but quickly ulcerates to form the characteristic chancre with a clean base and raised edges.
    - Chancres occur at the site of inoculation, typically sites of intimate contact including the genitals and oropharynx, though they can occur at any site on the skin or mucous membranes.
    - Lesions are typically nontender.
    - Regional lymph nodes may be enlarged.
    - Chancres heal spontaneously over a period of weeks but can leave a scar.
  - Differential diagnosis: other ulcerative genital diseases, including genital herpes, HIV, trauma, aphthous ulcers, malignancy, fixed drug eruption, primary EBV, and Behcet disease. In patients with the right exposure and travel history, chancroid, lymphogranuloma venereum, and donovanosis.
- Secondary syphilis (Fig. 4-11B)
  - Secondary syphilis is typically the first symptomatic phase of syphilis infection.
    - Systemic symptoms can include fevers, myalgias and joint pains, malaise, sore throat, and headaches.
    - Rash typically appears about 8 weeks after infection. The rash can be diverse in appearance, usually beginning on the upper trunk, palms and soles, and flexural surfaces of the extremities. Initial lesions are macular but can progress to papules by 3 months.

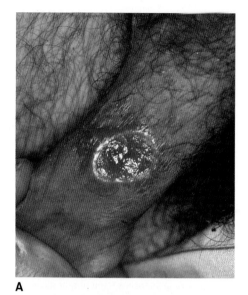

A

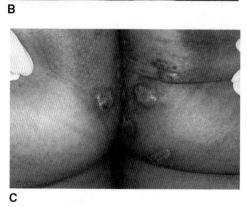

B

C

Figure 4-11. Syphilis. **A:** Primary chancre. **B:** Secondary syphilis. **C:** Condyloma lata. (Courtesy of Arthur Eisen, MD.)

- ○ Generalized lymphadenopathy can occur, as opposed to the regional lymphadenopathy of primary syphilis.
- The most common presentation (~80%) is a nonpruritic papulosquamous eruption. Lesions can range from 1 to 20 mm with color variability from pink to violaceous to red-brown.
  - ○ Differential diagnosis: pityriasis rosea, guttate psoriasis, viral exanthems, lichen planus, pityriasis lichenoides chronica, primary HIV, drug eruption, nummular eczema, and folliculitis[26]
- Mucosal lesions can vary from aphthous appearance to gray plaques.
  - ○ Differential diagnosis of mucosal lesions: lichen planus; chronic aphthae; hand, foot, and mouth disease; herpangina; and perleche.[26]
- Condyloma lata occur in anogenital regions (Fig. 4-11C).
  - ○ Differential diagnosis: HPV, bowenoid papulosis, condyloma acuminata, and squamous cell carcinoma[26]
- Some less common manifestations include annular plaques with central hyperpigmentation, granulomatous nodules, necrotic lesions with scale crust, and necrotic, ulcerated, and crusted lesions with constitutional symptoms ("malignant" syphilis).[26] Patchy alopecia results from toxic telogen effluvium.
- Latent syphilis
  - Patients are by definition asymptomatic during the latent stage.
  - Latent syphilis occurs after spontaneous resolution of secondary syphilis.
    - ○ Early latent syphilis is defined as the year following the onset of latency.
    - ○ If time of latency cannot be determined and neurosyphilis is not present, patients are considered to be in the late latent stage.
    - ○ Diagnosis is often incidental by serologic testing.
- Tertiary syphilis
  - In those who progress to tertiary syphilis, about half will develop gummas in various organs (skin, bones, liver, heart, testis, brain, respiratory tract, and others).
    - ○ When present in the skin, gummas are erythematous, nodular, or noduloulcerative plaques, frequently with an arciform pattern.
    - ○ Differential diagnosis: lupus vulgaris, chromoblastomycosis, endemic mycoses, leishmaniasis, SLE, mycosis fungoides, sarcoidosis, and benign and malignant tumors.[26]
  - The complications of tertiary syphilis are cardiovascular and neurologic, including aortic aneurysms, tabes dorsalis, general paresis (formerly generalized paresis of the insane), and a form of dementia.
- Congenital syphilis
  - Maternal-fetal transmission can occur via the transplacental route or via infective birth canal.
  - Perhaps, one of the most important reasons to recognize syphilis in adults is to prevent its transmission to a fetus because of the severe consequences.
    - ○ When transmitted via transplacental route, there is an approximately 10% risk of spontaneous abortion, 10% risk of stillbirth, and 20% risk of infant death.[26]
  - Twenty percent of children develop congenital syphilis, with its own set of severe consequences.
    - ○ Early congenital syphilis has wide-ranging manifestations including marasmic syphilis, a rash similar in appearance to secondary syphilis, bloody or purulent mucinous nasal discharge ("snuffles"), perioral and perianal fissures, lymphadenopathy, hepatosplenomegaly, osteochondritis, anemia, thrombocytopenia, pneumonitis, hepatitis, nephropathy, and neurosyphilis.[26]
    - ○ Rash tends to be more bullous and erosive as compared to adults.

- Late congenital syphilis is the equivalent of tertiary syphilis in adults.
- Hutchinson triad is a combination of interstitial keratitis, neural deafness, and Hutchinson teeth.

16.3. Evaluation

- In general, in patients with a high index of suspicion for syphilis, a single negative darkfield microscopy examination does not rule out syphilis. Darkfield microscopy is used for diagnosis of primary or secondary syphilis.
  - If microscopy is negative and suspicion is still high, repeat specimen collection and darkfield microscopy should be performed, in addition to serologic testing.
  - Positive serologic testing should be confirmed with treponemal tests. Treponemal tests include TPHA, MHA-TP, TPPA, FTA-ABS, SPHA, and FTA-ABS-19S-IgM (for congenital syphilis). Antibody titers correlate with disease activity.
    - Treponemal tests can confirm reactive nontreponemal tests but generally remain positive for life (except in very early treated syphilis) and therefore are not useful in monitoring treatment response.
    - Treponemal tests do not differentiate from other treponemes or spirochetes.
    - Sensitivity of treponemal tests varies based on the stage: 70% to 100% in primary, 100% in secondary and latent, and 95% in late.[27]
      - In patients with high pretest probability for syphilis, but negative serologic tests, the prozone phenomenon must be kept in mind (falsely negative serologic testing that occurs in the presence of high antibody titers).
  - All patients who present with ocular or neurologic symptoms should have a lumbar puncture performed to rule out CNS involvement, as this changes treatment.
- Latent syphilis
  - Diagnosis is established by positive serologic titers.
  - Treatment response is assessed by monitoring titers of RPR or VDRL. Titers should decline fourfold or greater in 12 to 24 months to be considered successful treatment. In the absence of a fourfold decline, treatment is considered a failure and examination of the CSF should be performed.
- Tertiary syphilis
  - Diagnosis is made with positive serologic tests.
  - All patients suspected of having tertiary syphilis require a lumbar puncture to guide treatment.
- Congenital syphilis
  - Diagnosis is by PCR, serologic titers that are at least fourfold higher than the mother's titers, or FTA-ABS-19S-IgM testing.
- All patients diagnosed with syphilis should be tested for HIV infection.

16.4. Treatment

- Primary, secondary, and early-latent syphilis
  - Adults: Benzathine penicillin G 2.4 million units IM as a single dose.
  - Children ≥1 month of age: Benzathine penicillin G 50,000 units/kg IM, up to the adult dose of 2.4 million units in a single dose.
  - In penicillin-allergic adults, doxycycline 100 mg orally twice daily for 14 days is likely the best alternative.
    - Pregnant patients with penicillin allergies should be desensitized and treated with penicillin.[28]

- Late latent syphilis
  - Adults: Benzathine penicillin G 2.4 million units IM as 3 doses administered at 1-week intervals.
  - Children ≥1 month of age: Benzathine penicillin G 50,000 units/kg IM, up to the adult dose of 2.4 million units, administered as 3 doses at 1-week intervals
  - In penicillin-allergic adults, doxycycline 100 mg orally twice daily for 28 days is likely the best alternative.
    ○ Pregnant patients with penicillin allergies should be desensitized and treated with penicillin.[28]
- Tertiary syphilis (gummatous and cardiovascular)
  - Adults: Benzathine penicillin G 2.4 million units IM as 3 doses administered at 1-week intervals.
  - Pregnant patients with penicillin allergies should be desensitized and treated with penicillin.[28]
- Neurosyphilis
  - Adults: Aqueous crystalline penicillin G 18 to 24 million units per day, administered as 3 to 4 million units IV every 4 hours or continuous infusion, for 10 to 14 days
  - In penicillin-allergic patients, desensitization should be considered. Ceftriaxone 2 g IM or IV for 10 to 14 days is an alternative regimen based on limited data.[28]
- Congenital syphilis
  - Neonate with proven or highly probable disease or born to mother with untreated early syphilis
    ○ Preferred treatment: Aqueous crystalline penicillin G 100,000 to 150,000 units/kg/d, administered as 50,000 units/kg/dose IV every 12 hours during the first 7 days of life and every 8 hours thereafter for a total of 10 days
    ○ Alternative treatment: Procaine penicillin G 50,000 units/kg/dose IM in a single daily dose for 10 days[28]
  - Neonate with no signs of disease born to mother with treated syphilis
    ○ Benzathine penicillin G 50,000 units/kg/dose IM in a single dose[28]

17. TUBERCULOSIS

17.1. Background
- Tuberculosis affects approximately a third of the world population, predominating in developing countries with high rates of poverty and malnutrition.
- Similarly to syphilis, the manifestations of tuberculosis are protean. Cutaneous manifestations of tuberculosis occur in only 1% to 4% of patients.[29]

17.2. Clinical Presentation
- Cutaneous manifestations of TB occur via exogenous inoculation, endogenous spread, and hematogenous dissemination and due to hypersensitivity to the tubercle bacilli.
- Exogenous inoculation
  - Cutaneous TB can occur by exogenous inoculation. In developing countries, this typically occurs through open wounds on barefoot feet over grounds covered with tuberculous sputum.[30] This results in tuberculosis verrucosa cutis, a warty lesion that is typically asymptomatic. Before verrucous evolution, lesions progress through a stage of erythematous papules with a surrounding purple inflammatory halo. Differential diagnosis: warts, chromomycosis, syphilis, and hypertrophic lichen planus.[26]

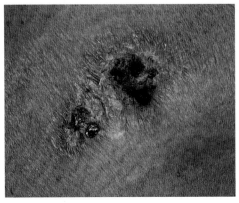

Figure 4-12. Cutaneous tuberculosis. (Courtesy of Arthur Eisen, MD.)

- Tuberculous chancre can also occur via exogenous inoculation, typically via trauma in previously nonsensitized patients. Lesions are reddish-brown nodules that develop into painless ulcers. Tissue culture is the main method of diagnosis. Differential diagnosis: sporotrichosis, endemic mycoses, cat-scratch disease, nocardiosis, tularemia, and syphilis[26] (Fig. 4-12).
- Endogenous spread
  - Scrofuloderma results from contiguous involvement of the skin from underlying tissues such as lymph nodes, joints, or bones. Lesions initially are ulcerated purple plaques with a purulent exudate, progressing to disfiguring scars when healed. Concurrent pulmonary TB is common.[31] The face and neck are the most frequently affected. Diagnosis is made with biopsy showing caseating granulomas in the lower dermis, acid-fast bacilli, and TB on culture. Differential diagnosis: bacterial abscesses, malignancy, endemic mycoses, hidradenitis suppurativa, acne conglobata and, when the inguinal lymph nodes are involved, sexually transmitted infections such as lymphogranuloma venereum.
  - Lupus vulgaris occurs more frequently in women than men. Classically, lupus vulgaris appears as head and neck–predominant, well-demarcated, reddish-brown plaques that can reach over 10 cm. Lesions can be seen on the legs and buttocks, more commonly in tropical countries.[32] As plaques enlarge peripherally, there can be central discoloration and atrophy. Diascopy of the lesions in patients with light-toned skin reveals classic "apple jelly" quality, common to other granulomatous processes such as sarcoidosis. Biopsy reveals caseating granulomas in the upper dermis. Differential diagnosis: sarcoidosis, discoid lupus, endemic mycoses, syphilis, and leishmaniasis.
- Hematogenous dissemination
  - Tuberculous gummas are the result of hematogenous dissemination and typically occur on the trunk and extremities of malnourished children and immunocompromised adults. Culture is often negative, and therefore, diagnosis is made when clinical suspicion is high and there is a response to anti-TB therapy. Differential diagnosis: other forms of bacterial abscesses.

- In patients with miliary TB, a sporotrichoid pattern can occur. Differential diagnosis: sporotrichosis, *Mycobacterium marinum* infection, leishmaniasis, nocardiosis, and less frequently endemic mycoses.[33]
- The dermatologic manifestation of miliary TB is known as tuberculosis cutis miliaris disseminata.[34] Miliary TB can result in sheets of white-topped papules. Alternatively, bluish papules can be present that progress through vesiculopustules, necrosis, and ulceration.[18] Patients have severe systemic symptoms. Differential diagnosis: varicella, PLEVA, rickettsialpox, and enteroviral exanthems.[26]
- Orificial TB occurs in patients with impaired cell-mediated immunity and results in painful, yellow papules on the mucosal surfaces, typically oral, nasal, anal, or vaginal. Orificial TB is a marker of severe visceral TB disease. Differential diagnosis: herpes simplex, aphthous stomatitis, pemphigus, and histoplasmosis.[26]
- Lupus vulgaris can also occur via hematogenous dissemination.
- Hypersensitivity reactions
  - A variety of cutaneous manifestations of TB occur as a result of hypersensitivity reactions to the bacillus; these are referred to as the tuberculids. The tuberculids typically result from chronic hematogenous dissemination of the bacillus in patients with moderate to high levels of immunity. The forms include erythema induratum of Bazin (EIB), lichen scrofulosorum, papulonecrotic tuberculid, and nodular tuberculid.[29]
  - EIB predominates on the lower extremities in the form of multiple painful, indurated nodules. These nodules can ulcerate with chronicity. EIB tends to appear on the posterior surfaces of the legs and can occur in flares every 3 to 4 months.[35] Diagnosis of TB in patients with EIB is often difficult. EIB is not well understood and may also occur in infections with nontuberculous mycobacteria. Differential diagnosis: erythema nodosum. EIB differs from erythema nodosum on pathology as it is a lobular panniculitis with vasculitis, whereas erythema nodosum is a septal panniculitis without vasculitis.
  - Lichen scrofulosorum is rare and occurs mostly in children. Lesions are 1 to 2 mm skin-colored papules found on the trunk that are otherwise asymptomatic. Cultures for TB are negative, but noncaseating perifollicular granulomas can be seen in the papillary dermis.[29]
  - Nodular tuberculid appears as blue or dusky-red nodules on the shins. Histology demonstrates granulomatous inflammation at the subcutaneous fat/lower dermis junction.[36,37]
  - Papulonecrotic tuberculid presents as a symmetric eruption of dusky-red papules on the extensor surfaces of the limbs. Though typically asymptomatic, papules can progress to ulcers and scarring.[31] Lesions frequently recur without TB treatment.
  - All forms of tuberculid respond quickly to antituberculous therapy.
  - TB can manifest with erythema nodosum, particularly in young females. The differential diagnosis for erythema nodosum is broad but includes streptococcal infection, sarcoidosis, endemic mycoses, and irritable bowel disease.

17.3. Evaluation

- Tuberculosis is suggested by history, physical examination, and imaging findings.
- Diagnosis can be achieved with induced sputum or bronchoscopy when there is concurrent pulmonary disease.
- Negative PPD or interferon-gamma release assay is suggestive but does not rule out infection.
- TB can cause a false positive on RPR testing.

- Dermal biopsy can demonstrate acid-fast bacilli or caseating granulomas, but not universally.
- PCR is becoming more widely available but is still not sensitive enough to preclude diagnosis of cutaneous TB when there is high suspicion.
- Definitive diagnosis sometimes cannot be achieved. When clinical suspicion is high, response to antituberculous treatment can confirm the diagnosis.

17.4. Treatment

- The mainstay of treatment is four-drug RIPE therapy (rifampin, isoniazid, pyrazinamide, ethambutol) for 8 weeks followed by two drug therapy (based on sensitivities), typically isoniazid and rifampin, for 6 to 9 months in most cases.
- Bone or joint involvement requires 9 to 12 months of treatment.
- In cases of drug resistance, treatment should be tailored to the resistance pattern of the organism. Consultation with an infectious diseases specialist is advised.
- All patients with a diagnosis of tuberculosis should be reported to the state health department as they require directly observed therapy (DOT).
- Treatment of patients with multidrug-resistant tuberculosis or those who are coinfected with HIV should be left to experts in those areas.

TICK-BORNE ILLNESSES

- Ticks are second only to mosquitoes as vectors of bacterial, viral, and protozoal diseases.
- In the United States, a number of tick-borne illnesses are recognized including Lyme disease, Rocky Mountain spotted fever, human monocytic ehrlichiosis, and babesiosis. Ticks may also bite without transmitting disease.

18. LYME DISEASE

18.1. Background

- Lyme disease is the most commonly reported vector-borne disease in the United States. The number of reported cases have increased from 10,000 in 1992 to 30,000 currently, with the true number of annual cases estimated to be as high as 300,000.[38]
- Multisystem disease caused by *Borrelia* species of spirochetes, a gram-negative organism transmitted by the *Ixodes* tick.
- *Borrelia burgdorferi* is the predominant etiologic organism in the United States with white-footed mice and white-tailed deer being the natural hosts.[39]
- Factors associated with transmission of *B. burgdorferi* from ticks to humans: duration of tick feeding and geographic proportion of infected ticks. The rate of transmission of microbe to human via tick saliva is low in the first 24 hours of attachment and increases dramatically after 48 hours.[40]
- The species of *Ixodes* tick vector varies by geographical location with *Ixodes scapularis* (also known as *Ixodes dammini*) predominant in the Eastern United States and Great Lakes region and *Ixodes pacificus* in the Western United States. In the Northeast and Midwest United States, approximately 10% to 20% of nymphal stage *I. scapularis* and 30% to 40% of adult ticks are infested with *B. burgdorferi*.[38]
- The incidence of Lyme disease parallels the emergence of the *Ixodes* tick, with most cases reported between May and November.

18.2. Clinical Features

- Lyme disease has been classically divided into three stages of disease: early localized disease, early disseminated disease, and late Lyme disease.
- The most common manifestation of early localized diseases is erythema migrans that develops at the site of the tick bite within 4 to 20 days (Fig. 4-13).
  - The lesion begins as an erythematous macule and gradually expands over the course of days to weeks, and while the most common description is a targetoid lesion, in approximately two-thirds of patients, the lesions either are uniformly erythematous or have enhanced central erythema.[40,41]
  - Lesions of erythema migrans favor the trunk, axilla, groin, and popliteal fossa and are seen in approximately 60% to 90% of diagnosed individuals.
- Systemic manifestations of the initial stage include flu-like illness, fatigue, headache, and malaise.
- In approximately 20% of patients, erythema migrans will be the only manifestation of Lyme disease even if left untreated.
- Within the first few weeks, spirochetes disseminate hematogenously to other tissues. Secondary annular lesions develop at distant sites. This stage can also be associated with Lyme neuroborreliosis (LNB) presenting as meningoradiculitis or meningitis and carditis presenting as atrioventricular conduction disturbances or rarely myocarditis or pancarditis.[42]

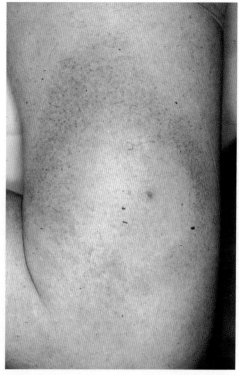

Figure 4-13. Lyme disease. (Courtesy of Arthur Eisen, MD.)

- Late manifestations of untreated infection include arthritis, encephalopathy, peripheral neuropathy, and encephalomyelitis.[43]

18.3. Diagnosis

- There are no standardized diagnostic criteria for Lyme disease.
- The diagnostic gold standard is the isolation of *Borrelia* by culture with subsequent PCR-based or other confirmation of its identity. Culture is expensive and requires special media and laboratory techniques, and results require several weeks. Therefore, culture is not useful for clinical decision making.
- PCR from tissue or fluid specimens can be used to confirm infection but is generally performed only for research purposes.
- For serologic testing, the CDC recommends a two-tier approach consisting of a sensitivity enzyme immunoassay (usually ELISA), followed by immunoblotting for positive or indeterminate tests.
  - In patients with erythema migrans, serologic testing is often of little use due to poor sensitivity, with only 29% of patients with a positive IgM or IgG antibody response.[44] Of patients tested during the acute EM phase, those with evidence of disseminated disease had a higher percentage test positive for an antibody response versus those without dissemination (43% vs. 17%).[44]
  - Serologic testing is most sensitive in patients with early disseminated disease with neurologic or cardiac manifestations or in those with late manifestations including arthritis (nearly 100%). Serologic tests should not be used to screen patients with nonspecific symptoms and a low probability of infection due to the poor positive predictive value.[45]

18.4. Differential Diagnosis

- Southern tick-associated rash illness (STARI) is a Lyme-like illness, transmitted by the Lone Star tick, and causes skin lesions indistinguishable from erythema migrans. Other entities that can be confused with EM include tinea, nummular eczema, granuloma annulare, contact dermatitis, fixed drug eruption, and erythema multiforme.

18.5. Treatment

- Cure rates exceed 90% when early-stage disease is treated with appropriate antibiotics. The Infectious Diseases Society of America provides treatment recommendations based upon where in the spectrum of disease activity patients fall and should be consulted prior to initiating treatment. Patients with early-stage disease with erythema migrans can be treated with doxycycline or amoxicillin for 14 days in the absence of neurologic or cardiac manifestations.
- Areas of Uncertainty
  - In a minority of patients who receive appropriate antibiotics for Lyme disease and have resolution of objective signs of infection, subjective symptoms persist. These patients are classified as having post-Lyme disease symptoms if they persist for <6 months and as post–Lyme disease syndrome if they persist for more than 6 months.[43] The etiology of this syndrome is unknown. Randomized, placebo-controlled trial of prolonged antibiotic therapy for patients with persistent subjective symptoms after appropriate initial treatment for Lyme disease has shown minimal or no benefit and increased risk of adverse effects.[45,46] As such, prolonged antibiotics for subjective symptoms are not recommended in patients whose objective signs of Lyme disease have resolved.

19. SOUTHERN TICK-ASSOCIATED RASH ILLNESS

19.1. Background

- A Lyme disease–like illness observed since the mid-1980s with a rash indistinguishable from the rash of early Lyme disease.[47]
- This Lyme-like disease has been described in the Southeastern United States in association with *Amblyomma americanum,* or the Lone Star tick; however, the exact etiologic organism remains uncertain.

19.2. Clinical Features

- Erythema migrans–like lesions due to STARI versus those due to *B. burgdorferi* infection have many clinical differences:
  - STARI skin lesions tend to be smaller, more circular, with greater likelihood of central clearing and less commonly seen in multiples.[48]
  - Less likely to have regional lymphadenopathy and tender or pruritic rashes.
  - Fewer symptoms at the time of rash onset.
- As the etiology remains uncertain with no definitive tests available, the clinical sequelae have not been definitively established.
- It is likely that the arthritis associated with STARI is less severe than that seen with Lyme disease.

19.3. Diagnosis

- Diagnosis must be made on clinical evidence.
- Patients with STARI do not seroconvert with serologic testing for Lyme disease.

19.4. Treatment

- Treatment of STARI is similar to treatment of early Lyme disease, with doxycycline 100 mg orally twice daily.

20. ROCKY MOUNTAIN SPOTTED FEVER

20.1. Background

- *Rickettsia rickettsii* is the etiologic agent of Rocky Mountain spotted fever (RMSF).
- Rickettsiae are small, obligately intracellular, gram-negative bacteria.
- Epidemiologically important vectors of *R. rickettsii* in N. America and C. America include the Rocky Mountain wood tick (*Dermacentor andersoni*), the American dog tick (*Dermacentor variabilis*), the Cayenne tick (*Amblyomma cajennense*), and the brown dog tick (*Rhipicephalus sanguineus*).[49]
- In the United States, RMSF still occurs predominantly in the Midwestern and Southeastern states including Oklahoma, Missouri, Arkansas, Tennessee, and North Carolina.

20.2. Clinical Features

- Abrupt onset of high fever often accompanied by headache, nausea, vomiting, anorexia, and malaise.
- A rash begins on the 2nd to 4th day following appearance of fever. Only rarely is an eschar identified at the infection site (Fig. 4-14 A, B).

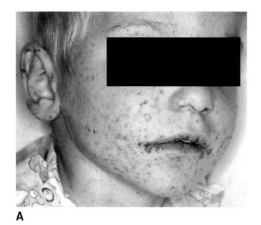

A

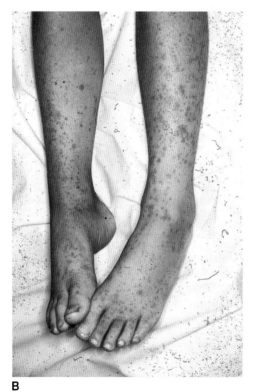

B

Figure 4-14. A,B: Rocky Mountain spotted fever. (Courtesy of Arthur Eisen, MD.)

- Rash appears as small pink macules, typically on wrists, ankles, and forearms. Evolves into maculopapules.
- Lesions evolve into petechiae or purpura in 50% to 60% of patients.
- Severe manifestations may include pulmonary edema, cerebral edema, myocarditis, renal failure, disseminated intravascular coagulopathy, and gangrene.
- Cutaneous findings are absent in 10% to 15% of patients.

20.3. Diagnosis

- Diagnosis is based on clinical and epidemiologic criteria such as signs, symptoms, and exposure history.
- Empiric treatment is given based on clinical suspicion rather than waiting for confirmatory test results.
- Serologic diagnosis is usually retrospective because antibodies do not develop until at least day 7 of illness.
- Rickettsiae can be identified by immunofluorescence or immunohistochemistry in a biopsy specimen of a maculopapular lesion.

20.4. Treatment

- Drug of choice is doxycycline. Chloramphenicol is a less effective alternative, having a higher rate of fatal outcomes.
  - Chloramphenicol is recommended for treatment of RMSF during pregnancy.
  - Despite currently available effective treatment and advances in medical care, an estimated 5% to 10% of US patients die.

REFERENCES

1. Howley PM, Douglas RL. Papillomaviruses. In: Knipe DM, Howley PM, eds. *Fields virology.* 5th ed. Philadelphia, PA: Lippincott Williams & Wilkins; 2001:2299–2354.
2. Rubben A, Kalka K, Spelten B, et al. Clinical features and age distribution of patients with HPV 2/27/57-induced common warts. *Arch Dermatol Res* 1997;289(6):337–340.
3. Rinaldi MG. Dermatophytosis: epidemiological and microbiological update. *J Am Acad Dermatol* 2000;43(5 suppl):S120–S124.
4. Abdel-Rahman SM, Farrand N, Schuenemann E, et al. The prevalence of infections with *Trichophyton tonsurans* in schoolchildren: the CAPITIS study. *Pediatrics* 2010;125(5):966–973.
5. Masri-Fridling GD. Dermatophytosis of the feet. *Dermatol Clin* 1996;14(1):33–40.
6. Miller MA, Hodgson Y. Sensitivity and specificity of potassium hydroxide smears of skin scrapings for the diagnosis of tinea pedis. *Arch Dermatol* 1993;129(4):510–511.
7. Gupta R, Warren T, Wald A. Genital herpes. *Lancet* 2007;370(9605):2127–2137.
8. Xu F, Sternberg MR, Kottiri BJ, et al. Trends in herpes simplex virus type 1 and type 2 seroprevalence in the United States. *JAMA* 2006;296(8):964–973.
9. Roberts CM, Pfister JR, Spear SJ. Increasing proportion of herpes simplex virus type 1 as a cause of genital herpes infection in college students. *Sex Transm Dis* 2003;30(10):797–800.
10. Freeman EE, Weiss HA, Glynn JR, et al. Herpes simplex virus 2 infection increases HIV acquisition in men and women: systematic review and meta-analysis of longitudinal studies. *AIDS (London, England)* 2006;20(1):73–83.
11. Corey L, Wald A, Patel R, et al. Once-daily valacyclovir to reduce the risk of transmission of genital herpes. *N Engl J Med* 2004;350(1):11–20.
12. Hope-Simpson RE. The nature of herpes zoster: a long-term study and a new hypothesis. *Proc R Soc Med* 1965;58:9–20.

13. Brown GR. Herpes zoster: correlation of age, sex, distribution, neuralgia, and associated disorders. *South Med J* 1976;69(5):576–578.

14. Stevens DL, Bisno AL, Chambers HF, et al. Practice guidelines for the diagnosis and management of skin and soft tissue infections: 2014 update by the Infectious Diseases Society of America. *Clin Infect Dis* 2014;59(2):e10–e52.

15. Crawford SE, Boyle-Vavra S, Daum RS. Community associated methicillin-resistant *Staphylococcus aureus*. In: Hooper D, Scheld M, eds. *Emerging Infections*. vol. 7. Washington, DC: ASM Press; 2007:153–179.

16. Herold BC, Immergluck LC, Maranan MC, et al. Community-acquired methicillin-resistant *Staphylococcus aureus* in children with no identified predisposing risk. *JAMA* 1998;279(8):593–598.

17. Liu C, Bayer A, Cosgrove SE, et al. Clinical practice guidelines by the infectious diseases society of America for the treatment of methicillin-resistant *Staphylococcus aureus* infections in adults and children: executive summary. *Clin Infect Dis* 2011;52(3):285–292.

18. Cohen J, Opal SM, Powderly WG, eds. *Cohen & powderly: infectious diseases*. 3rd ed. United Kingdom: Elsevier Limited; 2010.

19. Andreasen TJ, Green SD, Childers BJ. Massive infectious soft-tissue injury: diagnosis and management of necrotizing fasciitis and purpura fulminans. *Plast Reconstr Surg* 2001;107(4):1025–1035.

20. Prevention of Invasive Group A Streptococcal Infections Workshop Participants. Prevention of invasive group A streptococcal disease among household contacts of case patients and among postpartum and postsurgical patients: recommendations from the Centers for Disease Control and Prevention. *Clin Infect Dis* 2002;35(8):950–959.

21. Linner A, Darenberg J, Sjolin J, et al. Clinical efficacy of polyspecific intravenous immunoglobulin therapy in patients with streptococcal toxic shock syndrome: a comparative observational study. *Clin Infect Dis* 2014;59(6):851–857.

22. Gjestland T. The Oslo study of untreated syphilis; an epidemiologic investigation of the natural course of the syphilitic infection based upon a re-study of the Boeck-Bruusgaard material. *Acta dermato-venereologica Supplementum* 1955;35(suppl 34):3–368; Annex I-LVI.

23. Buchacz K, Patel P, Taylor M, et al. Syphilis increases HIV viral load and decreases CD4 cell counts in HIV-infected patients with new syphilis infections. *AIDS (London, England)* 2004;18(15):2075–2079.

24. Sellati TJ, Wilkinson DA, Sheffield JS, et al. Virulent *Treponema pallidum*, lipoprotein, and synthetic lipopeptides induce CCR5 on human monocytes and enhance their susceptibility to infection by human immunodeficiency virus type 1. *J Infect Dis* 2000;181(1):283–293.

25. Fleming DT, Wasserheit JN. From epidemiological synergy to public health policy and practice: the contribution of other sexually transmitted diseases to sexual transmission of HIV infection. *Sex Transm Infect* 1999;75(1):3–17.

26. Bolognia JL, Jorizzo JL, Schaffer JV, eds. *Dermatology*, 3rd ed. Philadelphia, PA: Elsevier; 2012.

27. Larsen SA, Steiner BM, Rudolph AH. Laboratory diagnosis and interpretation of tests for syphilis. *Clin Microbiol Rev* 1995;8(1):1–21.

28. Workowski K. 2010 Sexually Transmitted Diseases Treatment Guidelines. In: Edited by CDC DoSTDPTG. http://www.cdc.gov/std/treatment/2010/genital-ulcers.htm#a5: CDC; 2010.

29. Lai-Cheong JE, Perez A, Tang V, et al. Cutaneous manifestations of tuberculosis. *Clin Exp Dermatol* 2007;32(4):461–466.

30. Gruber PC, Whittam LR, du Vivier A. Tuberculosis verrucosa cutis on the sole of the foot. *Clin Exp Dermatol* 2002;27(3):188–191.

31. Barbagallo J, Tager P, Ingleton R, et al. Cutaneous tuberculosis: diagnosis and treatment. *Am J Clin Dermatol* 2002;3(5):319–328.

32. Frankel A, Penrose C, Emer J. Cutaneous tuberculosis: a practical case report and review for the dermatologist. *J Clin Aesthet Dermatol* 2009;2(10):19–27.

33. Premalatha S, Rao NR, Somasundaram V, et al. Tuberculous gumma in sporotrichoid pattern. *Int J Dermatol* 1987;26(9):600–601.

34. Rietbroek RC, Dahlmans RP, Smedts F, et al. Tuberculosis cutis miliaris disseminata as a manifestation of miliary tuberculosis: literature review and report of a case of recurrent skin lesions. *Rev Infect Dis* 1991;13(2):265–269.

35. Mascaro JM Jr, Baselga E. Erythema induratum of bazin. *Dermatol Clin* 2008;26(4): 439–445, v.

36. Friedman PC, Husain S, Grossman ME. Nodular tuberculid in a patient with HIV. *J Am Acad Dermatol* 2005;53(2 suppl 1):S154–S156.

37. Jordaan HF, Schneider JW, Abdulla EA. Nodular tuberculid: a report of four patients. *Pediatr Dermatol* 2000;17(3):183–188.

38. Lyme Disease Data [http://www.cdc.gov/lyme/stats/]

39. Hengge UR, Tannapfel A, Tyring SK, et al. Lyme borreliosis. *Lancet Infect Dis* 2003;3(8):489–500.

40. Piesman J. Dyanamics of *Borrelia burgdorferi* transmission by nymphal *Ixodes dammini* ticks. *J Infect Dis* 1993;167(5):1082–1085.

41. Nadelman RB, Nowakowski J, Forseter G, et al. The clinical spectrum of early Lyme borreliosis in patients with culture-confirmed erythema migrans. *Am J Med* 1996;100(5): 502–508.

42. Borchers AT, Keen CL, Huntley AC, et al. Lyme disease: a rigorous review of diagnostic criteria and treatment. *J Autoimmun* 2015;57:82–115.

43. Feder HM Jr, Johnson BJ, O'Connell S, et al. A critical appraisal of "chronic Lyme disease". *N Engl J Med* 2007;357(14):1422–1430.

44. Steere AC, McHugh G, Damle N, et al. Prospective study of serologic tests for lyme disease. *Clin Infect Dis* 2008;47(2):188–195.

45. Wormser GP, Dattwyler RJ, Shapiro ED, et al. The clinical assessment, treatment, and prevention of lyme disease, human granulocytic anaplasmosis, and babesiosis: clinical practice guidelines by the Infectious Diseases Society of America. *Clin Infect Dis* 2006;43(9):1089–1134.

46. Klempner MS, Hu LT, Evans J, et al. Two controlled trials of antibiotic treatment in patients with persistent symptoms and a history of Lyme disease. *N Engl J Med* 2001;345(2):85–92.

47. Blanton L, Keith B, Brzezinski W. Southern tick-associated rash illness: erythema migrans is not always Lyme disease. *South Med J* 2008;101(7):759–760.

48. Feder HM Jr, Hoss DM, Zemel L, et al. Southern Tick-Associated Rash Illness (STARI) in the North: STARI following a tick bite in Long Island, New York. *Clin Infect Dis* 2011;53(10):e142–e146.

49. Parola P, Paddock CD, Socolovschi C, et al. Update on tick-borne rickettsioses around the world: a geographic approach. *Clin Microbiol Rev* 2013;26(4):657–702.

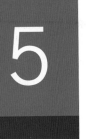

5

Reactive Disorders and Drug Eruptions

Shivani V. Tripathi, MD and Milan J. Anadkat, MD

Reactive disorders and drug eruptions encompass a broad range of dermatologic conditions in which a systemic insult manifests in the skin. While some of the clinical findings are specific, others are not and require clinicopathologic correlation.

1. STASIS DERMATITIS

- Stasis dermatitis is considered part of the clinical spectrum of chronic venous insufficiency.
  - *Chronic venous insufficiency + eczematous dermatitis = stasis dermatitis*
- Typically seen on lower extremities. However, stasis dermatitis may rarely involve the upper limbs in patients with congenital arteriovenous (AV) malformations or in patients with AV fistulas for dialysis.[1]

1.1. Background

- Epidemiology
  - Stasis dermatitis is reported in 1% to 20% of women and 1% to 17% of men.[2]
- Risk factors include pregnancy, increased age, family history of venous disease, obesity, and professions that require continuous periods of standing.
- Venous hypertension can be the result of pump failure, poor valve function, and valve obstruction. Valve insufficiency in venous hypertension along with eczematous changes leads to the chronic condition of stasis dermatitis.

1.2. Clinical Presentation (Fig. 5-1)

- Stasis dermatitis is a late manifestation of chronic venous disease, which includes the following physical exam findings:
  - **Cushion-like pitting edema** of the medial aspects of the shin and calf around and proximal to the ankle, corresponding to the location of the major communicating veins. Varicosities can also be present in the lower legs.
  - **Hyperpigmentation** develops with intermittent episodes of hemosiderin deposits present on the skin, called stasis purpura.
  - **Atrophie blanche** (whitish atrophic scar) can develop in severe cases of vascular insufficiency. It is not specific to venous insufficiency. The exam finding is an ivory-white depressed atrophic plaque that can be star shaped or polyangular.[3]
- Chronic venous insufficiency can also lead to an "inverted wine bottle appearance" or *lipodermatosclerosis* of the affected area. In lipodermatosclerosis, the adipose tissue and deep dermis become sclerotic and adherent with a circular cuff that develops around the distal calf.

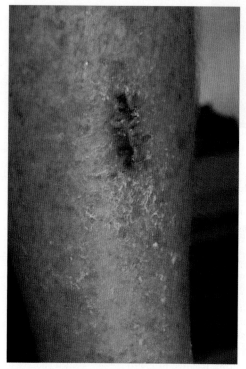

Figure 5-1. Venous stasis (as noted on recent postoperative patient). (Courtesy of M. Laurin Council, MD.)

- Stasis dermatitis can mimic cellulitis. As the edema worsens, it can begin to involve more of the calf leading to erythema and inflammation. Stasis dermatitis is the most frequent condition that is mistaken for cellulitis, leading to unnecessary hospital admission.[4] However, unlike cellulitis, the skin findings related to stasis dermatitis develop slowly and are more likely to be bilateral. Scaling and itching are common in stasis dermatitis but are rarely seen in cellulitis.
- Chronic rubbing and scratching can lead to thickening of the skin called *lichenification*.
- Vascular papules that develop from the edema can present over the changes of stasis dermatitis, called *acroangiodermatitis* or pseudo-Kaposi sarcoma. These may be mistaken for classic Kaposi sarcoma (KS) on clinical exam, but lack the histopathologic findings of KS.
- In acute exacerbations, eczematous changes with scaly, exudative, and weeping plaques can develop.
- Complications
  - Contact sensitization, possibly due to repeated application of various topical treatments at the affected site.
    - Common culprits—balsam of Peru, lanolin, rubber or latex products, bandages, topical antibiotics (Neosporin), topical corticosteroids

- Venous leg ulcers
- **Autoeczematization**—an acute, pruritic, papulovesicular eruption that develops at sites distant from the primary cutaneous findings. It typically involves the forearms, thighs, trunks, and face. Also called an "id reaction."
- **Superinfection**—due to the disrupted skin barrier, bacteria and fungi can colonize the areas affected by stasis dermatitis leading to impetiginized skin, cellulitis, or erysipelas with common pathogens such as *Staphylococcus aureus* and *Streptococcus pyogenes*.

1.3. Evaluation

- **Skin Exam**—erythema, scaling, hyperpigmentation, and varicosities typically present.
- Erythema, scaling, and hyperpigmentation. Varicosities typically present. Edema may be pitting or nonpitting. Unlike cellulitis, the presentation is typically chronic and nontender.[5]
- Doppler ultrasound can be helpful showing venous incompetency and diagnosing deep venous thrombosis.
- If the diagnosis is uncertain, skin biopsy can be considered. Poor wound healing after biopsy is likely due to already compromised circulation.
  - Histopathology will demonstrate a superficial perivascular lymphocytic infiltrate, epidermal spongiosis, serous exudate, scale, and crust, in the acute setting. The more chronic lesions may show epidermal acanthosis with hyperkeratosis, hemosiderin deposits, and dilated capillaries.
- Bacterial culture and/or potassium hydroxide preparation can be useful when superinfection of the area is suspected.
- Patch testing for contact sensitization can be useful in patients who develop worsening of disease despite skin care and topical therapy.

1.4. Treatment

- Improving stasis dermatitis begins with treating underlying venous insufficiency.
  - Leg elevation
  - Compression therapy[6]
  - Medical and surgical management of venous disease[7]
- Symptomatic treatment involves addressing pruritus, dryness, and inflammation.
  - Gentle skin care with lukewarm showers and mild soaps, avoiding washcloth use, and regular application of emollients to damp skin after bathing (petrolatum jelly).
  - Mid- to high-potency topical steroids, including triamcinolone 0.1% ointment or clobetasol 0.05% ointment, should be applied twice daily during acute flare.

2. PETECHIAE, PURPURA, AND CUTANEOUS VASCULITIS

- Cutaneous vasculitis results almost exclusively from inflammation of the small or medium-sized blood vessels in the skin. Vasculitis is a histopathologic finding with a range of clinical manifestations and associations, and presentation is determined by the size of the vessel involved.[8,9]
- Vascular injury presents as visible red or purple lesions, which is evidence of hemorrhage into the skin and mucous membranes. The cutaneous manifestations of vasculitis involve purpuric lesions that can be divided based on clinical exam findings: size of lesion and raised versus flat lesion.[10]

- Petechiae and ecchymoses are flat and are differentiated based on size of the lesions.
- **Petechiae**—nonblanchable and nonpalpable pinpoint macules resulting from capillary inflammation and extravasation of red blood cells (Fig. 5-2A).
- **Palpable purpura**—a common manifestation of small-vessel vasculitis that can initially present as erythematous papules and plaques progressing to raised, non-blanchable lesions. Palpable purpura can be any size, but is differentiated by the fact that it is raised (Fig. 5-2B).
- Retiform purpura is also raised, but has a more geometric, net-like presentation. Retiform purpura can be either noninflammatory or inflammatory.
- Vasculitis is DIFFERENT than vasculopathy.
  - *Vasculitis* is defined by inflammatory injury to the vasculature, while *vasculopathy* is a noninflammatory occlusive injury to the vessel.

2.1. Background

- Nonpalpable purpuric lesions—petechiae and ecchymosis[11]
  - **Petechiae (size <4 mm)**
    Causes of petechiae—thrombocytopenia, abnormal platelet function, other
    - *Thrombocytopenia*—idiopathic, drug-induced, thrombotic, disseminated intravascular coagulation
    - *Abnormal platelet function*—congenital or hereditary platelet function defects. Examples: acquired platelet dysfunction (aspirin, nonsteroidal anti-inflammatory drugs [NSAIDS], renal insufficiency, monoclonal gammopathy), thrombocytosis secondary to myeloproliferative disorders
    - *Nonplatelet etiologies*—elevations in intravascular pressures (Valsalva, etc.), fixed increase in pressure (stasis) or intermittent pressure (blood pressure cuff), trauma (often linear), perifollicular (scurvy/vitamin C deficiency), mild inflammatory conditions (pigmented purpuric eruptions, hypergammaglobulinemic purpura of Waldenstrom)
  - **Ecchymosis (size ≥1 cm)**
    Causes of ecchymosis—procoagulant or poor dermal support or platelet dysfunction + minor trauma
    - Procoagulant—anticoagulant use, hepatic insufficiency, vitamin K deficiency, disseminated intravascular coagulation
    - Poor dermal support—actinic purpura, corticosteroid therapy (topical or systemic), vitamin C deficiency (scurvy), systemic amyloidosis (light chain related, some familial), Ehlers-Danlos syndrome
    - Platelet dysfunction—von Willebrand disease, medication induced, metabolic disease, acquired or congenital thrombocytopenia
- Two major causes of purpura are microvascular occlusion syndromes and vasculitis.
- **Vasculitis** is defined by the size of the affected vessel (small, medium, mixed, or large).
  - *Small vessel (leukocytoclastic vasculitis)*—Henoch-Schönlein purpura, acute hemorrhagic edema of infancy, urticarial vasculitis, erythema elevatum diutinum, malignancy related, infection (Group A Strep, Neisseria meningococcus, human immunodeficiency virus, hepatitis C), medication (anti–tumor necrosis factor, hydralazine, minocycline, NSAIDs, quinolones), autoimmune connective tissue disease (systemic lupus erythematosus [SLE], rheumatoid arthritis, Sjögren's), inflammatory bowel disease

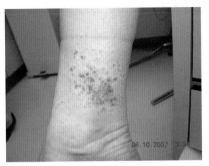

A

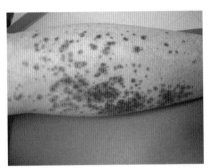

B

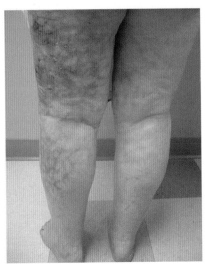

C

Figure 5-2. A: Petechiae. **B:** Vasculitis.
C: Vasculopathy.

- *Small to medium-sized vessels*—ANCA-associated vasculitides (Churg-Strauss syndrome, granulomatosis with polyangiitis, microscopic polyarteritis), essential cryoglobulinemic vasculitis
  - Secondary causes—infections, inflammatory disorders (autoimmune connective tissue disease), drug exposure, neoplasms
- *Medium sized vessel vasculitis*—polyarteritis nodosa (PAN)
- *Large-vessel vasculitis*—Takayasu arteritis, giant cell arteritis
- **Palpable purpura**
  - Vessel inflammation results in vessel wall damage and extravasation of erythrocytes seen on exam. Vasculitis may be a primary process or may be secondary to an underlying disease.
  - Palpable purpura is the pathognomonic lesion of small-vessel vasculitis/leukocytoclastic vasculitis.
  - Immune complex disease.
    - Idiopathic, infection, or drug-associated IgG or IgM complexes.
    - Idiopathic IgA complexes (Henoch-Schonlein purpura) or IgA complexes associated with drugs or infection.
    - Hypergammaglobulinemic purpura of Waldenstrom.
    - Urticarial vasculitis (Fig. 5-2C).
    - Pustular vasculitis.
    - Mixed cryoglobulinemia.
  - Pauci-immune leukocytoclastic vasculitis.
    - ANCA associated—granulomatosis with polyangiitis, microscopic polyangiitis, Churg-Strauss.
    - Others—erythema elevatum diutinum Sweet syndrome (acute febrile neutrophilic dermatosis).

2.2. Clinical Presentation

- All forms of purpura do not blanch when pressed, as they are due to vascular extravasation as opposed to areas of vascular dilatation.
- **Small to medium-sized vessel involvement**—subcutaneous nodules, purpura, and livedo racemosa (fixed livedo reticularis/that does not resolve with warming)[12]
  - Typically presents 7 to 10 days after exposure to an inciting agent with a single group of lesions made up of palpable purpura, erythematous papules, vesicles, or urticarial lesions.
  - Initial lesion is a purpuric macule or partially blanching urticarial papule.
  - Diameter can range from 1 mm to multiple centimeters.
  - Lesions of cutaneous small-vessel vasculitis favor dependent areas as well as areas affected by trauma (pathergy) or under tight-fitting clothing.
  - Typically asymptomatic, but can be associated with pain, burning, and pruritus.
  - Residual postinflammatory hyperpigmentation can persist for months or more.
  - Constitutional symptoms may accompany episodes of cutaneous small-vessel vasculitis.[13]
- **Medium-sized vessel disease** presents with livedo reticularis, retiform purpura, subcutaneous nodules, claudication, ulceration, and necrosis.
  - Lesions favor dependent sites as well as areas under tight-fitting clothing.
  - Lesions are typically asymptomatic, but may be associated with burning, pain, and pruritus.

2.3. Evaluation

- Leukocytoclastic vasculitis secondary to drug and infectious disorders accounts for many cases of cutaneous vasculitis, and a history should be obtained of new medications and constitutional symptoms in relation to the onset cutaneous findings.[13]
- **Targeted history and physical exam assessment**
  - Drug-induced vasculitis typically occurs 7 to 10 days after the introduction of the medication at fault.
  - Weight loss, joint pain, photosensitivity, mucosal ulcerations, Raynaud phenomenon, xerostomia, and xerophthalmia can suggest an underlying connective tissue disease.
  - Weight loss, night sweats, and fevers can suggest malignancy.
  - Levamisole-tainted cocaine can lead to retiform purpura[14]; patients with this finding should be questioned with regard to recreational drug use.
  - Patients should be asked whether they have experienced a change in urine to determine renal function, or new-onset pulmonary symptoms to determine if vasculitis could be associated with systemic findings.
- A punch biopsy can be particularly helpful in diagnosing leukocytoclastic vasculitis. In addition to a biopsy for hematoxylin and eosin (H&E), a biopsy for direct immunofluorescence (DIF) can be particularly important in the diagnosis of IgA vasculitis, vasculitis related to cryoglobulinemia, and hypocomplementemic vasculitis.[15,16]
  - Smaller lesions can be sampled with a 4-mm punch biopsy. Larger lesions may require a 6-mm punch or a wedge biopsy. Lesions between 24 and 48 hours old are most likely to be diagnostic.
  - Location of skin biopsy—in livedo racemosa, a biopsy should be taken from the pale center of the lesion. If an ulcer is present, a biopsy for H&E staining should be taken from the edge of the ulcer, while a biopsy for DIF should be taken from within the lesion.
    - Small-vessel involvement (venules and arterioles)—angiocentric and/or angioinvasive inflammatory infiltrates, disruption of the vessel walls by inflammatory infiltrates, and fibrinoid necrosis.
    - Medium-sized vessel involvement (small arteries and veins)—inflammatory infiltrate of the muscular vessel wall and fibrinoid necrosis.
- **Laboratory testing**
  - Primary studies—complete blood count with differential, liver function tests, blood urea nitrogen/creatinine level, and urinalysis with microscopy
  - Secondary studies—hepatitis B and C serologies, serum complement levels (CH50, C3, C4), antinuclear antibody (ANA), anti-dsDNA, anti-Ro, anti-La, anti-RNP, anti-Sm, rheumatoid factor, serum cryoglobulins, antineutrophil cytoplasmic antibodies (ANCAs), serum and urine protein electrophoresis and immunofixation (SPEP & UPEP), and human immunodeficiency virus
  - Chest x-ray in patients with cutaneous vasculitis and pulmonary symptoms, as ANCA-associated vasculitis can affect small and medium vessels of the lungs

2.4. Treatment

- Treatment of vasculitis depends on the underlying etiology. As most cases of leukocytoclastic vasculitis can be attributed to underlying infection or drug, removing the eliciting agent is the first step.

3. URTICARIA

- **Definition**—intensely pruritic, pink or pale swelling of the superficial dermis ranging in size from a few millimeters in diameter to multiple centimeters (wheal). Lesions can be numerous or single. The hallmark of a wheal is that it appears and disappears rapidly—within 24 hours. Urticaria can also present with angioedema, in which the swellings occur deeper in the dermis and in the subcutaneous or submucosal tissue. Angioedema can affect the mouth and, rarely, the bowel. Angioedema tends to be painful rather than itchy, and lesions can often last for 2 to 3 days.[17]
- Several causes of urticaria
  - Allergy
  - Autoimmunity
  - Drugs
  - Dietary pseudoallergens
  - Infections
  - Note—C1 esterase inhibitor deficiency should be considered a cause of recurrent angioedema without wheals
- Urticaria is typically categorized as **acute** (present for <6 weeks) or **chronic** (recurrent, with signs and symptoms recurring most days of the week for 6 weeks or longer).

3.1. Background

- Epidemiology—approximately 25% of the general population will experience hives during their lifetime.[18]
- Cutaneous mast cells, located in the superficial dermis, are the primary effectors of urtricaria. Mast cell granules have preformed mediators of inflammation: histamines and cytokines.[19]
- Classic immediate hypersensitivity reactions involve binding of an allergen to mast cell receptor–bound IgE. Other nonimmunologic stimuli, such as opiates and neuropeptides (e.g., substance P), can activate mast cell degranulation independent of the high-affinity IgE receptor.
- Urticarial vasculitis is thought to involve circulating immune complexes (type III hypersensitivity reaction).
- Common causes—infections; allergic reactions to medications, foods, or insect stings and bites; reactions to medications that lead to nonallergic mast cell activation (e.g., narcotics); and NSAIDs.
- Infections—acute urticaria may develop during or following viral or bacterial infection. Over 80% of cases of acute urticaria in children are associated with an infectious process.[20]

3.2. Clinical Presentation (Fig. 5-3)

- The individual lesions of classic urticaria last for ≤24 hours and resolve without sequelae, but often return episodically.
- In urticarial-like dermatoses (i.e., bullous pemphigoid), the lesions can last many days and may present with other cutaneous findings, such as blistering, to help differentiate from classic urticaria.
- Clinical classifications of urticaria and angioedema
  - Classic urticaria
  - Physical urticarias
  - Urticarial vasculitis

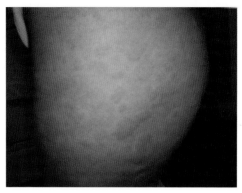

Figure 5-3. Urticaria (hives).

- Contact urticaria
- Angioedema (without urticaria)
- Distinctive urticarial syndromes
- Chronic urticaria—symptoms last for 6 or more weeks. Chronic urticaria is applied to continuous urticaria occurring at least twice a week off treatment.
- Urticaria occurring less frequent than twice per week is termed recurrent or episodic urticaria.
- Acute urticaria is common in young children with atopic dermatitis.
- Chronic urticaria incidence peaks in the fourth decade, is more common in the evening or is present upon waking, can significantly affect quality-of-life measures, and can have premenstrual exacerbations in women.
- **Physical urticarias**
  - Induced by exogenous physical stimuli.
  - May severely affect quality of life, especially delayed pressure urticaria and cholinergic urticaria.
  - Classification
    - Urticaria due to mechanical stimuli
      - Dermatographism (Fig. 5-4)
      - Delayed pressure urticaria (vibratory angioedema, inherited, acquired)
    - Urticaria due to temperature changes and stress
      - Cholinergic urticaria
      - Stress (adrenergic urticaria)
      - Cold
        - Primary cold urticaria (cold contact urticaria)
        - Secondary to cryoglobulins
      - Solar urticaria
      - Aquagenic urticaria
- Constitutional symptoms such as fatigue may be present, but recurrent fevers and arthritis warrant an additional workup to rule out urticarial vasculitis or urticarial syndrome (Muckle-Wells or Schnitzler's).
- Chronic urticaria has been associated with autoimmune thyroid disease.
- Patients with histamine-releasing autoantibodies have a very strong association with HLA-DR4 and associated alleles HLA-DQ8.

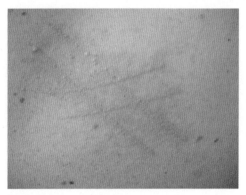

Figure 5-4. Dermatographism.

- An association with *Helicobacter pylori* gastritis and urticaria has been shown, with studies showing higher frequency of remission when the infection was eradicated than when it was not.[21]
- **Dermatographism**
  - Immediate dermatographism—divided into simple and symptomatic.
  - Simple immediate dermatographism occurs in about 5% of normal people in response to moderate stroking of the skin and may be regarded as an exaggerated physiologic response.
  - Symptomatic dermatographism is the most common of the physical urticarias.
    - Linear wheals at sites of scratching and at other sites of friction.
    - Young adults.
    - Pruritus can coexist and present concurrently with wheals.
    - Worst in the evening and usually resolves in an hour.
- **Delayed pressure urticaria**
  - Development of deep erythematous edema at sites of sustained pressure to the skin, after a delay of 30 minutes to 12 hours.
  - Swellings are usually pruritic, painful, or both and may persist for days.
  - Waistline, below the elastic of socks, feet in tight shoes, palms after manual work, and genitalia after intercourse.
  - Systemic features like fatigue, arthralgias, etc., may be present.
  - Mean duration is 6 to 9 years.
- **Vibratory angioedema**
  - Vibratory stimulus induces localized swelling and erythema within minutes.
  - Jogging, rubbing with a towel, and using machinery like a lawnmower.
  - Familial form with autosomal dominant inheritance.
- **Stress exposure**
  - Cholinergic urticaria—transient papular wheals measuring 2 to 3 mm in size and surrounded by an obvious flare, occurring within 15 minutes of sweat-inducing stimuli (physical activity, hot baths, emotional stress). Moving from a hot to cold room; eating spicy food. Pruritus can follow the development of the monomorphic wheals. Cold urticaria, symptomatic dermatographism, or aquagenic urticaria may be associated with cholinergic urticaria.

- Adrenergic urticaria—sudden stress induces small pink wheals surrounded by blanched vasoconstricted skin.
- Local heat contact urticaria—one of the rarest forms of urticaria. Within minutes of contact with heat from any source, itching and whealing occur at the precise location of contact with heat such as hot water or even sunlight. Symptoms can last for an hour.
- Cold urticaria
  - Primary cold urticaria
    - Itching, burning, and hives occur minutes after the exposure to a cold environment or object.
    - Can follow respiratory infection or arthropod bites and has been associated with HIV.
  - Secondary cold urticaria
    - Can be seen with serum abnormalities like cryoglobulinemia and cryofibrinogenemia or associated with Raynaud phenomenon and purpura.
    - Wheals can last 24 hours or more.
    - Serum cryoglobulins and cryofibrinogens should be measured.
    - Underlying cause may be hepatitis B or C, lymphoproliferative diseases, and infectious mononucleosis.
- Solar urticaria
  - Itching and whealing within minutes to UV exposure or visible wavelengths of solar radiation and may penetrate light clothing. Systemic symptoms are also possible.
  - Primary solar urticaria
    - Mediated by an immediate type I hypersensitivity reaction to a cutaneous or circulating irradiation-induced neoantigen.
    - Secondary solar urticaria is seen in patients with certain types of porphyria.
- Aquagenic urticaria—contact with water of any temperature induces an urticarial eruption resembling cholinergic urticaria. Lesions occur most frequently on the upper part of the body and last for an hour or less. Other physical urticarias, as well as aquagenic pruritus, must be excluded.
- Urticarial vasculitis—cutaneous lesions resemble urticaria clinically, but last longer than 24 hours, are painful instead of itchy, and show evidence of small-vessel vasculitis/leukocytoclastic vasculitis on histopathology.
- Contact urticaria
- Urticarial syndromes
  - Muckle-Wells syndrome—rare autosomal dominant condition characterized by mutation in the NALP3 (CIAS1) gene that produces the protein cryopyrin. Burning and itching plaques can last up to 2 days and develop as a result of drop in body temperature. Fever, headaches, and leukocytosis may also be present. The spectrum can also include chronic infantile neurologic cutaneous and articular (CINCA) syndrome, associated with sensorineural deafness and amyloidosis.
  - Familial Mediterranean fever—autosomal recessive, eastern European and Middle Eastern descent. Patients may present with peritonitis, pleurisy, or synovitis.
  - Schnitzler syndrome—nonpruritic urticarial eruption, recurrent fevers, bone pain, arthritis and arthralgias, as well as monoclonal gammopathy, which can progress to a lymphoproliferative disorder.

3.3. Evaluation

- **Differential diagnosis**—arthropod bites, febrile neutrophilic dermatosis (Sweet syndrome), prebullous pemphigoid (urticarial bullous pemphigoid), acute facial contact dermatitis, urticarial drug reactions, and mastocytosis.
- **Comprehensive history**—duration of disease, frequency of attacks, duration of individual lesions, associated illness, previous treatments, known allergies or adverse reactions, personal and familial medical history, occupation and leisure activities, and quality-of-life measures.
- **Labs**—urticaria that is responsive to antihistamines does not typically necessitate an extensive work-up, but in complicated cases basic laboratory tests (CBC, CMP, etc), skin biopsy for lesions lasting more than 24 hours, question of food additives and drugs, and occasionally skin tests for allergies might be indicated.[22,23]
- **Acute urticaria** workup—IgE-mediated reactions to environmental allergens related to acute and contact urticaria can be confirmed by skin prick testing and radioallergosorbent test (RAST) of the blood.
- **Chronic urticaria**—complete blood count and white cell differential (to detect eosinophilia related to intestinal parasitosis) and erythrocyte sedimentation rate (typically normal in chronic urticaria, but may be raised in urticarial vasculitis). Thyroid function, TSH, and free T4 (the presence of thyroid autoantibodies is higher in patients with chronic urticaria and could be an indicator of autoimmune urticaria).
- **Physical urticarias**—symptomatic dermatographism can be tested by stroking the skin of the back lightly with the rounded edge of a wooden spatula. Provocation tests for cholinergic urticaria include exercise to the point of sweating in an overheated environment or partial immersion in a hot bath at 42°C for 10 minutes. Cold contact urticaria is confirmed by the development of whealing at the site of application of an ice cube in a glove for 20 minutes. Phototesting confirms the diagnosis of solar urticaria, with development of wheals within minutes of exposure to sunlight.
- **Urticarial vasculitis**—lesional skin biopsy is essential and should be done on lesions that last more than 24 hours to confirm the histologic presence of leukocytoclastic vasculitis. Vasculitis screen: serum complement assays and exclusion of SLE. Systemic involvement: complete blood count; ESR; urinalysis; tests for renal and liver function; serum complement levels of C3, C4, and CH50 (if C4 is low, anti-C1q); pulmonary function tests; and chest x-ray.
- **Test for associated diseases**—serum antibodies for SLE and Sjögren syndrome, serum protein and immunofixation electrophoreses, cryoglobulins, hepatitis B and C and Epstein-Barr viral serologies, and *Borrelia* antibody tests.
- **Angioedema without wheals**—the types of angioedema can be differentiated with complement and, in some cases, genetic testing.

3.4. Treatment

- Initial treatment of new-onset urticaria should focus on short-term relief. Any life-threatening symptoms of airway obstruction from angioedema are considered a medical emergency and should be treated appropriately with subcutaneous epinephrine.
- A majority of urticaria is nonemergent, and two-thirds of new-onset urticaria will be self-limited and resolve spontaneously. Treatment with an antihistamine can help to address the short-term discomfort and prevent recurrent episodes of urticaria.
  - **H1 antihistamines**: Second-generation H1 antihistamines are preferred (cetirizine, loratadine, and fexofenadine). Older, first-generation H1 antihistamines

(diphenhydramine, chlorpheniramine, and hydroxyzine) are lipophilic and cross the blood-brain barrier, leading to more sedation when compared with second-generation H1 antihistamines.[24]

- **H2 antihistamines**: Some data suggest a synergistic effect with the combination of H1 antihistamines with H2 antihistamines (ranitidine, famotidine, cimetidine) in treating acute urticaria.[25] This combination is not currently the standard treatment for acute urticaria.

- **Chronic urticaria (CU)** may require additional treatment when it is refractory to antihistamines. Additionally, patients who require repeated courses of oral glucocorticoids are also candidates for additional therapies. In patients with autoinflammatory syndromes (i.e., Muckle-Wells, familial cold autoinflammatory syndrome, and neonatal-onset multisystem inflammatory disease), therapies will differ.
  - Omalizumab, a monoclonal antibody against immunoglobulin E (IgE), is safe and effective, but can be cost prohibitive for many patients. However, this medication is typically recommended over immunosuppressive (cyclosporine, tacrolimus, or methotrexate) treatments and other anti-inflammatory agents (dapsone, sulfasalazine, or hydroxychloroquine).[26,27]

4. VIRAL EXANTHEMS

- An exanthem is an acutely appearing rash that affects many locations on the skin simultaneously and may be associated with fever or other systemic symptoms (Table 5-1). Viral infection is the most common etiology for exanthems.
- The Greek word *exanthema* means "a breaking out."
- Enanthem is an eruption on the mucous membranes ("a breaking in").
- Various viruses cause common morbilliform eruptions. A morbilliform eruption is a group of macules and papules resembling a measles rash. With characteristic lesions and distinctive prodromes, the diagnosis can be easier. However, a nonspecific rash might lead to a less feasible diagnosis.[28]
- Common culprits of exanthem
  - **Varicella (aka chickenpox)**
  - **Measles** (aka 1st disease, rubeola)
  - **Rubella** (aka 3rd disease, German measles, 3-day measles)
  - **Erythema infectiosum** (fifth disease)—Parvovirus B19
  - **Roseola infantum (sixth disease)**—human herpesvirus (HHV)-6 and HHV-7
  - **Pityriasis rosea**—HHV-7
  - **Hand, foot, and mouth disease**—coxsackievirus A type 16, but also associated with other strains of coxsackievirus (A5, A7, A9, A10, B2, B5) and enterovirus 71

4.1. Background

- **Varicella**
  - Caused by the varicella zoster virus (VZV), a deoxyribonucleic acid (DNA) virus in the herpes family.
  - Vaccination for VZV was introduced in 1995. There has been a decline in primary varicella infection since that time.
  - Two doses of the vaccination are recommended for all individuals who are not already immune.[29]
  - Spread by airborne respiratory droplets or contact with blister fluid, the virus first colonizes the upper respiratory tract. Replication takes place in the regional

Table 5-1	Viral Exanthems			
Name	Etiology	Incubation	Presentation	Associations Treatment / Prevention
Measles, Rubeola, first disease	Paramyxovirus, measles virus	8–12 d	Prodrome: fever, irritability, malaise, coryza, conjunctivitis, and Koplik spots Morbilliform eruption that is cranial to caudal, starting at the hairline and involving the rest of the body by day 3	Cough, coryza, conjunctivitis Patients should be isolated for 4 d after the onset of eruption, and for the immunocompromised, for the entire duration of the disease. MMR (measles, mumps, rubella) vaccination
Rubella, German measles, third disease	Togavirus/ rubella virus	Spread by respiratory droplets 14–21 d	Mild exanthema in children, starts on face then generalizes Associated with cervical lymphadenopathy, Forchheimer spots	If contracted in the first trimester of pregnancy, fetus can have severe ocular, cardiac, and pulmonary abnormalities.
Erythema infectiosum, slapped cheek disease, fifth disease	Parvovirus B19	Spread by respiratory secretions, blood products, and vertical transmission 4–14-d incubation	Bright erythematous patches on cheeks; tends to avoid trunk, and can also present with purpuric papules on hands/feet of young adults (papular purpuric gloves and socks syndrome)	If infected during pregnancy, can lead to complications and aplastic crisis in those with sickle cell disease

Name	Etiology	Incubation	Presentation	Associations / Treatment / Prevention
Roseola infantum	HHV-6	Present in most individuals after 6 mo	9- to 12-mo-old infant, onset of high fever (40°C) lasting for 3 d Defervescence and appearance of morbilliform exanthema	Erythematous papules on mucosa of soft palate and uvula
Pityriasis rosea	HHV-6 and HHV-7 suspected		Begins with a salmon-colored "herald patch" Evolves into a generalized eruption after 1–2 wk with a duration of 6–8 wk Bilateral and symmetric macules with a collarette of scale along the cleavage lines	Self-resolving
Hand, foot, and mouth	Coxsackie A16	1 wk	Macular lesions→blisters, vesicles on buccal mucosa, tongue, hard palate Tender macules and vesicles on palms and soles	

lymph nodes over 2 to 4 days before the virus spreads to the liver and spleen. After 1 week, secondary viremia disseminates, producing the typical skin lesions.[30]
- Incubation period is 10 to 21 days.
- Systemic symptoms include fever, headache, upper respiratory symptoms, and gastrointestinal disturbance. Adults can experience prodromal symptoms for up to 2 days and can have more severe systemic complications (CNS infection/encephalitis, pneumonia, and hepatitis). There is a greater possibility of severe side effects with exposure during pregnancy for the affected mother and fetus.

- **Measles**
  - Caused by the measles virus, a single-stranded, negative-sense enveloped ribonucleic acid (RNA) virus in the Paramyxoviridae family.
  - Spreads by respiratory droplets and is highly contagious.
  - Most common in children ages 3 to 5 years old.
  - Children/adolescents who were never vaccinated are highly susceptible; common in developing countries.
  - Presents in late winter/spring.

- **Rubella**
  - School-age children, adolescents, and young adults.
  - Outbreaks occur most frequently in late winter and early spring.
  - Spreads through direct or droplet contact from nasopharyngeal secretions.
  - Noncongenital rubella can be subclinical, and incidence has decreased with vaccination.

- **Erythema infectiosum**
  - Erythema infectiosum is only one of the clinical presentations of Parvovirus B19, ranging from asymptomatic and benign to life threatening.
  - Most common in children 4 to 10 years old, but can affect all ages.
  - Outbreaks late winter to early spring.
  - Increasing prevalence of antibodies with age (50% of young adults and 90% of elderly population).
  - Transmission via contact with respiratory tract secretions, percutaneous exposure to blood or blood products, and vertical transmission from mother to fetus.
  - Incubation period from exposure to onset of rash, usually between 1 and 2 weeks.
  - Individuals are most infectious prior to the onset of rash.

- **Roseola infantum (sixth disease, exanthem subitum)**
  - Has a multivirus etiology and is most commonly caused by the human herpesvirus (HHV)-6 and less commonly by HHV-7.[31,32]
  - Called roseola infantum because it affects infant and older babies and is the most common exanthema before age 2.
  - The infection results in immunity, and there is no vaccination for roseola.
  - Seroprevalence of HHV-6 in the adult population is 95%.

- **Pityriasis rosea**
  - Most common in children and young adults.
  - Most cases occur in the spring.
  - Acute self-limiting eruption of fine scaling lesions.
  - Duration of 6 to 8 weeks.
  - Usually begins with a single, larger, "herald patch," which is seen in 50% to 90% of cases a week or more before the numerous smaller lesions, which are distributed in a "Christmas tree"-like pattern.

- Recurrence of pityriasis rosea (PR) is rare, and the disease is not considered transmissible.
- During pregnancy, it can be associated with miscarriage during the first 15 weeks, or premature delivery.[33]
- A viral etiology is suggested, particularly for HHV-6 and HHV-7, but has not been confirmatory.[34,35]
- **Hand, foot, and mouth disease**
  - Sore mouth, malaise, and fever.
  - Macular lesions on buccal mucosa, tongue, and hard palate, which develop into vesicles that erode and have an erythematous halo.
  - Uncommonly, patient may develop an aseptic meningitis. This is more likely with enterovirus-71.

4.2. Clinical Presentation

- **Varicella (chickenpox; see Chapter 4, Fig. 4-7A)**
  - Pruritic and erythematous eruption that develops into small blisters on the torso, face, scalp, axilla, and extremities and with an enanthem in the oral mucosa.
  - Systemic symptoms present with the rash, including fever, decreased appetite, arthralgia, myalgias, and URI symptoms.
  - Individuals are infectious 1 to 2 days prior to the appearance of the rash and until the blisters have dried and become scabs. Though blisters usually dry and become scabs within 4 to 5 days, there are typically several crops of blisters in different stages of healing, so infected individuals should stay home and away from others until ALL blisters have crusted over.
- **Measles (1st disease; see Fig. 5-5)**
  - Incubation period—8 to 12 days from exposure to onset of symptoms.
  - Contagious for 3 to 5 days prior to rash onset and 4 days after the appearance of rash.
  - **Prodrome**—fever, malaise, conjunctivitis, cough, coryza (head cold with nasal congestion, rhinorrhea sore throat), Koplik spots (enanthem that consists of punctate blue-white lesions with an erythematous rim on the buccal mucosa that manifests 2 to 3 days before full body rash).
  - **Exanthem**—erythematous macules and papules that start on the face and spread cranial to caudal. Also move centrifugally, starting centrally and moving outward to cover the entire body in 2 to 3 days.
  - **Recovery**—constitutional symptoms begin to improve 2 days after the rash presents, with rash progressively improving and lasting about a week.
  - **Complications**—otitis media, pneumonia (most common fatal complication in children and most common overall in adults), laryngotracheobronchitis (croup), and diarrhea.
- **Rubella**
  - **Prodrome**—low-grade fever, headache, sore throat, conjunctivitis, rhinorrhea, cough, and lymphadenopathy, occasionally with arthritis.
  - **Exanthem**—pruritic pink to red macules and papules that start on the face and then spread to trunk and extremities within 24 hours. Within 2 to 3 days, the rash clears, starting at the head and neck first.
  - **Enanthem**—petechial lesions on the soft palate and uvula (Forchheimer sign).
  - **Complications**—encephalitis, thrombocytopenia, peripheral neuritis, optic neuritis, myocarditis, pericarditis, hepatitis, orchitis, and hemolytic anemia.

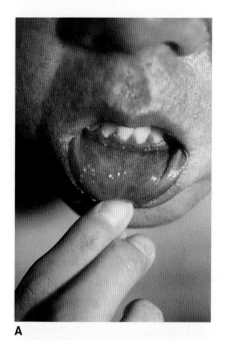

A

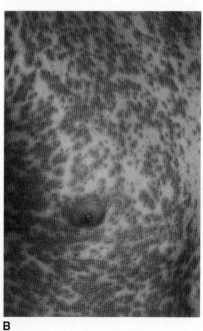

B

Figure 5-5. A,B: Measles. (From Mallory SB, Bree A, Chern P. *Illustrated Manual of Pediatric Dermatology.* New York: Taylor and Francis Publishing; 2005.)

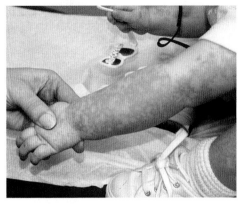

Figure 5-6. Erythema infectiosum.

- **Erythema infectiosum (fifth disease); see Figure 5-6**
  - Caused by Parvovirus B19
  - Can lead to serious complications in pregnancy (hydrops fetalis and fetal death) and aplastic crisis in patients with sickle cell disease
  - **Prodrome**—low-grade fever, malaise, headache, pruritus, coryza, myalgias, and joint pain
  - **Exanthem**—bright red cheeks (slapped cheeks), and, as the facial rash fades over 1 to 4 days, a symmetric, erythematous, reticular (lace-like) rash appears on the torso and extremities, lasting 5 to 9 days
- **Papular purpuric gloves and socks syndrome**
  - ○ Caused by parvovirus B19.
  - ○ Painful, pruritic papules, petechiae, and purpura of hands and feet.
  - ○ Also presents with enanthem (oral erosions).
  - ○ Patients with the rash are viremic and contagious.
- **Roseola infantum**
  - **HHV-6 infection in children**—(a) subclinical infection, (b) acute febrile illness without rash, and (c) sudden rash/exanthema subitum.
  - **Prodrome**—high fever (39°C to 40°C), palpebral edema, cervical lymphadenopathy, and mild upper respiratory tract symptoms. As fever subsides, exanthem appears.
  - **Exanthem**—macules and papules with a surrounding white halo, beginning on the trunk and spreading to the neck and proximal extremities.
- **Pityriasis Rosea**
  - Initially a pink patch develops and expands becoming well-demarcated with a collarette of scale, known as the herald patch typically on the back though can be anywhere on the body.
  - A generalized eruption develops over 1 to 2 weeks on lines of tension in a symmetric distribution on neck, torso and extremities sparing face, hands, and feet know as the "Christmas tree" pattern lasting approximately 2 months.
  - Atypical variants are seen as well (inverse PR, non-symmetric distribution, etc.).
- **Hand, Foot, Mouth Disease**
  - Prodrome for 1 to 3 days including low-grade fever, anorexia, malaise, cough, sore throat, abdominal pain.
  - Enanthem can precede the exanthem.

- Oral lesions begin as red macules evolving into blisters that can be painful and tender.
- Skin findings are located on the hands, feet, and buttock as red macules that develop central grey vesicles.
- Unlike oral lesions, cutaneous lesions are typically asymptomatic.

4.3. Evaluation

- Diagnosis relies on clinical findings, viral cultures, or serologic cultures.
- **Varicella**
  - Diagnosis suspected based on history and physical exam.
  - Tzanck smear (scraping of base of vesicle for H&E staining) shows multinucleated giant cells and epithelial cells with eosinophilic intranuclear inclusion bodies.
  - A vesicular fluid culture can be helpful, but is positive <40% of the time.
  - DIF serologic testing, VZV PCR, and VZV serology to determine evidence of immunity, with the latex agglutination test being the most popular serologic assay for determining immunity and exposure.
- **Measles**
  - Diagnosis is suspected from presence of high fever, Koplik spots, conjunctivitis, upper respiratory tract infectious symptoms, and typical exanthem.
  - If suspected, serologically confirm with antimeasles IgM and IgG, isolation of measles virus, or identification of measles RNA.
  - Report immediately to local or state health department without waiting for diagnostic test results.
- **Rubella**
  - Suspected from clinical exam
  - Diagnosis confirmed with serology: rubella-specific IgM antibody or a fourfold rise in antibody titer in acute and convalescent-phase serum
- **Erythema infectiosum**
  - Detection of serum parvovirus B19–specific IgM antibody indicates that infection has likely occurred within the previous 2 to 4 months.

4.4. Treatment

- **Varicella**
  - Vaccination is available and was approved by the U.S. Food and Drug Administration in 1995 for prophylactic use in healthy children and adults: 1 dose for children 12 to 18 months and 2 doses in a 4- to 8-week interval in those over 13 years.[36]
  - Treatment for a healthy child is supportive, while an adult or an immunocompromised individual typically requires systemic therapy.[37]
  - **Supportive care for a healthy child (<12 years)**
    - Acetaminophen for fever.
    - Do not give aspirin as this can lead to Reye syndrome (fatal multiorgan failure, specifically brain and liver).
    - Calamine lotion to relieve pruritus.
    - Antiviral treatment, acyclovir, for severe cases.
    - Cool oatmeal baths.
    - Rest and hydration.
    - Keep nails short to prevent excessive itching, which can lead to scarring and bacterial superinfection.
  - Complications linked to VZV infection include secondary bacterial infection, pneumonia, encephalitis, cerebellar ataxia, transverse myelitis, and Reye syndrome.
  - The virus remains dormant in nerves and can reactivate as herpes zoster (shingles).

- *Treatment in immunocompetent adults*
  - ○ Since individuals >12 years are likely to have more severe reactions, oral acyclovir, 800 mg 5 times daily for 1 week, has been shown to decrease the duration of lesions, if started within 24 hours of the appearance of symptoms.
- *Treatment in immunocompromised individuals*
  - ○ IV acyclovir therapy is indicated in these patients because of the possible life-threatening complications.
  - ○ Foscarnet can be used in individuals with acyclovir-resistant VZV.
- **Measles**
  - Uncomplicated measles is self-limiting, lasting 10 to 12 days.
  - In majority of cases, treatment is supportive.
  - Malnutrition, immunosuppression, and lack of substantial supportive care worsen prognosis.
  - Vitamin A supplementation has been shown to benefit measles.
- **Rubella**
  - Report suspected cases to the local health department.
  - Droplet precautions and minimal to no contact (especially school/daycare) for 1 week AFTER the onset of rash.
- **Erythema infectiosum (fifth disease)**
  - No specific treatment for uncomplicated Parvovirus B19 infection and supportive therapy for fatigue, malaise, pruritus, and arthralgias
  - Typically resolves within 5 to 10 days, but can last for months depending on environmental exposures

5. DRUG ERUPTIONS

- Adverse drug reactions can commonly present with cutaneous manifestations, and determining the cause of a drug eruption depends on the chronicity of the offending agent and the clinical manifestations. Below is the list of some of the most commonly encountered drug eruptions that will be reviewed in this section.
  - Exanthematous eruption
  - Urticaria, angioedema, anaphylaxis
  - Photosensitivity
  - Fixed drug eruption
  - Acute generalized exanthematous pustulosis (AGEP)
  - Drug-induced hypersensitivity syndrome (DIHS), also referred to as drug reaction with eosinophilia and systemic symptoms (DRESS)
  - Anticoagulant-induced skin necrosis
  - Reactions to chemotherapy
  - Stevens-Johnson syndrome (SJS)
  - Toxic epidermal necrolysis (TEN)
- DIHS, AGEP, SJS and TEN include some of the more severe drug reaction. Though rare, these are associated with the greatest morbidity and mortality.

5.1. Background

- Skin is one of the most common targets for adverse drug eruptions, and antibiotic and anticonvulsants are reported to produce adverse events in 1% to 5% of patients.
- Women, the elderly, and those who are immunosuppressed from human immunodeficiency virus have a greater risk of developing adverse drug reactions.
  - Those with a CD4+ <200 have a 10- to 50-fold greater chance of developing an adverse eruption compared to the general population.

5.2. Clinical Presentation

- **Exanthematous eruption or morbilliform drug eruptions**
  - Most common adverse drug reaction affecting the skin; very commonly seen in hospitalized patients.
  - Classically begins 7 to 14 days after the start of a new medication, but can also occur earlier, or even after the drug is discontinued.
  - Begin as erythematous macules that evolve into confluent papules on the trunk and upper extremities; face, palms, soles, and mucous membranes are typically spared. The eruption resolves without sequelae in 1 to 2 weeks.
  - Commonly associated drugs: aminopenicillins, sulfonamides, cephalosporins, and anticonvulsants.
- **Urticaria and angioedema**
  - Urticaria presents with transient, pruritic, edematous, and erythematous plaques. Lesions may appear anywhere on the body and typically last several hours, unlike urticarial vasculitis, which lasts more than 24 hours and can leave hyperpigmentation at the lesion site.
  - Drugs are responsible for fewer than 10% of cases.
  - Medications may cause an immunologically based urticaria, especially antibiotics (most commonly penicillins or cephalosporins) and monoclonal antibodies used in treatment for neoplastic or inflammatory diseases.
  - Angioedema is a transient edema of the deep subcutaneous and submucosal tissue, and about 50% of cases are associated with urticaria. New users of angiotensin-converting enzyme (ACE) can experience angioedema, at a rate of 1 to 2 per 1,000.
  - Angioedema presents with acute subcutaneous swelling of the face (eyelids, lips, ears, nose), and buccal mucosa and tongue may also occur. Edema of the larynx, epiglottis, and surrounding tissue may lead to impaired swallowing and upper airway obstruction.
  - Drugs implicated in angioedema: penicillins, ACE inhibitors, NSAIDs, radiographic contrast media, and monoclonal antibodies.
  - About 1 in 5,000 exposures to penicillin can progress to anaphylaxis.
- **Photosensitivity**
  - The combination of light and drug can lead to several forms of cutaneous inflammation. Photosensitivity is typically divided into two major types: phototoxic (more common) and photoallergic.
  - A phototoxic drug eruption presents as an exaggerated sunburn and occurs in a short exposure time. The area will heal with hyperpigmentation.
  - Common offenders include tetracyclines (doxycycline), the NSAIDs, and fluoroquinolones. Additionally, amiodarone, psoralens, and phenothiazines can also lead to phototoxic eruptions.
  - Photoallergic drug eruptions are more chronic and pruritic than phototoxic drug eruptions. Lesions clinically may resemble dermatitis or lichen planus. The offending agent should be immediately removed to prevent long-term sequelae.
  - Common offenders include thiazide diuretics, sulfonamide antibiotics, and sulfonylureas. Additionally, quinine, quinidine, tricyclic antidepressants, and antimalarials are also culprits in photoallergic reactions.
- **Fixed drug eruption (Fig. 5-7)**
  - Eruptions develop 1 to 2 weeks after first exposure and within 24 hours of subsequent exposures.
  - Clinically, these present as one or a few round sharply demarcated erythematous and edematous plaques with a violaceous hue, dusky color, central blister or a detached epidermis.

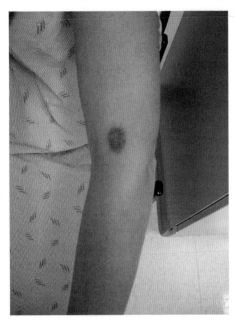

Figure 5-7. Fixed drug eruption.

- Favored locations include the lips, hands, feet, and genitalia, but can occur anywhere, and a reexposure to the offending agent leads to lesions *recurring at exactly the same location as previously affected sites,* hence the name "fixed drug." Additional sites may subsequently develop.
- Commonly associated drugs: sulfonamides, NSAIDs, barbiturates, tetracyclines, and carbamazepines.
- **Acute generalized exanthematous pustulosis (AGEP, Fig. 5-8)**
  - Characterized by multiple, nonfollicular sterile pustules, <5 mm in size, overlying areas of edematous erythema.

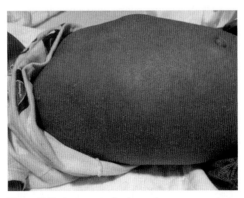

Figure 5-8. Acute generalized exanthematous pustulosis.

- The patient presents with a high fever that typically begins the same day as the pustular eruption, but may present a few days prior. The eruption begins on the face, axilla, and groin and then disseminates over the course of a few hours.
- The rash may also present with edema of face and hands, vesicles, bullae, and purpura and can involve mucous membranes.
- The main differential for AGEP is pustular psoriasis. A history can distinguish the two entities, with acute onset of the rash and use of a causative drug more consistent with AGEP. Additionally, skin biopsy findings are more likely to show dermal edema, keratinocyte necrosis, and exocytosis of eosinophils in AGEP versus acanthosis in pustular psoriasis.
- The time frame between drug administration and skin eruption is short, typically <2 days, and the rash lasts 1 to 2 weeks.
- Antibiotics are primarily indicated in AGEP, particularly beta-lactams (penicillins, aminopenicillins, cephalosporins) and macrolides. Other common culprits are calcium channel blockers (diltiazem) and antimalarials. Although less common, other drugs have been implicated.
- **Drug rash with eosinophilia and systemic symptoms (DRESS)**
  - **Can also be referred to as drug-induced hypersensitivity syndrome (DIHS).**
  - Develops 2 to 6 weeks after exposure to the drug.
  - Skin involvement begins as a morbilliform eruption, which later becomes edematous with follicular accentuation.
  - Symptoms last even after discontinuation of the medication, typically up to 2 weeks.
  - Systemic symptoms include fever >38°C, absolute eosinophilia >1,500, multi-organ involvement, lymphocyte activation (lymphocytosis, atypical lymphocytes, lymphadenopathy), and viral reactivation (predominately HHV-6, but also cytomegalovirus, Epstein-Barr virus, and HHV-7).
  - Edema affecting the face or upper extremities is a characteristic finding.
  - Lymphadenopathy and arthralgias.
  - Severe liver involvement can occur, and this finding is associated with 10% of deaths in DIHS/DRESS.[38]
  - Potential acute visceral complications of DIHS/DRESS include colitis, encephalitis, aseptic meningitis, interstitial nephritis, interstitial pneumonitis, sialadenitis, and myocarditis.
  - Potential delayed complications of DIHS/DRESS include syndrome of inappropriate secretion of antidiuretic hormone (SIADH), thyroiditis, diabetes mellitus, myocarditis, and rarely systemic lupus. Monitoring for these sequelae should occur during and for months after withdrawal of the offending agent.[39]
  - The most common drug culprits include aromatic anticonvulsants (phenobarbital, carbamazepine, and phenytoin), lamotrigine (especially when coadministered with valproate), and sulfonamides.[40,41]
  - Minocycline, allopurinol (especially in those with renal failure and HLA-5801), gold salts, dapsone, and abacavir (used to treat HIV) can also lead to DIHS/DRESS.
  - Defects in drug metabolism (as in the detoxification of anticonvulsants and sulfonamides) have been seen in patients with DRESS. Immune mechanisms and the role of viral reactivation (HHV-6 and HHV-7) have also been implicated.
- **Anticoagulant-induced skin necrosis**
  - Warfarin necrosis begins 2 to 5 days after therapy and coincides with the expected drop in protein C function.
  - Presents with erythematous, painful plaques that develop into hemorrhagic blisters and necrotic ulcers due to occlusive thrombi in the skin and subcutaneous tissues.

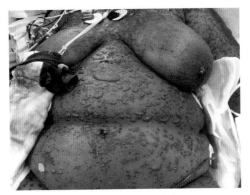

Figure 5-9. Toxic epidermal necrolysis. (Courtesy of Amy Musiek, MD.)

- Most commonly affected areas include breasts, thighs, and buttock.
- Patients with protein C deficiency are at higher risk of developing warfarin necrosis.
- Heparin-induced cutaneous necrosis is due to antibodies that bind to complexes of heparin and platelet factor 4, leading to platelet aggregation and consumption, which cause thrombosis and cutaneous necrosis at site of injection and distant locations.
- **Stevens-Johnson syndrome (SJS)/ toxic epidermal necrolysis (TEN) (Fig. 5-9)**
  - Rare, life-threatening, acute mucocutaneous diseases.
  - Keratinocyte cell death results in separation of significant areas of skin at the dermal-epidermal junction (denudation) and also affects the mucous membranes.
  - SJS—skin detachment is <10% body surface area (BSA), and SJS-TEN overlap 10% to 30% BSA, TEN >30% BSA.
  - Initial symptoms can include fever, stinging eyes, and pain upon swallowing. These can occur 1 to 3 days prior to the onset of skin findings.
  - Skin findings will present initially on the trunk before spreading to the neck, face, and extremities, with palms and soles involved though distal arms are spared. Oral, ocular, and genital mucosal involvement occurs in most patients, and 25% of TEN patients have respiratory tract involvement.
  - The skin lesions are usually tender and the mucosal erosions are painful. First, the skin lesions appear as erythematous, dusky, red, or purpuric macules of irregular size and shape. The addition of mucosal involvement, as well as tenderness, suggests progression to SJS and TEN.
  - The Nikolsky sign—tangential mechanical pressure with a finger on erythematous zones, which leads to detachment of the epidermis and confirms diagnosis.
  - Asboe-Hansen sign—placing pressure adjacent to the blister extends it laterally. Denudation or loss of the epidermal layer leaves a wet and bright red erosion.
  - Pathology findings are similar between erythema multiforme and SJS/TEN, so clinical characteristics are what helps to distinguish the two.
  - Medications most commonly associated with SJS/TEN: allopurinol, aminopenicillins, antiretroviral drugs, barbiturates, carbamazepine, chlormezanone, phenytoin antiepileptics, lamotrigine, phenylbutazone, piroxicam, sulfadiazine, sulfasalazine, and trimethoprim-sulfamethoxazole (see Table 5-2).[42,43]

- Occurs within 7 to 21 days after first exposure of the causative agent, but can occur within 2 days after reexposure.

5.3. Evaluation

- Begin with obtaining a list of all the medications a patient is taking: prescription, nonprescription, and alternative medications. Note the dates of drug administration and the doses.
- Identify the time between initiation of the drug and onset of drug eruption (Table 5-2) (AGEP has a shorter time of onset vs. DIHS).
- The SCORTEN scale is a TEN severity grading system that can help to predict mortality.[44]
  - SCORTEN—age >40 years, heart rate >120 beats per minute, malignancy, BSA on day 1 above 10%, serum urea level (>10 mmol/L), serum bicarbonate level (<20 mmol/L), and serum glucose level (>14 mmol/L). Each prognostic factor is a point, and 0 to 1 point portends a 3.2% mortality rate, whereas ≥5 portends a 90% mortality rate.

Table 5-2	Drug Eruptions	
Name of drug eruption	**Onset from medication exposure**	**Responsible medications**
Exanthematous eruption	4–14 d	Aminopenicillins Sulfonamides Cephalosporins Anticonvulsants Allopurinol
Urticaria Anaphylaxis	Minutes to hours	Penicillins Cephalosporins NSAIDs Monoclonal antibodies Contrast media
Fixed drug eruption	First exposure: 1–2 wk Reexposure: <48 h, usually 24 h	TMP-SMX NSAIDs Tetracyclines Pseudoephedrine
Acute generalized exanthematous pustulosis (AGEP)	<4 d	B-lactam antibiotics Macrolides Calcium channel blockers
Drug-induced hypersensitivity syndrome (DRESS)	15–40 d	Anticonvulsants Sulfonamides Allopurinol Minocycline Lamotrigine
Stevens-Johnson syndrome (SJS) Toxic epidermal necrolysis (TEN)	7–21 d	Sulfonamides Anticonvulsants NSAIDs Allopurinol

5.4. Treatment

- Depends on the severity of eruption
  - Discontinuation of inciting medication in severe eruptions—AGEP, DIHS, SJS, and TEN.
  - DRESS—systemic steroids are needed, and patients must avoid medications that cross-react. This is particularly important for aromatic anticonvulsants (phenytoin, carbamazepine, phenobarbitone).
  - AGEP—topical or systemic steroids.
  - SJS/TEN—wound care, electrolyte balance, steroids, and IVIG.
  - Photosensitizing eruptions—can continue treatment in phototoxic drug eruptions, but avoid UVR exposure, encourage photoprotection.

REFERENCES

1. Deguchi E, Imafuku S, Nakayama J. Ulcerating stasis dermatitis of the forearm due to arteriovenous fistula: a case report and review of the published work. *J Dermatol* 2010;37(6):550–553.
2. Beebe-Dimmer JL, Pfeifer JR, Engle JS, et al. The epidemiology of chronic venous insufficiency and varicose veins. *Ann Epidemiol* 2005;15(3):175–184.
3. Barron GS, Jacob SE, Kirsner RS. Dermatologic complications of chronic venous disease: medical management and beyond. *Ann Vasc Surg* 2007;21(5):652–662.
4. Keller EC, Tomecki KJ, Alraies MC. Distinguishing cellulitis from its mimics. *Cleve Clin J Med* 2012;79(8):547–552.
5. David CV, Chira S, Eells SJ, et al. Diagnostic accuracy in patients admitted to hospitals with cellulitis. *Dermatol Online J* 2011;17(3):1.
6. Partsch H. Compression therapy: clinical and experimental evidence. *Ann Vasc Dis* 2012;5(4):416–422.
7. Word R. Medical and surgical therapy for advanced chronic venous insufficiency. *Surg Clin North Am* 2010;90(6):1195–1214.
8. Gonzalez-Gay MA, Garcia-Porrua C, Pujol RM. Clinical approach to cutaneous vasculitis. *Curr Opin Rheumatol* 2005;17(1):56–61.
9. Jennette JC, Falk RJ. The role of pathology in the diagnosis of systemic vasculitis. *Clin Exp Rheumatol* 2007;25(1 suppl 44):S52–S56.
10. Jennette JC, Falk RJ, Bacon PA, et al. 2012 revised International Chapel Hill Consensus Conference Nomenclature of Vasculitides. *Arthritis Rheum* 2013;65(1):1–11.
11. Carlson JA, Ng BT, Chen K-R. Cutaneous vasculitis update: diagnostic criteria, classification, epidemiology, etiology, pathogenesis, evaluation and prognosis. *Am J Dermatopathol* 2005;27(6):504–528.
12. Xu LY, Esparza EM, Anadkat MJ, et al. Cutaneous manifestations of vasculitis. *Semin Arthritis Rheum* 2009;38(5):348–360.
13. Chen K-R, Carlson JA. Clinical approach to cutaneous vasculitis. *Am J Clin Dermatol* 2008;9(2):71–92.
14. Chung C, Tumeh PC, Birnbaum R, et al. Characteristic purpura of the ears, vasculitis, and neutropenia—a potential public health epidemic associated with levamisole-adulterated cocaine. *J Am Acad Dermatol* 2011;65(4):722–725.
15. Hoffman GS, Calabrese LH. Vasculitis: determinants of disease patterns. *Nat Rev Rheumatol* 2014;10(8):454–462.
16. Marzano AV, Vezzoli P, Berti E. Skin involvement in cutaneous and systemic vasculitis. *Autoimmun Rev* 2013;12(4):467–476.
17. Beltrani VS. Urticaria and angioedema. *Dermatol Clin* 1996;14(1):171–198.
18. Williams KW, Sharma HP. Anaphylaxis and urticaria. *Immunol Allergy Clin North Am* 2015;35(1):199–219.
19. Kaplan AP, Greaves M. Pathogenesis of chronic urticaria. *Clin Exp Allergy* 2009;39(6):777–787.

20. Sackesen C, Sekerel BE, Orhan F, et al. The etiology of different forms of urticaria in childhood. *Pediatr Dermatol* 2004;21(2):102–108.

21. Federman DG, Kirsner RS, Moriarty JP, et al. The effect of antibiotic therapy for patients infected with *Helicobacter pylori* who have chronic urticaria. *J Am Acad Dermatol* 2003;49(5):861–864.

22. Zuberbier T. A Summary of the New International EAACI/GA2LEN/EDF/WAO Guidelines in Urticaria. *World Allergy Organ J* 2012;5(suppl 1):S1–S5.

23. Joint Task Force on Practice Parameters. The diagnosis and management of urticaria: a practice parameter part I: acute urticaria/angioedema part II: chronic urticaria/angioedema. Joint Task Force on Practice Parameters. *Ann Allergy Asthma Immunol* 2000;85(6 Pt 2): 521–544.

24. Zuberbier T, Asero R, Bindslev-Jensen C, et al. EAACI/GA(2)LEN/EDF/WAO guideline: management of urticaria. *Allergy* 2009;64(10):1427–1443.

25. Fedorowicz Z, van Zuuren EJ, Hu N. Histamine H2-receptor antagonists for urticaria. *Cochrane Database Syst Rev* 2012;(3):CD008596.

26. Romano C, Sellitto A, De Fanis U, et al. Maintenance of remission with low-dose omalizumab in long-lasting, refractory chronic urticaria. *Ann Allergy Asthma Immunol* 2010;104(1):95–97.

27. Kaplan A, Ledford D, Ashby M, et al. Omalizumab in patients with symptomatic chronic idiopathic/spontaneous urticaria despite standard combination therapy. *J Allergy Clin Immunol* 2013;132(1):101–109.

28. Biesbroeck L, Sidbury R. Viral exanthems: an update. *Dermatol Ther* 2013;26(6):433–438.

29. Magel GD, Mendoza N, Digiorgio CM, et al. Vaccines in dermatological diseases. *G Ital Dermatol Venereol* 2011;146(3):225–233.

30. Heininger U, Seward JF. Varicella. *Lancet* 2006;368(9544):1365–1376.

31. Stone RC, Micali GA, Schwartz RA. Roseola infantum and its causal human herpesviruses. *Int J Dermatol* 2014;53(4):397–403.

32. Yamanishi K, Okuno T, Shiraki K, et al. Identification of human herpesvirus-6 as a causal agent for exanthem subitum. *Lancet* 1988;1(8594):1065–1067.

33. Drago F, Broccolo F, Javor S, et al. Evidence of human herpesvirus-6 and –7 reactivation in miscarrying women with pityriasis rosea. *J Am Acad Dermatol* 2014;71(1):198–199.

34. Drago F, Broccolo F, Rebora A. Pityriasis rosea: an update with a critical appraisal of its possible herpesviral etiology. *J Am Acad Dermatol* 2009;61(2):303–318.

35. Wolz MM, Sciallis GF, Pittelkow MR. Human herpesviruses 6, 7, and 8 from a dermatologic perspective. *Mayo Clin Proc* 2012;87(10):1004–1014.

36. Andrei G, Snoeck R. Advances in the treatment of varicella-zoster virus infections. *Adv Pharmacol* 2013;67:107–168.

37. Gershon AA, Gershon MD. Pathogenesis and current approaches to control of varicella-zoster virus infections. *Clin Microbiol Rev* 2013;26(4):728–743.

38. Lee T, Lee YS, Yoon S-Y, et al. Characteristics of liver injury in drug-induced systemic hypersensitivity reactions. *J Am Acad Dermatol* 2013;69(3):407–415.

39. Ushigome Y, Kano Y, Ishida T, et al. Short- and long-term outcomes of 34 patients with drug-induced hypersensitivity syndrome in a single institution. *J Am Acad Dermatol* 2013;68(5):721–728.

40. Husain Z, Reddy BY, Schwartz RA. DRESS syndrome: part I. Clinical perspectives. *J Am Acad Dermatol* 2013;68(5):693.e1–693.e14; quiz 706–708.

41. Husain Z, Reddy BY, Schwartz RA. DRESS syndrome: part II. Management and therapeutics. *J Am Acad Dermatol.* 2013;68(5):709.e1–709.e9; quiz 718–720.

42. Schwartz RA, McDonough PH, Lee BW. Toxic epidermal necrolysis: part I. Introduction, history, classification, clinical features, systemic manifestations, etiology, and immunopathogenesis. *J Am Acad Dermatol* 2013;69(2):173.e1–173.e13; quiz 185–186.

43. Schwartz RA, McDonough PH, Lee BW. Toxic epidermal necrolysis: part II. Prognosis, sequelae, diagnosis, differential diagnosis, prevention, and treatment. *J Am Acad Dermatol* 2013;69(2):187.e1–187.e16; quiz 203–204.

44. Bastuji-Garin S, Fouchard N, Bertocchi M, et al. SCORTEN: a severity-of-illness score for toxic epidermal necrolysis. *J Invest Dermatol* 2000;115(2):149–153.

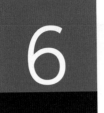

6 Disorders of Pigmentation

Shaanan Shetty, MD and Caroline Mann, MD

Disorders of pigmentation can manifest as light or dark areas of the skin or as hyperpigmentation or depigmentation of the entire skin surface. Although not typically harmful, these changes can have significant psychosocial impact on affected patients.

1. VITILIGO

- Vitiligo is an acquired condition characterized by areas of depigmentation due to loss of melanocytes.

1.1. Background

- Epidemiology
  - Can occur at any age but most commonly occurs during second and third decade
  - Prevalence estimated to be 0.5% to 2% overall and equal in men and women[1,2]
- Pathogenesis
  - There are likely multiple pathogenic mechanisms, which all lead to the loss of melanocytes. The autoimmune destruction of melanocytes is the mechanism that has the most supporting evidence.
  - Other hypotheses include defects in melanocyte adhesiveness, deficiency in factors needed for melanocyte survival, and defective melanocyte defense against oxidative stress.

1.2. Clinical Presentation

- Clinical Features
  - Completely depigmented macules and patches with well-defined, convex borders (Fig. 6-1).
  - Can be subtle in light-skinned individuals and is accentuated or becomes initially apparent with tanning.
  - Often occur in areas of trauma (Koebner phenomenon).
  - Common locations include perioral skin, periocular skin, elbows, knees, digits, and flexor wrists.
  - Loss of pigment in hairs within areas of vitiligo can occur as well (leukotrichia).
- Classification
  - Three main types: localized, generalized, and universal.
  - The most common type is generalized, and the most common subtype is vulgaris.
    - Localized
      - Focal—single area of involvement without a segmental distribution
      - Segmental—unilateral and involving one segment of the body. Often has abrupt midline demarcation. Most commonly seen in a trigeminal dermatome
      - Mucosal

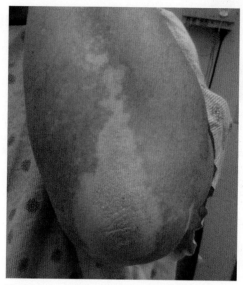

Figure 6-1. Depigmented patch on the elbow.

- ○ Generalized
    - – Vulgaris—scattered and widely distributed patches
    - – Acrofacial—involving distal extremities and face
    - – Mixed—combinations of segmental, acrofacial, and vulgaris subtypes
  - ○ Universal—involvement of >80% body surface area
- Variants
  - Blue vitiligo—vitiligo that develops in areas with postinflammatory hyperpigmentation. The presence of dermal melanin gives lesions a blue-gray appearance.
  - Inflammatory vitiligo—lesions have erythematous raised borders.
  - Trichrome vitiligo—an intermediate hypopigmented zone is present between normal skin and depigmented skin.
  - Vitiligo ponctué—small discrete macules that can occur within normal or hyperpigmented skin.
- Course
  - Course varies significantly between individuals—slow progression is most common.
  - Without treatment, complete repigmentation is rare. Some degree of repigmentation can occur spontaneously or with sun exposure.

1.3. Evaluation

- Diagnosis
  - Can usually be made based on physical exam and history alone.
  - A Wood's lamp can help in evaluating extent of involvement.
  - Biopsy may be useful in less obvious cases.
- Associated disorders
  - Associated with higher frequency of other autoimmune disorders, most frequently autoimmune thyroiditis (Hashimoto thyroiditis in particular)[3]

1.4. Treatment

- Younger patients and patients with dark skin are most likely to respond to treatment.
- The face, neck, and trunk are generally the most responsive areas, while the distal extremities and lips are often the least responsive.
- Repigmentation tends to spread from the hair follicle or the periphery of lesions.
- Corticosteroids
  - Topical corticosteroids are often used as first-line therapy.
  - They are most useful for localized areas of involvement.
  - Side effects can be minimized by not using them continuously.
  - More effective when combined with phototherapy.
  - Systemic steroids may stop rapidly spreading vitiligo and induce repigmentation. Their role in treatment is unclear given their side effects.
- Topical calcineurin inhibitors
  - Efficacy similar or slightly less than corticosteroids
  - More effective when combined with phototherapy
- Phototherapy
  - Generally useful for more extensive cases. Administered 2× to 3×/week and may require 6 months to 2 years of treatment.
  - Narrowband UVB
    - Often first-line therapy for generalized vitiligo.
    - Compared to PUVA, NBUVB has shorter treatment times, no GI side effects, less phototoxic reactions, and no need for posttreatment photoprotection.
  - Psoralen plus ultraviolet light therapy (PUVA)
    - Increased risk for melanoma and nonmelanoma skin cancers. Should limit to 1,000 J/cm^2 or 200 to 300 treatments total
  - Excimer laser or lamp
    - Wavelength is close to NBUVB.
    - Allows treatment of targeted areas.
    - May be more effective than NBUVB.[4]
- Surgical Therapies
  - Should be considered in patients with stable lesions that have been unresponsive to other treatments.
  - If vitiligo occurs in areas of trauma (koebnerization), surgical therapy may actually worsen vitiligo.
  - Blister grafting and punch grafting are techniques where the patient's own tissue is transferred from uninvolved to involved sites.
  - Autologous melanocyte suspension transplant is a technique where melanocytes with or without keratinocytes are harvested from uninvolved sites and transferred to involved sites.
- Depigmentation
  - 20% monobenzyl ether of hydroquinone (MBEH) can be useful for patients with widespread involvement and few uninvolved sites.
  - Loss of pigmentation can occur at sites other than those that are treated.
  - Depigmentation is usually permanent though repigmentation can sometimes occur with sun exposure.
- Camouflage
  - May be helpful in providing temporary or long-term relief.
  - Options include makeup, self-tanning agents, and tattoos.

2. MELASMA

- Characterized by hyperpigmented macules and patches with irregular borders most commonly on the face.
- Primarily affects young to middle-aged women with darker skin types.
- Exacerbating factors include pregnancy, oral contraceptive pills, and sunlight.

2.1. Background

- Epidemiology
  - Most common in darker skin types including individuals of African, Asian, and Hispanic descent
  - More common in women than men
- Pathogenesis
  - Triggering factors including sunlight, pregnancy, and oral contraceptive pills lead to increased melanin production through unknown mechanisms.

2.2. Clinical Presentation

- Characterized by light to dark brown or brown-gray macules and patches with irregular borders (Fig. 6-2).
- The face is most commonly affected and can display the following patterns:
  - Centrofacial (most common)—forehead, cheeks, nose, upper lip, chin
  - Malar—cheeks/nose
  - Mandibular—along jawline
- Less common sites of involvement include the extensor forearms and mid upper chest.
- Often first appears or is first noticed with significant UV exposure or with pregnancy.

2.3. Treatment

- Sun protection, including sun-protective clothing, broad-spectrum sunscreen, and sun avoidance, can help prevent melasma. It is also essential for any other treatment to be effective.

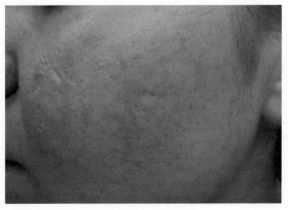

Figure 6-2. Light brown macules on the cheek.

- A Wood's lamp may be used to assess whether melanin is present in the epidermis or dermis. Epidermal pigmentation enhances with Wood's lamp exposure and may be more responsive to treatment.
- Hydroquinone
  - Hydroquinone inhibits tyrosinase and is available in concentrations from 2% to 4%. Prolonged use can lead to hyperpigmentation (exogenous ochronosis).
- Combination products
  - Several combination products exist, many of which include hydroquinone.
  - The combination of tretinoin 0.05%, hydroquinone 4%, and fluocinolone acetonide 0.01% appears to be more effective than any combination of two of these agents.[5]
- Topical retinoids
  - Mechanisms of action thought to include increased keratinocyte turnover, decreased melanosome transfer, and allowing other agents to more easily penetrate stratum corneum[6]
  - Can take >2 years to see improvement
- Azelaic acid
  - Inhibits tyrosinase
- Chemical peels
  - May be useful for patients who do not respond to skin-lightening agents.
  - Chemical peels can cause irritation, leading to postinflammatory hyperpigmentation. Often used concomitantly with skin-lightening agents to decrease this risk
- Laser/light therapies
  - Should be used in refractory cases and with caution in darker skin types as it may lead to postinflammatory hyperpigmentation.
  - Several types of lasers have been evaluated but with variable results.

3. OCULOCUTANEOUS ALBINISM

- Characterized by decreased or absent melanin with a normal number of melanocytes in the skin, hair, and eyes starting at birth.
- Due to defects in melanin synthesis pathway leading to decreased melanin.
- Well-characterized forms inherited in an autosomal recessive manner.
- Approximately 1 in 20,000 people affected worldwide.
- Ocular findings can include decreased visual acuity, photophobia, strabismus, and nystagmus.
- Patients are sensitive to sunlight with increased risk for skin cancers, particularly in those with minimal or no pigmentation.
- Photoprotection should be strongly encouraged.

3.1. Subtypes
- Subtypes can be differentiated based on clinical features and genetic testing.
- OCA types 1 and 2 are the most common forms worldwide.
- OCA type 1A is the most severe form and is due to a complete loss of tyrosinase activity. Characterized by lack of pigment in skin and hair with blue eyes at birth. Pigmentation does not increase with age.
- OCA type 1B is due to decreased levels of tyrosinase. Usually with lack of pigment in skin and hair with blue eyes at birth. May eventually have increased pigment in skin, hair, and eyes.

- OCA type 2—due to mutations in the OCA2 gene. Has a variable clinical phenotype—can vary from almost normal pigmentation to almost no pigmentation. Pigment tends to increase with age.
- OCA type 3—due to mutations in tyrosinase-related protein 1 (TYRP1) gene. Most common phenotype known as "rufous" and is characterized by ginger-red hair and reddish-brown skin.
- OCA type 4—due to mutation in SLC45A2 gene with a variable clinical phenotype.

4. DERMAL MELANOCYTOSIS

4.1. Congenital Dermal Melanocytosis (Mongolian Spot)

- Characterized by blue to bluish-gray patch or patches up to several centimeters in size
- Most common locations include the lumbosacral area, buttocks, and back
- Usually present at birth or soon after
- Due to presence of increased dendritic melanocytes in the deep dermis
- Most common in individuals with darker skin types including those of Asian and African descent
- Generally fades during childhood

4.2. Nevus of Ota

- Characterized by brown or blue-gray macules and patches in the V1 or V2 distribution of the face. Usually unilateral but can also be bilateral.
- Predominantly affects individuals with more pigmented skin including those of Asian and African descent.
- Most common ages of onset include infancy and puberty.
- Majority of reported cases have occurred in women.
- Characterized histologically by dendritic melanocytes in the upper dermis.
- Cutaneous lesions consist of macules and patches that can be brown, gray, or blue in color.
- Most patients also have involvement of the ipsilateral sclera.
- Lesions tend to be persistent.
- Melanoma develops rarely within these lesions, most often in the choroid. Most common presentation of melanoma in the skin is a subcutaneous nodule.[7]
- Q-switched lasers have been used to treat these lesions.
- Acquired nevus of Ota-like macules (Hori nevus) is characterized by brown or slate-gray macules acquired primarily in the bilateral maxillary area.[8]

4.3. Nevus of Ito

- Has similar clinical appearance and histology as nevus of Ota but with a different distribution.
- Lesions occur in distribution of lateral cutaneous brachial and posterior supraclavicular nerves and involve the supraclavicular, scapular, shoulder, and lateral neck regions.

5. DRUG-INDUCED PIGMENTATION

- Many medications and heavy metals can cause pigmentation changes.
- Pigmentation can be due to a combination of increased melanin, drug complex deposition, or heavy metal deposition.

- Involvement can be widespread or focal and can involve extracutaneous sites including the nails, mucosa, and sclera.
- In some cases, drug discontinuation leads to resolution.

5.1. Commonly Implicated Drugs/Metals

- Chemotherapeutic drugs: bleomycin, busulfan, cyclophosphamide, dactinomycin, daunorubicin, 5-fluorouracil, hydroxyurea, methotrexate
- Heavy metals: arsenic, bismuth, gold, iron, lead, silver
- Antimalarials: chloroquine, hydroxychloroquine, and quinacrine
- Tricyclic antidepressants/phenothiazines: amitriptyline, chlorpromazine, clomipramine, desipramine, imipramine, thioridazine
- Others: amiodarone, clofazimine, diltiazem, hydroquinone, imatinib, minocycline, zidovudine

5.2. Notable Drugs/Metals and Their Pattern of Involvement

- Antimalarials—gray to blue-black pigmentation most commonly involving shins. Can also involve face, oral mucosa, and subungual areas. Quinacrine can cause yellow to yellow-brown discoloration of skin and sclera.
- Amiodarone—photosensitivity leading to slate-gray to violaceous hyperpigmentation in sun-exposed areas.
- Hydroquinone—continuous topical application can lead to paradoxical hyperpigmentation (exogenous ochronosis).
- Minocycline—three patterns classically described. Type I with blue-black discoloration in areas of scarring and inflammation including acne scars. Type II characterized by blue-gray pigmentation of the shins. Type III described as a generalized "muddy brown" discoloration that is worse in sun-exposed areas.
- Prostaglandin analogues—ophthalmic solutions used for glaucoma can lead to periocular hyperpigmentation.
- Silver (argyria)—diffuse slate-gray pigmentation that is accentuated in sun-exposed areas.
- Zidovudine (AZT)—hyperpigmentation most commonly in nails. Diffuse hyperpigmentation can occur as well. More commonly affects darker skin types.

6. ERYTHEMA DYSCHROMICUM PERSTANS

- Characterized by slowly progressive appearance of gray or gray-brown oval-shaped macules and patches symmetrically distributed on the trunk, neck, and proximal extremities.
- Lesions typically measure up to several centimeters in size.
- During initial appearance of lesions, lesions may have a small rim of raised erythema at the periphery.
- Most commonly affects children and young adults and is most prevalent in Latin American patients with type III and type IV skin.
- Lesions may eventually fade over months to years and more commonly fade in children than in adults.[9]
- Treatment is generally ineffective though may be more helpful in the early inflammatory phase. Reported treatments include clofazimine and dapsone.

7. IDIOPATHIC GUTTATE HYPOMELANOSIS

- Common disorder characterized by hypopigmented small, sharply defined macules most commonly on shins and forearms.
- Lesions typically <5 mm in size and most prominent on darker skin types.
- Most common in individuals over the age of 40 with increased prevalence with increasing age.
- UV exposure thought to play a role in pathogenesis.
- Repigmentation does not occur.

8. PITYRIASIS ALBA

- Characterized by hypopigmented, slightly scaly macules that are poorly defined
- Most commonly located on the cheeks but can also be present on the neck, trunk, and upper arms
- Occurs in children and adolescents, particularly those with an atopic diathesis
- Tends to be more pronounced in patients with darker skin types
- Thought to be due to postinflammatory hypopigmentation
- Emollients and topical steroids often used for treatment

9. POSTINFLAMMATORY PIGMENT ALTERATION

9.1. Postinflammatory Hyperpigmentation

- Characterized by hyperpigmented macules and patches.
- Pigment in the epidermis is more likely to present as shades of brown. Dermal pigmentation often has a blue or gray appearance, though it can also have a brown appearance when melanin is in the superficial dermis.
- Can be caused by a variety of inflammatory skin conditions (e.g., acne, insect bites, contact dermatitis, atopic dermatitis, psoriasis, lichen simplex chronicus, lichen planus, fixed drug eruption, discoid lupus).
- Histopathologically, melanin is deposited in the epidermis, the dermis, or both.
- More common in patients with darker skin types, particularly types IV and V.
- The primary condition leading to hyperpigmentation may or may not be evident. The size, shape, and distribution of the hyperpigmentation can often help determine the primary cause.
- Treatment
  - Treatment should first aim at managing the underlying cause.
  - Increased epidermal melanin is more likely to resolve, while dermal melanin may last for years.
  - Epidermal melanin may respond to hydroquinone along with other skin-lightening agents including azelaic acid and combinations of hydroquinone with corticosteroids and retinoids.
  - Dermal pigmentation is not usually responsive to topical treatments.
  - Photoprotection can minimize further hyperpigmentation.

9.2. Postinflammatory Hypopigmentation

- Presents with hypopigmented macules and patches with lesion size, shape, and distribution often reflecting the underlying etiology.
- Less common than postinflammatory hyperpigmentation.

- Common causes include psoriasis, seborrheic dermatitis, atopic dermatitis, discoid lupus, and lichen sclerosus et atrophicus.
- Can occur after the underlying cause or present with it.
- More noticeable in patients with darker complexions.
- Treatment should aim at treating the underlying cause initially.
- UVB phototherapy or sun exposure can be helpful as well.

REFERENCES

1. Krüger C, Schallreuter KU. A review of the worldwide prevalence of vitiligo in children/adolescents and adults. *Int J Dermatol* 2012;51(10):1206–1212.
2. Kyriakis KP, Palamaras I, Tsele E, et al. Case detection rates of vitiligo by gender and age. *Int J Dermatol* 2009;48(3):328–329.
3. Alkhateeb A, Fain PR, Thody A, et al. Epidemiology of vitiligo and associated autoimmune diseases in Caucasian probands and their families. *Pigment Cell Res* 2003;16(3):208–214.
4. Casacci M, Thomas P, Pacifico A, et al. Comparison between 308-nm monochromatic excimer light and narrowband UVB phototherapy (311–313 nm) in the treatment of vitiligo—a multicentre controlled study. *J Eur Acad Dermatol Venereol* 2007;21(7):956–963.
5. Taylor SC, Torok H, Jones T, et al. Efficacy and safety of a new triple-combination agent for the treatment of facial melasma. *Cutis* 2003;72(1):67–72.
6. Ortonne JP. Retinoid therapy of pigmentary disorders. *Dermatol Ther* 2006;19(5):280–288.
7. Patel BC, Egan CA, Lucius RW, et al. Cutaneous malignant melanoma and oculodermal melanocytosis (nevus of Ota): report of a case and review of the literature. *J Am Acad Dermatol* 1998;38(5 Pt 2):862–865.
8. Ee HL, Wong HC, Goh CL, et al. Characteristics of Hori naevus: a prospective analysis. *Br J Dermatol* 2006;154(1):50–53.
9. Silverberg NB, Herz J, Wagner A, et al. Erythema dyschromicum perstans in prepubertal children. *Pediatr Dermatol* 2003;20(5):398–403.

7 Benign Skin Lesions

Shayna Gordon, MD and M. Laurin Council, MD

Benign skin lesions are frequently encountered during the dermatologic exam. Although removal is often not necessary, it may be indicated for the treatment of symptomatic lesions. Additionally, when atypia or malignancy is suspected, a biopsy is indicated for definitive diagnosis.

1. NEVI

1.1. Background

- Melanocytic nevi can be congenital or acquired proliferations of pigmented cells (melanocytes). An acquired melanocytic nevus, often referred to as a mole, is a very common benign lesion with several subtypes, including junctional, compound, intradermal, blue, halo, and Spitz (Fig. 7-1).[1]

1.2. Clinical Presentation

- **Junctional Nevi**
  - Junctional nevi are tan or brown uniform macules with smooth regular borders. They are usually <6 mm in diameter. The term "junctional" refers to the histologic location of lesional melanocytes along the dermoepidermal junction (Fig. 7-1A).
- **Compound Nevi**
  - Compound nevi are raised brown or tan papules. Histologically, melanocytes are found in both the dermis and the epidermis, hence the term "compound" (Fig. 7-1B).
- **Intradermal Nevi**
  - Intradermal nevi are usually skin-colored, tan or light brown, well-demarcated, dome-shaped papules. The melanocytes of these nevi are located entirely within the dermis (Fig. 7-1C).
- **Blue Nevi**
  - Blue nevi clinically appear as solitary, blue-black papules (Fig. 7-1D). Two histologic variants exist: the common blue and the cellular blue nevus. Common blue nevi typically arise on the head and neck, whereas cellular blue nevi are usually on the trunk or extremities. Atypical cellular blue nevi can be difficult to distinguish histologically from melanoma.
- **Halo Nevi**
  - Halo nevi appear as brown macules or papules with a surrounding halo of depigmentation. The depigmentation is a result of an immune response to the melanocytes in the region. Histologically, a brisk lymphocytic infiltrate may be seen around the nevus. Occasionally, the nevus will regress entirely.

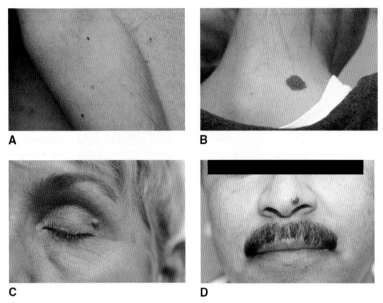

Figure 7-1. Spectrum of benign nevi. **A:** Junctional nevi. **B:** Compound nevus. **C:** Intradermal nevus. **D:** Blue nevus. (**C**, Courtesy of Eva Hurst, MD.)

- **Spitz Nevi**
  - Spitz nevi are solitary pink papules usually on face or scalp of a child or adolescent. Histologically, they are characterized by a distinct variant of the melanocyte, the Spitz cell. Atypical Spitz nevi can be difficult to distinguish histologically from melanoma. Because Spitz nevi are rare in adulthood, some advocate for complete excision of these lesions.

1.3. Evaluation

- Most nevi are benign and require only observation. Lesions with asymmetry, border irregularity, color variation, and diameter >6 mm or lesions that are changing should be biopsied to rule out atypia or malignancy.
- A nevus that is different than the patients' other nevi is referred to as the "ugly duckling sign" and may necessitate a biopsy to rule out atypia or malignancy.

1.4. Treatment

- In general, any lesion deemed suspicious should be removed via deep shave or excisional biopsy and examined histologically to rule out malignancy.
- Surgical removal of benign lesions may be performed for cosmesis.

2. SEBORRHEIC KERATOSIS

2.1. Background

- Seborrheic keratoses are common acquired benign epidermal lesions.

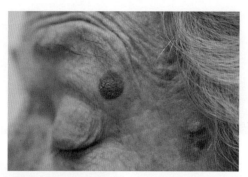

Figure 7-2. Seborrheic keratosis. (Courtesy of Eva Hurst, MD.)

2.2. Clinical Presentation

- The classic lesion typically demonstrates a verrucous or waxy surface with a "stuck on" appearance (Fig. 7-2). Lesions may be skin-colored, tan, or brown and can appear anywhere sparing the palms and soles. Generally, these lesions appear after the third decade and increase in number with age.
- There are few histologic and clinically distinct variants of seborrheic keratoses.
  - Dermatosis papulosa nigra is a form of seborrheic keratosis that occurs in darker-pigmented individuals and presents as small dark brown or black papules on the face and neck. This condition tends to be familial.[2]
  - Stucco keratoses appear as rough, white papules that are easily scraped off and are frequently located on the lower extremities.
  - Rarely, the sudden appearance of multiple seborrheic keratoses may be a paraneoplastic manifestation of an internal malignancy, known as the sign of Leser-Trelat.[3]

2.3. Evaluation

- Diagnosis can usually be made clinically, but a biopsy should be performed for confirmation of clinically suspicious lesions.

2.4. Treatment

- No treatment is necessary for seborrheic keratoses; however, removal may be requested for cosmesis, to decrease irritation or to rule out malignancy. Cryotherapy with liquid nitrogen is effective for most seborrheic keratoses, with the exception of extremely thick lesions. Repeat treatments may be necessary. Lesions can also be removed by curettage with or without electrocautery.

3. ACROCHORDONS

3.1. Background

- Acrochordons, or skin tags, are pedunculated fibrous papules commonly occurring in skin folds (Fig. 7-3).

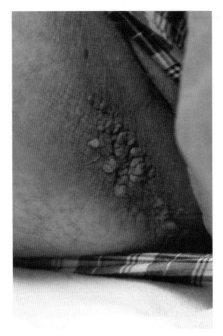

Figure 7-3. Plaque of acrochordons.

3.2. Clinical Presentation

• Clinically, acrochordons appear as skin-colored or tan 1- to 5-mm pedunculated papules. They frequently appear in areas of friction. The axilla is the most common location, but these lesions can also appear along the neckline, eyelids, and inguinal and inframammary creases. Obesity is often a predisposing factor.[4] Lesions are usually asymptomatic but may become irritated and tender if traumatized by friction, jewelry, or clothing.[5]

3.3. Evaluation

• Diagnosis can be made clinically, but a biopsy should be performed for confirmation of clinically suspicious lesions.

3.4. Treatment

• Asymptomatic lesions require no treatment. If lesions are irritated, or if removal is warranted for cosmesis, acrochordons can be removed via snip excision, using curved iris scissors. Electrosurgery or cryotherapy can also be used for removal.

4. ANGIOMAS

4.1. Background

• Cherry angiomas are mature capillary proliferations.

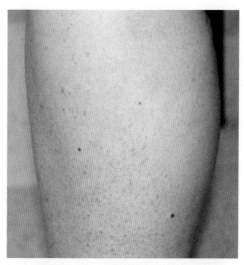

Figure 7-4. Angiomas.

4.2. Clinical Presentation

• Cherry angiomas appear as 0.5-mm to 5-mm, bright red to maroon macules or papules and are most commonly located on the trunk or proximal extremities (Fig. 7-4). Lesions are usually asymptomatic but may bleed with trauma. Generally, cherry angiomas develop after the third decade, and the number of lesions increases with age.

4.3. Evaluation

• Diagnosis can be made clinically, but a biopsy should be performed for confirmation of clinically suspicious lesions.

4.4. Treatment

• Patients may request removal of angiomas if they are cosmetically undesirable or chronically traumatized. Removal can be done by shave removal, electrodessication, or laser ablation with the pulsed dye laser.[6]

5. DERMATOFIBROMA

5.1. Background

• A dermatofibroma is an area of focal dermal fibrosis. It is controversial whether the lesions are spontaneous benign neoplasms or rather a reactive fibrous hyperplasia due to injury or arthropod bite.[7]

5.2. Clinical Presentation

• Dermatofibromas clinically appear as firm, discrete, asymptomatic nodules ranging in size from 3 to 10 mm in diameter (Fig. 7-5). Dermatofibromas can vary in color from pink to brown, often with a ring of hyperpigmentation. Most commonly, they appear on the lower legs and are usually asymptomatic, but occasionally tender.

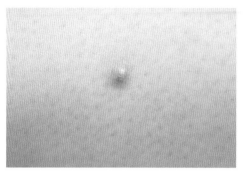

Figure 7-5. Dermatofibroma.

• A helpful diagnostic test is the "dimple sign," in which the lesion dimples when lateral pressure is applied.

5.3. Evaluation
• Diagnosis can be made clinically, but a biopsy should be performed of atypical or clinically suspicious lesions.

5.4. Treatment
• Treatment is not required unless the lesion is changing or symptomatic.

6. LENTIGINES

6.1. Background
• Lentigines are hyperpigmented benign macules caused by a proliferation of melanocytes at the dermoepidermal junction (Fig. 7-6).

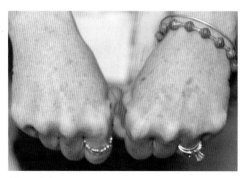

Figure 7-6. Lentigines.

6.2. Clinical Presentation

• Lentigines are tan or brown macules located in sun-exposed areas such as the dorsal hands, forearms, upper chest, and shoulders.[8]

6.3. Evaluation

• Diagnosis can be made clinically, but in cases of ambiguity, a biopsy should be performed to rule out lentigo maligna or melanoma in situ.

6.4. Treatment

• If there is no concern for malignancy, elective removal may be considered for cosmesis. Topical treatment with 2% to 4% hydroquinone, alone or in combination with a retinoid and steroid, may help lighten lesions. Laser destruction, chemical peels, and gentle freezing with liquid nitrogen are also effective. Strict photoprotection and the use of a high sun protection factor, and broad-spectrum sunscreen are necessary to prevent darkening of existing lentigines as well as the appearance of new lesions.

7. SEBACEOUS HYPERPLASIA

7.1. Background

• Sebaceous hyperplasia is a common and benign proliferation of sebaceous glands.

7.2. Clinical Presentation

• Sebaceous hyperplasia appears as a single lesion or as multiple soft white-yellow papules with a central umbilication (Fig. 7-7). Most lesions are 2 to 4 mm in diameter and appear on the forehead, cheeks, and nose of middle-aged and elderly patients.[9]

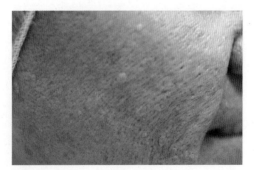

Figure 7-7. Sebaceous hyperplasia.

7.3. Evaluation

• Diagnosis can be made clinically, but a biopsy should be performed for confirmation of clinically suspicious lesions. Sebaceous hyperplasia can sometimes be confused clinically with basal cell carcinoma.

7.4. Treatment

• Treatment is not required but may be requested for cosmetic reasons. Elective removal may be accomplished with electrodessication, ablative laser surgery, cryosurgery, and shave excision with curettage.[10]

8. KELOIDS

8.1. Background

• Keloids and hypertrophic scars represent an excessive wound healing response after injury to the skin (Fig. 7-8).
• The distinction between the two entities is clinical: hypertrophic scars remain confined to the boundaries of the original injury, while keloids extend beyond the margins of the initial insult.

8.2. Clinical Presentation

• Keloids appear as firm, elevated, pink or dark brown nodules or plaques. The most common locations are the earlobes, upper chest, shoulders, and back. Keloids are more commonly found in individuals with darker skin types.[11] Lesions are usually asymptomatic but may be painful or pruritic.

8.3. Evaluation

• Diagnosis can be made clinically, but a biopsy should be performed of clinically suspicious lesions.

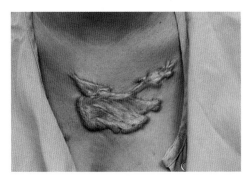

Figure 7-8. Keloid. (Courtesy of Eva Hurst, MD.)

8.4. Treatment

- Intralesional steroids may help flatten and soften hypertrophic scars and keloids and reduce any associated pruritus. Overtreatment with intralesional steroids can cause hypopigmentation and atrophy.[12] Keloids may be treated with excision, shave removal, or ablative laser, followed by serial injections with intralesional steroids to prevent recurrence.[13]

9. CYSTS

9.1. Background

- The most common types of cutaneous cysts are epidermal inclusion cysts (Fig. 7-9), pilar cysts, and milia cysts.

9.2. Clinical Presentation

- **Epidermal inclusion cysts**
  - Epidermal inclusion cysts are common subcutaneous lesions that range in size from several millimeters to several centimeters in diameter. A helpful diagnostic clue is a central punctum that may drain a foul-smelling, cheesy substance. When inflamed, epidermal inclusion cysts can become quiet painful, dramatically increase in size, and develop overlying erythema. At times, they may become secondarily infected.
- **Milia cysts**
  - Milia cysts are superficial epidermal inclusions cysts that are 1- to 2-mm white papules most commonly on the face of adults.
- **Pilar cysts**
  - Pilar (trichilemmal) cysts are firm mobile nodules commonly located on the scalp. They are typically seen in middle-aged women, and multiple lesions are frequent.

9.3. Evaluation

- Diagnosis can be made clinically, but surgical removal is indicated of large, growing, symptomatic, or clinically atypical lesions.

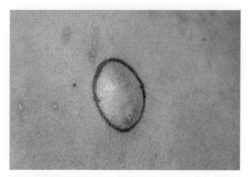

Figure 7-9. Epidermal inclusion cyst.

9.4. Treatment
- **Epidermal inclusion cysts**
  - Inflamed epidermal inclusion cysts can be treated with intralesional steroids to decrease inflammation and tenderness. Severely inflamed lesions may also be treated with antibiotics.[14] Surgical excision is typically reserved for noninflamed lesions, due to increased risk of complications in acutely inflamed cysts. If active infection is suspected, an incision and drainage, with culture, can be performed.
- **Milia cysts**
  - Milia can be removed for cosmesis by puncturing the skin with a no. 11 blade or 19-gauge needle and then applying gentle pressure with a comedone extractor. Smaller lesions may respond to topical retinoid treatment.
- **Pilar cysts**
  - Pilar cysts can be easily removed by simple excision. Like epidermal inclusion cysts, surgery is reserved for noninflamed lesions.

10. LIPOMAS

10.1. Background
- Lipomas are benign, subcutaneous tumors composed of mature fat cells (Fig. 7-10).

10.2. Clinical Presentation
- A lipoma clinically appears as a painless, round, soft, mobile, subcutaneous nodule, often with doughy consistency. They are slow growing, and usually 1 to 3 cm in diameter, but can grow up to >10 cm. They are most common in middle age and usually located on the shoulders, neck, trunk, and arms.
- Rarely, multiple lipomas can be associated with syndromes such as hereditary multiple lipomatosis, Banyan-Riley-Ruvalcaba, Gardner syndrome, adiposis dolorosa, and Madelung disease.[15]

10.3. Evaluation
- Lipomas can usually be diagnosed clinically, but if a lesion is symptomatic or changing, a biopsy should be performed for histopathologic diagnosis.

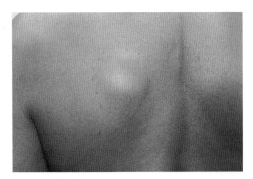

Figure 7-10. Lipoma.

10.4. Treatment

- Treatment for lipomas is not required but may be requested for cosmetic reasons. Most commonly, they are removed by simple surgical excision but can also be removed by liposuction.[16–18] Some histologic variants, such as the angiolipoma, may be painful. Surgical removal of these lesions can be performed.

REFERENCES

1. Witt C, Krengel S. Clinical and epidemiological aspects of subtypes of melanocytic nevi (Flat nevi, Miescher nevi, Unna nevi). *Dermatol Online J* 2010;16(1):1.
2. Lupo MP. Dermatosis papulosa nigra: treatment options. *J Drugs Dermatol* 2007;6(1):29–30.
3. Husain Z, Ho JK, Hantash BM. Sign and pseudo-sign of Leser-Trélat: case reports and a review of the literature. *J Drugs Dermatol* 2013;12(5):e79–e87.
4. Jindal A, Patel N, Shah R. Acrochordons as a cutaneous sign of metabolic syndrome: a case–control study. *Ann Med Health Sci Res* 2014;4(2):202.
5. Luba MC, Bangs SA, Mohler AM, et al. Common benign skin tumors. *Am Fam Physician* 2003;67(4):729–738.
6. Pancar GS, Aydin F, Senturk N, et al. Comparison of the 532-nm KTP and 1064-nm Nd: YAG lasers for the treatment of cherry angiomas. *J Cosmet Laser Ther* 2011;20:1–4.
7. Zelger BG, Zelger B. Dermatofibroma (fibrous histiocytoma): an inflammatory or neoplastic disorder? *Histopathology* 2001;38(4):379–381.
8. Praetorius C, Sturm RA, Steingrimsson E. Sun-induced freckling: ephelides and solar lentigines. *Pigment Cell Melanoma Res* 2014;27(3):339–350.
9. Dent CD, Hunter WE, Svirsky JA. Sebaceous gland hyperplasia. *J Oral Maxillofac Surg* 1995;53(8):936–938.
10. No D, McClaren M, Chotzen V, et al. Sebaceous hyperplasia treated with a 1450-nm diode laser. *Dermatol Surg* 2004;30(3):382–384.
11. Köse O, Waseem A. Keloids and hypertrophic scars: are they two different sides of the same coin? *Dermatol Surg* 2008;34(3):336–346.
12. Abdel-Meguid AM, Weshahy AH, Sayed DS, et al. Intralesional vs. contact cryosurgery in treatment of keloids: a clinical and immunohistochemical study. *Int J Dermatol* 2015;54(4):468–475.
13. Shockman S, Paghdal KV, Cohen G. Medical and surgical management of keloids: a review. *J Drugs Dermatol* 2010;9(10):1249–1257.
14. Poonawalla T, Uchida T, Diven DG. Survey of antibiotic prescription use for inflamed epidermal inclusion cysts. *J Cutan Med Surg* 2006;10(2):79–84.
15. Nguyen T, Zuniga R. Skin conditions: benign nodular skin lesions. *FP Essent* 2013;407:24–30.
16. Rao SS, Davison SP. Gone in 30 seconds: a quick and simple technique for subcutaneous lipoma removal. *Plast Reconstr Surg* 2012;130(1):236e–238e.
17. Amber KT, Ovadia S, Camacho I. Injection therapy for the management of superficial subcutaneous lipomas. *J Clin Aesthet Dermatol* 2014;7(6):46–48.
18. Ramakrishnan K. Techniques and tips for lipoma excision. *Am Fam Physician* 2002;66(8):1405.

8

Malignant Skin Lesions

David Y. Chen, MD, PhD, Amy Musiek, MD,
and Lynn A. Cornelius, MD

Malignant skin lesions are divided generally into melanoma and nonmelanoma types. Nonmelanoma skin cancers, particularly basal cell and squamous cell carcinomas (SCCs), are the most common cancers in humans, though this categorization includes a variety of rare cancers not discussed in this chapter. Correct identification of cancer type is of paramount importance to determining patient prognosis and appropriate management.

1. BASAL CELL CARCINOMA

• Basal cell carcinoma (BCC) is the most common cancer in the United States with over two million new cases each year. It is more common in men than in women, and its incidence is increasing in all age groups, particularly in women under 40 years of age.[1]

1.1. Background

• **Risk factors**—a confluence of genetic factors and environmental exposures determines risk of developing BCC. Environmental exposure to ultraviolet (UV) light from the sun or from tanning beds confers significant risk for development of BCC, both of which are preventable exposures. Approximately 98,000 additional cases of BCC in the United States each year are attributable to indoor tanning alone.[2] Additionally, a history of immunosuppression, increasing age, exposure to ionizing radiation or arsenic, and history of a prior nonmelanoma skin cancer increase risk. Genetic susceptibility to UV damage due to fair skin or hereditary disorders such as xeroderma pigmentosum (XP) confer independent risk for BCC. In another rare disorder, nevoid BCC syndrome (Gorlin syndrome), patients present with numerous, early-onset BCCs due to mutations in the patched 1 homolog (*PTCH1*) gene. Additional syndromes with early-onset BCC include Bazex-Dupre-Christol and Rombo syndromes. Therefore, patients with multiple or early BCC or extensive family history should be referred for dermatologic, and possibly genetic, evaluation.
• **Pathogenesis**—the hedgehog pathway is aberrantly activated in nearly all instances of BCC. Approximately 90% of spontaneous BCCs have mutations in *PTCH1*, while an estimated 10% harbor mutations in the downstream smoothened gene (*SMO*). Additionally, tumor protein P53 gene (*TP53*) is frequently mutated, and in spontaneous BCC, *PTCH1* and *TP53* mutations appear to be induced by UV irradiation. Tumor maintenance depends on continued hedgehog pathway signaling.[3]

1.2. Clinical Presentation

• **Clinical features**—BCC classically presents as a pink, translucent, or pearly papule or plaque with a rolled border and arborizing telangiectasias on sun-exposed skin (Fig. 8-1A). A number of common morphologic variants exist, including a

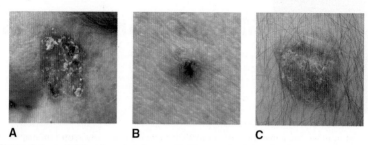

Figure 8-1. A: BCC with typical features. **B:** Pigmented BCC with arborizing telangiectasia and globular dark pigment. **C:** Superficial BCC with rolled borders at the periphery.

pigmented variant, which can sometimes be mistaken for melanoma (Fig. 8-1B). Additionally, BCCs may have a scar-like appearance and can frequently be ulcerated. Superficial BCC may present as a scaly red plaque that may resemble inflammatory lesion as seen in psoriasis, though a rolled border would be suggestive of BCC (Fig. 8-1C). Finally, an uncommon and relatively indolent variant of BCC, known as the fibroepithelioma of Pinkus, can have a verrucous surface and is commonly located on the lower back.

- **History**—patients may report a lesion that bleeds easily, does not heal, is slowly increasing in size, or is tender. It is a common scenario where the lesion has been neglected for months to years, given its relatively indolent nature.

1.3. Evaluation

- **Biopsy is required for complete evaluation**—though in many instances the diagnosis of BCC is strongly suspected based on clinical appearance, biopsy confirms the diagnosis and provides valuable information to the treating physician. Metatypical, infiltrative, morpheaform, sclerosing, or micronodular features on histology represent an aggressive growth pattern and influence treatment decisions. Any one of several biopsy techniques is acceptable including shave, punch, incisional, and excisional biopsies. BCCs rarely metastasize, and further workup, beyond a full skin examination, is generally not necessary.

1.4. Treatment

- Destructive and surgical measures are the mainstay of therapy for BCC. Curettage and electrodesiccation provides a rapid and effective method to treat BCCs with a nonaggressive histology and in a low-risk location and results in a cure rate in excess of 90%. Surgical excision of BCCs, where appropriate, with a 4-mm margin provides a cure rate of in excess of 95%. For superficial BCC, topical 5-fluorouracil can clear more than 90% of tumors, whereas imiquimod has been shown to clear over 80% of such BCCs. Photodynamic therapy (PDT) has demonstrated efficacy in clearing superficial BCC, though recurrence rates may be high. Cryotherapy and radiation therapy are also options for patients with low-risk BCCs who are poor surgical candidates.
- **Mohs micrographic surgery (MMS)**—allows for intraoperative evaluation of the entire peripheral and deep margin of the resected tumor specimen. BCCs with aggressive histologic characteristics, larger tumors (>2 cm) in any location, or any

BCC in a high risk location including the "mask areas" of the face or the genitals, tumors in an immunocompromised patient, and recurrent BCCs can be appropriately treated with MMS. In a randomized, controlled trial of over 600 high-risk facial or recurrent facial BCCs, MMS was demonstrated to be superior over surgical excision for primary (4.4% vs. 12.2%) and recurrent (3.9% vs. 13.5%) BCCs with 10-year follow-up.[4]

- **Locally advanced or metastatic BCC**—evaluation and management by a multidisciplinary team including dermatology, surgery, oncology, and radiation oncology services is highly recommended due to the numerous treatment modalities available that may be tailored to each patient's case. The recent advent of the small molecule inhibitor of smoothened (*SMO*) homolog, vismodegib, offers a new, effective option for this class of BCC. A multicenter, phase II clinical trial demonstrated significant clinical activity with objective response rates of 43% in locally advanced disease and 30% in metastatic disease.[5] A possible role for neoadjuvant vismodegib is currently under investigation. Despite the response rate, patients commonly experience alopecia, dysgeusia, ageusia, muscle spasms, fatigue, and other side effects that, in some instances, compel treatment cessation.

- **Prognosis**—the prognosis for patients with BCC is excellent. Most patients with localized BCC are cured by the aforementioned modalities. If left untreated, BCCs continue to enlarge and are locally destructive. Metastases occur in <0.1% of patients and typically occur in patients whose tumors have aggressive histologic features. Common sites for metastases include the lymph nodes, lungs, and bones. Although currently considered incurable, patients with metastatic BCC should be considered for systemic therapy with hedgehog pathway inhibitors like vismodegib or enrollment in a clinical trial.

- **Follow-up and prevention**—patients with a history of BCC have a 50% chance of developing a second BCC within 5 years. Therefore, close follow-up is recommended with full skin exam every 6 to 12 months. Avoidance of precipitating factors such as sun exposure, tanning beds, and ionizing radiation needs to be stressed in these patients.

2. SQUAMOUS CELL CARCINOMA AND ACTINIC KERATOSES

- SCC is the second most common type of skin cancer in the United States after BCC. The overwhelming majority of SCCs occur on chronically sun-exposed skin in older individuals. Men are twice as likely to develop SCC, and its incidence is more than 20 times higher in fair-skinned individuals than in patients with darker pigment types. Incidence increases with latitudes closer to the equator, reflecting the importance of UV exposure in the pathogenesis of SCC.

2.1. Background

- **Risk factors**—the major risk factor for development of SCC is exposure to UV radiation or the sun. Therapeutic sources of UV radiation such as psoralen with UV A (PUVA) greatly increase the risk for SCC as do cosmetic sources of UV radiation—indoor tanning accounts for approximately 72,000 excess cases of SCC each year.[2] Other risk factors include immunosuppression especially in the context of solid organ transplantation, fair skin, exposure to ionizing radiation, infection with certain human papillomavirus subtypes, burn scars, nonhealing ulcers, increased age, and hereditary disorders such as XP or recessive dystrophic epidermolysis bullosa.

- **Pathogenesis**—cutaneous SCCs are thought to arise from the premalignant actinic keratosis (AK) through progressive genomic aberrations induced by UV radiation and genomic instability. Mutations in tumor suppressor gene *TP53* is frequently observed as well as rat sarcoma viral oncogene homolog (*RAS*) mutations, seen in 21% of cutaneous SCCs. These mutations, resultant aberrant cellular networks, and interaction with stromal factors and the immune system are all contributing factors to development and maintenance of cutaneous SCC.[6]

2.2. Clinical Presentation

- **Clinical features**—SCC generally presents as a persistent, enlarging, erythematous, scaly papule or plaque on sun-exposed skin that may bleed and be tender (Fig. 8-2A). SCC may also present as a crusted or scaly nodule or a poorly healing ulcer. Specific presentations of SCC deserve mention. SCCs may develop within chronic ulcers of the lower leg, known as Marjolin ulcer, and are usually advanced at the time of diagnosis. On external genitalia, SCC may present as vegetative or verrucous nodules and plaques. SCC on sun-exposed skin is generally thought to exist on a continuum from precursor actinic keratosis, to SCC in situ, to invasive SCC. Actinic keratoses characteristically are well-defined, erythematous papules with adherent scale (Fig. 8-2B). In some instances, they may be less well-defined faint pink or tan patches with sandpaper-like scale that are more easily felt than seen. This may be difficult to distinguish from SCC in situ, which typically presents as an isolated, well-defined, red plaque with adherent scale (Fig. 8-2C).

2.3. Evaluation

- **Biopsy is required for complete evaluation**—in most cases, actinic keratoses can be clinically diagnosed with confidence by an experienced clinician. However, any suspicion of SCC should prompt biopsy to make a definitive diagnosis. Several biopsy techniques are adequate including shave, punch, incisional, or excisional biopsies. Histopathologic examination may differentiate in situ carcinoma from invasive carcinoma and provide further information to guide therapy by noting depth of invasion or aggressive histologic features such as perineural invasion. In addition to biopsy, a full dermatologic examination and palpation of the draining lymph nodes should be performed. In the absence of large tumors with aggressive

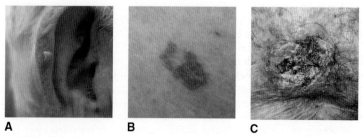

A **B** **C**

Figure 8-2. A: Squamous cell carcinoma. **B:** Hyperkeratotic papule, actinic keratosis. **C:** Red, minimally scaly plaque, SCC in situ. (**A and C**, courtesy of Arthur Z. Eisen, MD.)

histologic features, occurrence in a high-risk location, or clinical evidence for metastatic disease, further workup with imaging and laboratory studies is not indicated as outlined in the National Comprehensive Cancer Network (NCCN) guidelines for cutaneous SCC.

- **Staging of cutaneous squamous cell carcinomas**—is based on the tumor, node, metastasis (TNM) system, which has been revised in the seventh edition of the American Joint Committee on Cancer (AJCC) guidelines to include tumor thickness, as it may have prognostic value. One prospective study of SCC in 615 patients demonstrated no metastases in tumors <2.0 mm thick, while the rate increased to 4% in tumors 2.1 to 6.0 mm and 16% in tumors >6.0 mm.[7]

2.4. Treatment

- **Actinic keratoses**—several methods exist for treatment of actinic keratoses. The most commonly used is destruction with liquid nitrogen cryotherapy, which is effective and has few adverse effects other than temporary pain and localized redness and blistering associated with the treatment. Electrodessication and curettage destruction may be employed and is useful for treatment of hyperkeratotic lesions. For more numerous or diffuse lesions, several effective field therapies may be applied, including the following:
  - **5-fluorouracil**—an antimetabolite topical therapy that targets rapidly proliferating cells is available in multiple concentrations as a cream to be supplied to the patient for self-application. It is generally effective in clearing clinically apparent actinic keratoses as well as subtle lesions that may not be clinically obvious within the treatment field. Side effects range from mild irritation to severe inflammation. Care should be exercised in managing patient expectations. Testing small areas before wide application is one effective approach.
  - **Photodynamic therapy**—photosensitizers 5-aminolevulinic acid (ALA) and methyl aminolevulinate (MAL) cause preferential accumulation of protoporphyrin IX in neoplastic tissue, which is activated by blue or red visible light or pulsed dye laser to cause a reactive oxygen species–mediated phototoxic reaction. Clearance rates for actinic keratoses are similar to 5-fluorouracil application. Side effects include discomfort during treatment and ensuing mild irritation to severe inflammation.
  - **Other topical therapies**—have varying degrees of clearance. These include imiquimod, a Toll-like receptor7 (TLR7) agonist that causes inflammatory destruction, diclofenac gel, and ingenol mebutate.
- **Localized squamous cell carcinoma**—in situ or low-risk lesions in non–hair-bearing locations may be treated with curettage and electrodessication. Most lesions are removed surgically with 0.4-cm margins for lesions smaller than 2 cm in size and more than 0.6-cm margins for lesions larger than 2 cm or with ill-defined borders. Such margins provide cure rates of 90% to 95%. MMS can be employed for lesions that are at high risk for recurrence and metastasis such as SCC on the central face, ears, eyelids, lips, recurrent tumors, SCCs larger than 2 cm, SCCs with aggressive histologic subtypes, SCCs that develop in scars, or SCCs developing in immunocompromised patients. Additional therapies for SCCs include cryosurgery, radiation, and, rarely, intralesional chemo- or immunotherapy. Radiation therapy is generally reserved for patients who are poor surgical candidates and can be used as adjuvant therapy in patients with metastatic disease or resected high-risk SCCs, including those with extensive perineural invasion. However, patients with XP,

and other inherited disorders of nucleotide excision repair (NER), should never be treated with radiation.

- **Metastatic cutaneous squamous cell carcinoma**—platinum-based chemotherapy and epidermal growth factor receptor (EGFR) antagonists have demonstrated modest benefit for metastatic SCC. Referral to a multidisciplinary management team or clinical trial is recommended.
- **Prognosis**—the vast majority of cutaneous SCCs can be cured surgically. However, the incidence of local recurrence is 1% to 10% depending on the histologic variant and surgical modality and can be up to 20% in high-risk lesions in high-risk locations such as the ear. Overall, the incidence of metastasis in cutaneous SCC ranges from 2% to 6%, typically affecting the first draining lymph node. Certain SCCs have a more aggressive course and are designated as high risk, including lesions on the lips and ears, lesions larger than 2 cm, thick lesions, SCC in scars, recurrent SCC, SCC with perineural invasion, and SCCs in immunosuppressed patients (organ transplant and CLL) that carry high metastatic risk.
- **Follow-up and prevention**—patients with low-risk SCCs are followed up with full body skin examinations every 3 to 12 months for the first 2 years, every 6 to 12 months for the next 3 years, and annually thereafter. Patients with high-risk SCCs should be followed with total skin and lymph node examination every 1 to 3 months for the first year, every 2 to 4 months for the next year, then every 4 to 6 months for the next 3 years, and then every 6 to 12 months thereafter according to the 2014 NCCN guidelines for cutaneous SCC. Sun protection and sun avoidance need to be stressed in these patients. In high-risk patients, including solid organ transplant or otherwise immunosuppressed patients, precancerous actinic keratoses should be aggressively treated and threshold for biopsy of suspicious lesions should be low.
  - **Chemoprevention**—Patients with high risk of developing cutaneous SCC, particularly solid organ transplant patients, may benefit from the use of topical imiquimod, topical and oral retinoid, and topical 5-fluorouracil. Oral retinoid therapy may be associated with serum lipid abnormalities that may already be problematic in this patient population. In addition, the discontinuation of oral retinoid may be associated with a rebound development of SCCs.[8]

3. MELANOMA

- The Surveillance, Epidemiology and End Results Program (SEER) data demonstrate a steady rise in the incidence of cutaneous melanoma since 1975 and a continued average of 1.8% year-over-year increase between 2002 and 2011 (http://seer.cancer.gov). The American Cancer Society estimates that in the year 2014, approximately 76,100 cases of melanoma will be diagnosed, and 9,710 individuals will die of melanoma. The lifetime risk of being diagnosed with melanoma in the United States is approximately 1 in 50 for Whites, 1 in 1,000 for Blacks, and 1 in 200 for Hispanics. Overall, men account for more new cases of melanoma than do women (27.7 vs. 16.7 new cases per 100,000, SEER 18).

3.1. Background

- **Risk factors**—there are clear genetic and environmental determinants of melanoma risk. Although familial melanoma is much less common than sporadic cases, mutations in the cyclin-dependent kinase inhibitor 2A (*CDKN2A*) tumor suppressor gene are present with some frequency in families with multiple affected family members, or patients with multiple primary melanomas. Lower penetrance gene variants associated with increased melanoma risk include melanocortin 1 receptor (*MC1R*—the genetic determinant of pigmentation type), tyrosinase (*TYR*), cyclin-dependent kinase 4 (*CDK4*), microphthalmia transcription factor (*MITF*), BRCA1-associated protein 1 (*BAP1*), and others.[9] The discovery of new genetic risk determinants is being described with the application of next-generation sequencing, including a recent study that identified a nongenic polymorphisms affecting the regulatory region in telomerase (*TERT*) in a family with multiple family members with melanoma.[10] Despite identification of such genetic risk factors, the utility of their detection has not been established; genetic testing is not, therefore, a routine practice in the clinical setting as clinical examination of patients and family members remains the standard of care.

- The most significant environmental exposure that drives melanoma as well as nonmelanoma skin cancer risk is UV exposure. In fact, the World Health Organization (WHO) has classified UV radiation between 100 nm and 400 nm as a known carcinogen. UV exposure, in collaboration with genetic risk factors, including fair skin, red hair (*MC1R* variants), and UV sensitivity syndromes like XP, increases melanoma risk. Fair-complected individuals living in lower latitudes such as New Zealand and Australia, or those who electively expose themselves to excessive UV light through devices such as tanning beds, are at increased risk. To this point, a history of melanoma confers 10-fold risk of subsequent melanoma compared to the general population, likely reflecting a confluence of genetic factors and environmental exposure. Other risk factors include increased number of nevi (>50), history of greater than five clinically atypical nevi, large congenital nevi (>20 cm), and immunosuppression.

3.2. Clinical Presentation

- Cutaneous melanomas commonly arise in the absence of a clinically apparent precursor, though in some instances, benign nevi are associated with melanoma on histologic examination. Patients may report the appearance of a new skin lesion or change in an existing lesion and will occasionally note associated symptoms such as itching and bleeding. Nonpigmented, or amelanotic, primary lesions constitute approximately 5% of cutaneous melanomas (Fig. 8-3A).
- **Clinical features.** While evaluating a pigmented skin lesion, the ABCD morphologic criteria are helpful, but not absolute.
  - *Asymmetry*—one-half of the lesion does not match the other.
  - *Border irregularity*—the lesion has ragged or notched edges.
  - *Color variegation*—pigmentation is a heterogeneous mixture of tan, brown, or black. Red, white, or blue discolorations are particularly of concern.
  - *Diameter*—larger than 6 mm*.
  - *Evolution*—change in characteristics of a lesion noted by the patient or physician.
- Particular attention should be given to lesions that by clinical documentation (i.e., written or photographic records) or by patient report are evolving. Together, this set of criteria is sometimes known as the ABCDEs of melanoma. Lesions with one or more of these attributes should be brought to the attention of a physician, preferably a dermatologist, and evaluated for the possibility of melanoma (Fig. 8-3B). Other characteristics such as itching, bleeding, and the presence of ulceration should also prompt a careful evaluation for melanoma.

---

*This parameter serves as a guideline only; melanomas may present clinically as smaller lesions.

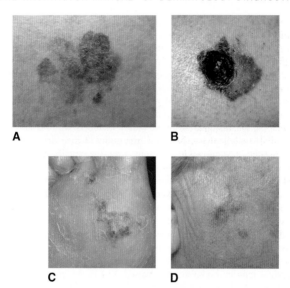

Figure 8-3. A: Multifocal, asymmetric, variably pigmented patch with border irregularity, representing typical in-situ melanoma. **B:** Melanoma with variegated coloration, irregular borders with eccentric pigment, gray veil, and nodular component. **C:** Acral lentiginous melanoma. **D:** Amelanotic melanoma. (**B and D,** courtesy of Arthur Z. Eisen, MD.)

3.3. Evaluation

- A comprehensive skin examination by a dermatologist, including scalp, hands and feet, genitalia, and oral cavity, is critical in evaluating and monitoring patients with multiple or atypical nevi, a history of excessive sun exposure, or a history of melanoma or nonmelanoma skin cancer.
- **Adequate biopsy is required for accurate diagnosis and staging**—the differential diagnosis of a pigmented skin lesion includes an atypical nevus as well as a benign growth such as melanocytic nevus, solar lentigo, seborrheic keratosis, angioma, and less commonly basal and SCCs. When melanoma or other malignant lesion is a consideration, biopsy is required to establish a diagnosis and should be done without delay.
  - **Excisional biopsy**—full-thickness removal of the entire clinical lesion with 1- to 3-mm margins with consideration of patterns of lymphatic drainage is optimal for diagnosis and accurate staging by Breslow thickness and ultimately treatment. Avoiding wider margins and interruption of lymphatic channels facilitates accurate sentinel lymph node mapping if later required.
  - **Incisional biopsy**—for large lesions or lesions on special sites like the palms and soles, face, ears, or digits, full-thickness incision or punch biopsy of the thickest clinical portion may be appropriate.
  - **Deep shave (saucerization)**—wide sampling is preferred in superficial lesions such as lentigo maligna, where atypical melanocytes may extend beyond the clinically observed lesion. Superficial shave biopsy is not recommended for any lesion suspected to be melanoma.
- **Histologic reporting and classification**—Breslow thickness in millimeters, presence or absence of histologic ulceration, dermal mitotic rate (events per square millimeter), and presence or absence of tumor at the lateral or deep margins

constitute the minimal elements that should be reported with the histologic evaluation of melanoma. Reports may include additional elements encouraged by the American Academy of Dermatology such as the presence or absence of regression, microsatellitosis, tumor infiltrating lymphocytes, lymphovascular invasion, neurotropism, and growth phase (radial vs. vertical). The pathologist may also report the histologic subtypes, which include superficial spreading melanoma, nodular melanoma, lentigo maligna melanoma, and acral lentiginous melanoma. Superficial spreading melanoma is the most common subtype constituting 75% of all melanomas, while lentigo maligna constitutes 10% to 15% and is thought to have an extended radial growth phase. Nodular melanomas are by definition in vertical growth phase (Fig. 8-3B). Acral lentiginous melanoma (Fig. 8-3C) is the least common type and characteristically arises on specialized sites like palmar, plantar, and subungual locations. Aside from the four dominant subtypes, there are rare variants including nevoid melanoma and desmoplastic melanoma. Though histologically distinct, the subtype does not affect staging and does not influence management or prognosis with the exception of a purely desmoplastic melanoma, where sentinel lymph node biopsy may not be indicated due to the decreased propensity of this subtype to develop regional, as opposed to local, metastases.

- **Staging**—for staging, the seventh edition of the American Joint Commission for Cancer (AJCC) staging system, updated in 2009, is used (Table 8-1). Though most of the staging criteria from the previous edition remained the same, the most recent edition incorporates sentinel lymph node biopsy and the detection of micrometastases. The most important prognostic factors in the staging of melanoma are the thickness of the primary lesion measured in millimeters (Breslow thickness), the presence of histologic ulceration, mitotic rate $>1/mm^2$, and the presence of regional lymph node involvement.

  - **Sentinel lymph node biopsy**—stage 0, I, and II melanomas are localized to the skin, while stage III melanoma denotes regional metastasis, which is detected by clinical exam or by sentinel lymph node biopsy. Lymphoscintigraphy and sentinel lymph node biopsy are performed at the time of wide local excision and offers prognostic value to patients with primary melanoma >1.0 mm, or a thinner melanoma with ulceration or increased mitotic rate. This is supported by multiple studies and recently reaffirmed in the final analysis of the Multicenter Selective Lymphadenectomy Trial-1 (MSLT-1). Generally, sentinel lymph node biopsy may be considered for primary for melanomas 0.76 to 1.0 mm based on the 2014 NCCN guidelines.

  - **Imaging**—routine imaging is not recommended in stage I or II disease unless used to evaluate specific clinical signs and symptoms. The exception is ultrasonography of a nodal basin for an indeterminate lymph node clinical exam, which can help guide decisions for fine needle aspiration (FNA) or lymph node biopsy. Positron emission tomography with computed tomography (PET-CT) offers no utility in detecting micrometastatic nodal disease. For stage III disease as determined by sentinel biopsy, clinically positive nodes, or in-transit metastases, baseline contrast-enhanced CT exam is recommended, with or without PET-CT or magnetic resonance imaging (MRI), based on clinical context. For suspected stage IV disease, in addition to CT of the chest, abdomen, and pelvis, gadolinium-enhanced brain MRI is recommended in the initial staging because of its increased sensitivity for detecting small posterior fossa lesions (<1 cm) compared to head CT. PET-CT is also appropriate for initial staging, but has no utility in the determination of brain metastases.

  - **Fine needle aspiration (FNA)**—suspected regional metastatic disease determined by clinical exam or imaging should be evaluated histologically by FNA or

Table 8-1 Revised 2009 American Joint Commission for Cancer (AJCC) Melanoma Staging and Classification

Stage	TNM classification	Tumor thickness (mm)	Features	% 5 Year survival[a]
0	In situ	0		
IA	T1a N0 M0	≤1.0		97
IB	T1b N0 M0	≤1.0	Ulcerated, or mitosis ≥1/mm2	92
	T2a N0 M0	1.01–2.0		
IIA	T2b N0 M0	1.01–2.0	Ulcerated	81
	T3a N0 M0	2.01–4.0		
IIB	T3b N0 M0	2.01–4.0	Ulcerated	70
	T4a N0 M0	>4.0		
IIC	T4b N0 M0	>4.0	Ulcerated	53
IIIA	T1–T4a N1a M0	Any	Microscopic node positive	78
	T1–T4a N2a M0			
IIIB	T1–T4b N1a M0		Microscopic node positive, ulcerated	59
	T1–T4b N2a M0			
	T1–T4a N1b M0		Macroscopic node positive	
	T1–T4a N2b M0			
	T1–4a N2c M0		In-transit metastases, negative nodes	
IIIC	T1–4b N1b M0		Macroscopic node positive, ulcerated	40
	T1–4b N2b M0			
	T1–4b N2c M0		In transit metastases, ulcerated	
	Any T N3 M0		In transit metastases with positive nodes	
IV	Any T any N M1		Distant skin, node or visceral metastases	15–20

[a]Observed survival rates from 2008 AJCC Melanoma Staging Database.
Data from Balch CM, et al. Final version of 2009 AJCC melanoma staging and classification. *J Clin Oncol* 2009;27(36):6199–6206.

core biopsy. In the appropriate context, FNA or core needle biopsy can be performed for suspected stage IV disease except when archival tissue is not available for genetic testing (i.e., for v-raf murine sarcoma viral oncogene homolog B, or BRAF, mutations). In this instance, open biopsy is preferred over FNA.

- **Lactate dehydrogenase (LDH)**—elevated serum levels of LDH are an independent predictor of poor outcome in stage IV disease. Monitoring LDH levels in patients with locoregional disease is not recommended.

3.4. Treatment

- **Wide local excision**—in stage 0, I, and II disease, wide local excision of the primary lesion with appropriate clinical margins provides the greatest chance of local control. Recommendations for excision margins come from randomized trials comparing conservative versus aggressive margins.[11] Margins of 0.5 to 1 cm are recommended for melanoma in situ. A margin of 1 cm is adequate for primary melanomas with a Breslow thickness of 1 mm or less, while melanomas between 1.01 and 2 mm thickness require a 1- to 2-cm margin. Any melanoma with a Breslow thickness of >2 mm requires a 2-cm clinical margin. More aggressive margins than those recommended have not been demonstrated to improve survival. Conversely, margins may need to be compromised in sensitive areas to preserve function, for example, periocular melanoma.

- **Nonsurgical therapy**—although surgical excision is the standard of care for in situ melanoma, topical imiquimod may be considered particularly for melanoma in situ (MIS) or lentigo maligna (MIS on chronically UV-exposed skin such as the face) when surgical cure is not achievable.

- **Advanced melanoma**—the field of melanoma therapy is rapidly advancing owing to seminal discoveries in key signaling pathways in melanoma as well as advances in immunotherapy; thus, moderate- to high-risk (stage IIB to IIIC) and metastatic melanoma may benefit from referral to a multidisciplinary management team. Considerations for moderate- and high-risk, resected melanomas include adjuvant therapy with interferon or newer agents under investigation. Around 50% of melanomas harbor activating mutations at $BRAF^{V600}$, which render these tumors exquisitely sensitive to inhibitors of the mutant kinase—vemurafenib and dabrafenib. Combination of these with inhibitors of the downstream kinase mitogen-activated protein kinase (MEK) demonstrated improved survival over monotherapy.[12] Immunomodulatory therapies like the CTLA-4 antagonist ipilimumab and PD-1 antagonists pembrolizumab and nivolumab have demonstrated promising results, while combination cytotoxic T-lymphocyte–associated protein 4 (CTLA-4) and programmed cell death 1 (PD-1) antagonists are currently under study.[13]

- **Follow-up**—patients with a history of melanoma should be followed closely with comprehensive skin and lymph node examinations. They should be taught skin self-examination, as they are at increased risk for a second primary melanoma, as well as recurrence of disease. In addition, these patients need to be counseled regarding the daily use of a broad-spectrum sunscreen that blocks both UVA and UVB. Patients should also be taught sun avoidance strategies such as avoiding the midday sun (10 AM to 4 PM) and wearing protective clothing. Patients diagnosed with melanoma of any stage are not eligible to donate blood, tissue, or solid organs.

  - Patients with stage 0 melanoma should be followed with periodic skin examinations for life. Current recommendations for stage IA to stage IIA with no evidence of disease are to have a history and physical examination (H&P) every 6 to 12 months for the first 5 years, then annual skin examinations for life. Routine imaging is not recommended and should be considered only as the clinical scenario dictates. Patients with stage IIB and greater melanoma with no evidence of disease warrant clinical examination every 3 to 6 months for the first 2 years after diagnosis, then every 3 to 12 months for 3 years, and then annually. According to NCCN guidelines, radiographic evaluation with chest x-ray, CT, or PET-CT every 4 to 12 months, as well as a brain MRI every 12 months, may be considered to assess for metastatic or recurrent disease. Routine radiologic screening in stage IIB and higher is not recommended if rendered no evidence of disease after 5 years, unless symptoms warrant imaging.

4. CUTANEOUS T-CELL LYMPHOMA

- Cutaneous T-cell lymphomas (CTCL) are a heterogeneous group of non-Hodgkin lymphomas that primarily involve the skin, though blood and viscera may also be affected. The two variants discussed in detail in this section are the most common clinical subtypes for the generalist to recognize—together, mycosis fungoides (MF) and Sézary syndrome (SS) constitute roughly 53% of cases of CTCL.[14]

4.1. Background

- The median age for diagnosis of MF is between ages 55 and 60 years with a preponderance of male to female by 2:1. The etiology is not known but may be due to chronic antigenic stimulation resulting in expansion of T helper cells.[14,15]

4.2. Clinical Presentation

- MF and SS may mimic benign conditions like eczema, psoriasis, vitiligo, folliculitis, and others. The mushroom-like tumors of late-stage MF were first described in 1806 by Alibert.[15] Despite the name, the preponderance of clinical MF is patch and plaque early-stage disease (Fig. 8-4A). Progression to tumors often takes months or years, and in many cases, advanced disease never develops (Fig. 8-4B). Alternatively, MF may progress to erythroderma, or generalized redness of the skin, which signals advanced disease and is one of the diagnostic criteria for SS (Fig. 8-4C). MF and SS are thought to be separate entities with most cases of SS arising without preceding classical MF. The clinical staging of MF is assessed by the presence of the following:
  - **Patches**—nonindurated areas of erythema, hyperpigmentation, or hypopigmentation. These areas may develop scale and involve larger, though discrete, areas of the body.
  - **Plaques**—indurated areas of erythema, hyperpigmentation, or hypopigmentation. Plaque stage tends to have a more generalized distribution than does patch stage.
  - **Tumors**—nodular or exophytic growths >1 cm.
  - **Erythroderma**—generalized redness of skin. This can exist concomitantly with plaques or tumors and is often associated with severe pruritus.
- **Secondary clinical characteristics**—while not specific to MF, features may suggest this diagnosis including alopecia, follicular-centered papules, and poikiloderma (hyper- and hypopigmentation with telangiectasias with associated atrophy). Generalized erythema with ectropion or palmoplantar hyperkeratosis is more frequently associated with Sézary syndrome.

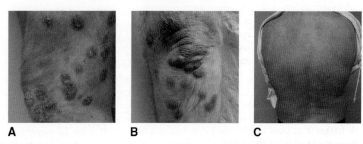

A   B   C

Figure 8-4. A: Scaly erythematous plaques of plaque stage MF. **B:** Erythematous nodules, some ulcerated in tumor stage MF. **C:** Erythroderma in a patient with SS.

4.3. Evaluation

- The most common scenario for initial presentation of MF is the patient with long-standing pruritic, nonspecific dermatitis in sun-protected areas that generally waxes and wanes but does not resolve despite repeated rounds of topical therapy. Clinical suspicion and careful clinicopathologic correlation is required to secure the diagnosis of MF, often requiring the integration of longitudinal clinical examinations, skin biopsies while off topical therapy, and laboratory evaluation. If there is clinical suspicion of CTCL, referral to a dermatologist with experience evaluating and treating this condition is strongly advised.

- **Physical examination**—full body skin and lymph node exam is required for accurate assessment and staging of disease. Determining the body surface area (BSA) involved by features discussed in the prior section will aid in staging.

- **Biopsy and laboratory examination**—in early-stage or erythrodermic MF, nondiagnostic biopsies are common. It may be helpful to acquire biopsies of different concurrent morphologies of the eruption as well as from anatomically distinct sites. If a single biopsy is done, it should be of the most indurated area. Repeated biopsies over time are indicated if CTCL remains the favored diagnosis despite nondiagnostic biopsies. Histopathologic examination is the cornerstone for diagnosis, while immunophenotyping and assessment of T-cell clonality are supportive.

  - **Histopathology**—larger, atypical lymphocytes with cerebriform nuclei infiltrate the upper dermis and may tag the dermal-epidermal junction or even aggregate in the epidermis (Pautrier microabscess).

  - **Immunophenotyping**—malignant cells typically express cluster of differentiation 3 (CD3) and CD4, while few cells will stain for CD8 and CD30. T-cell surface antigens CD2 and CD5 may be lost. Additionally, CD7, a marker for mature T cells, loss may be observed and may aid in distinguishing MF from a reactive lymphocytic infiltrate.

  - **T-cell receptor gene rearrangement studies**—polymerase chain reaction (PCR) analysis may be performed to assess clonality of the T-cell population in biopsy specimens. Caution is advised as nonmalignant conditions may demonstrate clonal T-cell populations, and conversely, not all CTCL has demonstrable clonality, particularly in low-stage MF.

- **Staging**—the International Society for Cutaneous Lymphomas and European Organization of Research and Treatment of Cancer (ISCL/EORTC) set revised guidelines for staging MF and SS type CTCL in 2007, based on the tumor, node, visceral metastasis, and blood (TNMB) involvement.[16] T staging represents patches or plaques<10% BSA (T1) or >10% BSA (T2), tumors (T3), or erythroderma (T4). Blood tumor burden with clonal population and Sézary cells at a concentration of 1,000 or greater cells per microliter (or its equivalent; see reference [16]) defines the B2 stage. Erythroderma and leukemic involvement of Sézary cells (T4B2) defines SS. Staging reflects prognosis with stage IA MF achieving life expectancy similar to matched control populations, while the 5-year survival for SS (stage IV) is 24%.[14]

4.4. Treatment

- Cutaneous T-cell lymphoma is a treatable, but not curable, disease. Early-stage MF (stages I to IIA) typically responds well to skin-directed therapies, including topical medications, light therapy, or total skin electron beam radiation therapy for extensive or recalcitrant disease.

- **Topical therapy**—midstrength or superpotent steroids, nitrogen mustards like mechlorethamine gel, and topical retinoids like bexarotene are effective as monotherapies for low-stage disease, or as adjuncts in higher-stage disease.
- **Light therapy**—narrowband UVB (NBUVB) and psoralen with UVA (PUVA) may provide long-term response in patch (NBUVB, PUVA) or plaque (PUVA) stage disease. Both treatments are typically administered multiple times a week with a slow taper based on clinical response.
- **Radiation therapy**—external beam radiation therapy (EBRT) is effective but is limited by systemic toxicity, including marrow suppression and more appropriate for localized tumor stage. Total skin electron beam therapy (TSEBT) results in 56% to 96% complete response with IA to IIA disease, though relapse rates are high (reviewed in Ref. 15). TSEBT may also be considered in generalized tumor stage.
- There is a wide array of treatment options for advanced stage MF and SS (stages IIB to IVB) with no sufficiently evidence-based treatment algorithms available.[17] Therapies range from oral retinoids to extracorporeal photopheresis, histone deacetylase inhibitors, interferons, single or multiagent chemotherapy, hematopoietic stem cell transplant, and investigational therapies. Benefits and risks of treatment approach are best addressed in the setting of a multidisciplinary specialty group including dermatology, oncology, and radiation oncology services.
- **Retinoids**—oral bexarotene at a dose of 300 mg/m^2 can be given as a monotherapy for refractory or advanced-stage MF (stages IIB to IVB). Central hypothyroidism, hypercholesterolemia, and hypertriglyceridemia are common side effects requiring concomitant management.
- **Histone deacetylase inhibitors**—include oral vorinostat and intravenous romidepsin, which are given either as monotherapy or in combination for refractory CTCL. The most common side effects include gastrointestinal disturbances. Romidepsin is also known to cause QT prolongation.

REFERENCES

1. Christenson L, Borrowman T, Vachon C, et al. Incidence of basal cell and squamous cell carcinomas in a population younger than 40 years. *JAMA* 2005;294(6):681–690.
2. Wehner M, Shive M, Chren M, et al. Indoor tanning and non-melanoma skin cancer: systematic review and meta-analysis. *BMJ* 2012;345:e5909.
3. Epstein E. Basal cell carcinomas: attack of the hedgehog. *Nat Rev Cancer* 2008;8(10):743–754.
4. Loo E, Mosterd K, Krekels G, et al. Surgical excision versus Mohs' micrographic surgery for basal cell carcinoma of the face: a randomised clinical trial with 10 year follow-up. *Eur J Cancer* 2014;50(17):3011–3020.
5. Sekulic A, Migden M, Oro A, et al. Efficacy and safety of vismodegib in advanced basal-cell carcinoma. *N Engl J Med* 2012;366(23):2171–2179.
6. Ratushny V, Gober M, Hick R, et al. From keratinocyte to cancer: the pathogenesis and modeling of cutaneous squamous cell carcinoma. *J Clin Invest* 2012;122(2):464–472.
7. Brantsch KD, Meisner C, Schönfisch B, et al. Analysis of risk factors determining prognosis of cutaneous squamous-cell carcinoma: a prospective study. *Lancet Oncol* 2008;9(8):713–720.
8. Harwood CA, Leedham-Green M, Leigh IM, et al. Low-dose retinoids in the prevention of cutaneous squamous cell carcinomas in organ transplant recipients: a 16-year retrospective study. *Arch Dermatol* 2005;141(4):456–464.
9. Bishop DT, Demenais F, Iles MM, et al. Genome-wide association study identifies three loci associated with melanoma risk. *Nat Genet* 2009;41(8):920–925.
10. Horn S, Figl A, Rachakonda PS, et al. TERT promoter mutations in familial and sporadic melanoma. *Science* 2013;339(6122):959–961.

11. Eggermont A. Randomized trials in melanoma; an update. *Surg Oncol Clin N Am* 2006;15(2):439–451.

12. Robert C, Karaszewska B, Schachter J, et al. Improved overall survival in melanoma with combined dabrafenib and trametinib. *N Engl J Med* 2015;372(1):30–39.

13. Wolchok J, Kluger H, Callahan M, et al. Nivolumab plus ipilimumab in advanced melanoma. *N Engl J Med* 2013;369(2):122–133.

14. Jawed S, Myskowski P, Horwitz S, et al. Primary cutaneous T-cell lymphoma (mycosis fungoides and Sézary syndrome): part I. Diagnosis: clinical and histopathologic features and new molecular and biologic markers. *J Am Acad Dermatol* 2014;70(2):205.e1205.e16.

15. Siegel RS, Pandolfino T, Guitart J, et al. Primary cutaneous T-cell lymphoma: review and current concepts. *J Clin Oncol* 2000;18(15):2908–2925.

16. Olsen E, Vonderheid E, Pimpinelli N, et al. Revisions to the staging and classification of mycosis fungoides and Sezary syndrome: a proposal of the International Society for Cutaneous Lymphomas (ISCL) and the cutaneous lymphoma task force of the European Organization of Research and Treatment of Cancer (EORTC). *Blood* 2007;110(6):1713–1722.

17. Jawed S, Myskowski P, Horwitz S, et al. Primary cutaneous T-cell lymphoma (mycosis fungoides and Sézary syndrome): part II. Prognosis, management, and future directions. *J Am Acad Dermatol* 2014;70(2):223.e1223.e17.

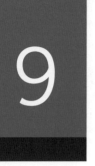

Disorders of the Hair and Nails

Katherine M. Moritz, MD and Ann G. Martin, MD

Disorders of the hair and nails are common dermatologic concerns, particularly of the female patient. While some of these conditions are idiopathic, others may signify an underlying systemic condition.

1. ANDROGENETIC ALOPECIA

- Progressive, androgen-dependent form of hair loss with distinctive patterns in males and females (Fig. 9-1)

1.1. Background
- Pathogenesis involves the conversion of terminal hairs into "miniaturized" or vellus hairs.
- 5-Alpha reductase is an enzyme in hair follicles that converts testosterone into dihydrotestosterone (DHT) and is implicated in the pathophysiology of androgenetic alopecia (AGA).
- Levels of 5-alpha reductase and DHT are increased in scalp hairs of men with AGA.[1]

1.2. Clinical Presentation
- "Male type" pattern usually involves thinning at frontotemporal and vertex scalp.
- "Female type" pattern typically preserves the anterior hairline and involves diffuse thinning at crown, often in a "Christmas tree" pattern.
- No inflammation is seen.

1.3. Evaluation
- Diagnosis is made by clinical history and examination.
  - Histopathology is not usually necessary except in women who present with an atypical pattern.
- Clinical history often includes a positive family history; however, a negative family history does not exclude the diagnosis.
- Associated comorbidities include metabolic disorder and benign prostatic hypertrophy; an association with cardiovascular disease remains controversial.[2]

1.4. Treatment
- Treatment of AGA is aimed at maintaining current hair density and does not return scalp to normal hair density or reverse areas of alopecia.

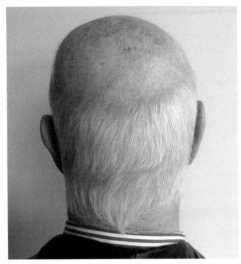

Figure 9-1. Androgenetic alopecia. (Courtesy of M. Laurin Council, MD.)

- Discontinuing effective treatment will cause progression of alopecia to the level it would have been without treatment.
- The two FDA-approved drugs for the treatment of AGA in men are topical 5% minoxidil applied 1 to 2 times daily and oral finasteride 1 mg qd.
- For female pattern hair loss, FDA-approved therapy includes both 2% and 5% topical minoxidil solution applied 1 to 2 times daily. The 5% concentration however demonstrated significantly superior efficacy over the 2% in a double-blind, placebo-controlled trial of 381 female patients with AGA.[3] Facial hypertrichosis is a more common side effect in women.
- See Table 9-1 for a list of most commonly used treatments.

Table 9-1	Treatments for Male and Female Pattern Hair Loss
Males	**Females**
Topical minoxidil 5%[a]	Topical minoxidil 2%[a] or 5%[a]
Finasteride 1 mg daily[a]	Finasteride 1 mg daily (in postmeno-
Dutasteride	pausal women)
Surgical treatment	Dutasteride 0.5–2.5 mg daily
Topical ketoconazole	Spironolactone 200 mg daily
Wigs, camouflages	Topical ketoconazole
	Surgical treatment
	Wigs, camouflages

[a]Indicates FDA approval for AGA.

2. ALOPECIA AREATA

- Nonscarring form of autoimmune alopecia mediated by T cells (Fig. 9-2).
- Alopecia areata (AA) has a lifetime prevalence of approximately 1.7%.[4]

2.1. Clinical Presentation

- Most commonly presents as round to oval, noncicatricial patches of alopecia, most commonly on scalp>beard>eyebrows>extremities.
  - Variable course, approximately 50% recover in 1 year without treatment; however, relapses are common.
  - Asymptomatic.
- Alopecia totalis is loss of all hair on the scalp; alopecia universalis is loss of all scalp and body hair.
  - Ophiasis pattern involves band-like alopecia in the parietooccipital scalp and is particularly refractory to treatment.
- May be associated with diffuse nail pitting as well as atopic disease and other autoimmune diseases.

2.2. Evaluation

- Diagnosis is usually based on clinical examination.
- Punch biopsy of acutely affected areas shows peribulbar mononuclear cell infiltrate.

2.3. Treatment

- Topical and intralesional corticosteroids are appropriate for patchy disease.
  - Intralesional triamcinolone acetonide 3 to 5 mg/mL can be injected every 4 to 8 weeks.
- Topical irritants such as anthralin 1% cream and topical immunotherapy such as squaric acid dibutyl ester may be first-line choices in treating widespread scalp involvement.
- Please refer to Table 9-2 for a more extensive list of treatments.

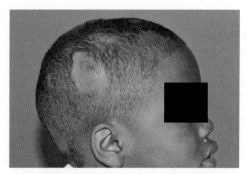

Figure 9-2. Alopecia areata. (Courtesy of Susan J. Bayliss, MD.)

Table 9-2	Treatments for Alopecia Areata

Topical and intralesional corticosteroids
Topical irritants (anthralin 1%)
Topical immunotherapy (squaric acid dibutyl ester and diphencyprone)
Topical minoxidil (2% and 5%)
PUVA (topical or oral)
Photodynamic therapy
Pulsed corticosteroids
Systemic cyclosporine
Targeted immunomodulators ("biologics")

3. TELOGEN EFFLUVIUM

• Excessive shedding of scalp hairs due to precipitating event

3.1. Background

• Hair loss normally occurs in an asynchronous manner to maintain a stable density of scalp hair.
• In telogen effluvium (TE), an inciting event drives an abnormally large amount of anagen (growing) phase hairs into telogen (resting) phase causing synchronous shedding.
  • Common causes include stress, surgery, fever, childbirth, infections, medications, and dietary changes.
  • See Table 9-3 for list of common causes of TE.

3.2. Clinical Presentation

• Diffuse hair loss usually begins approximately 3 months after particular stressor occurs and usually lasts for 3 to 6 months.

Table 9-3	Common Causes and Basic Laboratory Evaluation of Telogen Effluvium

Common causes	Lab workup
Stress	CBC, ferritin
Iron deficiency	ESR
Febrile illness	TSH
Postpartum	
Major surgery	
Hypothyroidism	
Malnutrition or crash diets	
Medications (includes initiation, cessation, or change in dose):	
• Oral contraceptives	
• Anticoagulants	
• Systemic retinoids	
• Anticonvulsants	
• Lithium	

- A chronic form of TE can affect women, usually age 30s to 60s, in which hair shedding may occur for years.
  - May be due to multifactorial causes; however, these patients generally have a good prognosis, and progression to baldness does not occur.

3.3. Evaluation
- If there is no clear cause, basic workup involves ruling out iron deficiency and hypothyroidism.

3.4. Treatment
- Treatment involves reassurance and eliminating any underlying cause if possible.
- Eventual hair regrowth can be expected.

4. ANAGEN EFFLUVIUM

- Diffuse loss of anagen (growth phase) hairs due to abrupt cessation of mitotic activity, most commonly from direct toxic effect from antineoplastic agents, radiation, or environmental toxins, particularly ingestion of heavy metals.[5]
- Given that 90% of human scalp hairs are in anagen phase at any time, a high volume of hair is rapidly lost, usually within a few weeks of insult.
- Treatment consists of reassurance and removal of toxin if possible.

5. TRICHOTILLOMANIA

- Impulse control disorder with repetitive self-induced manipulation of hair from scalp, eyebrows, eyelashes, beard, or other areas of the body (Fig. 9-3)
- Pts pull out or twist off hairs
- Can be an isolated disorder or part of an obsessive-compulsive disorder
- More common in females

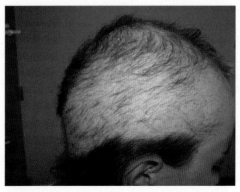

Figure 9-3. Trichotillomania. (Courtesy of Susan J. Bayliss, MD.)

5.1. Clinical Findings
- Single or multiple well-defined patches of alopecia, often with a geometric pattern
- Contain broken hairs of various lengths

5.2. Evaluation
- Diagnosis is by clinical history and exam.
- Punch biopsy may reveal hair casts, perifollicular hemorrhage, and a predominance of catagen hairs.

5.3. Treatment
- Treatment is difficult and involves specialized behavioral modification therapy.
- SSRIs and clomipramine have been used with partial success.[6]

6. CENTRAL CENTRIFUGAL CICATRICIAL ALOPECIA

- Most common form of scarring alopecia among black patients (Fig. 9-4)

6.1. Background
- Pathogenesis involves predisposition toward premature desquamation of the follicular internal root sheath.[7]
- Damage to the already abnormal hair follicle is exacerbated by use of chemical or thermal relaxers and straighteners.

6.2. Clinical Presentation
- Scarring alopecia of the crown and vertex scalp that progresses centrifugally from the center of the scalp.
  - Active inflammation in roughly circular perimeter surrounding central patch of alopecia.
- Often asymptomatic, however can be associated with burning and itching.
- Loss of follicular ostia is a marker of the cicatricial nature of the disease, and scattered tufted hairs are often seen within the alopecic area.
- Disease usually slowly progresses despite cessation of harsh hair care practices.

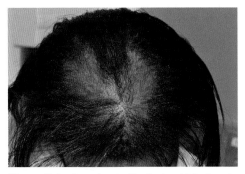

Figure 9-4. Central centrifugal cicatricial alopecia. (Courtesy of Susan J. Bayliss, MD.)

6.3. Evaluation

- Diagnosis is made by clinical history and exam.
- A punch biopsy should be done at the periphery of the spreading alopecic plaque where the active inflammation is occurring.

6.4. Treatment

- High-potency topical steroids may be first-line treatment, such as clobetasol propionate 0.05% solution or fluocinonide 0.05% solution applied twice daily to active areas.
- Monthly injections of triamcinolone acetonide 3 to 5 mg/mL to the hair-bearing areas surrounding the central alopecic patch help halt active inflammation.
- Topical or intralesional corticosteroids are usually given in conjunction with a tetracycline antibiotic such as doxycycline hyclate 50 to 100 mg b.i.d. for several months.
- Highly inflammatory or purulent cases may be due to bacterial superinfection and require antistaphylococcal therapy.

7. DISCOID LUPUS ERYTHEMATOSUS (SEE CHAPTER 10)

- Form of chronic cutaneous lupus erythematosus that often causes scarring alopecia
  - Majority of patients do not have systemic involvement; however, approximately 10% of patients will progress to develop systemic disease.

7.1. Background

- Pathogenesis of discoid lupus erythematosus (DLE) is unknown but involves perivascular and periadnexal lymphocytic inflammation and may be an immunologic reaction to an unknown antigenic trigger.

7.2. Clinical Presentation

- Patients present with erythematous alopecic plaques with follicular plugging and occasional scale on scalp, face, ears, neck, and other sun-exposed areas.
  - Progresses to depigmented, scarred atrophic plaques
- Pruritus and tenderness of lesions are common.

7.3. Evaluation

- Diagnosis requires histologic confirmation and cannot be made by clinical exam alone.
  - Punch biopsy should be done in area of active erythema, avoiding scarred or depigmented areas.
- A complete blood count, creatinine, urinalysis, antinuclear antibodies, and extractable nuclear antigens should be checked upon initial evaluation.

7.4. Treatment

- High-potency topical steroids and intralesional corticosteroids may be used as first-line treatment.
- Antimalarials such as hydroxychloroquine and chloroquine are often used in conjunction with topical corticosteroids.
- Strict avoidance of sun exposure as well as smoking cessation are imperative for treatment success.
  - See Table 9-4 for list of therapies.

Table 9-4	Treatments for Discoid Lupus Erythematosus

High-potency topical corticosteroids
- Clobetasol propionate 0.05% solution or ointment b.i.d.
- Fluocinonide 0.05% solution b.i.d.

Triamcinolone acetonide 3–5 mg/cc injections q 4–6 wk
Antimalarials
- Hydroxychloroquine 200 mg b.i.d. (6.5 mg/kg/d)
- Chloroquine (4.5 mg/kg/d)
- Quinacrine 100 mg qd

Other:
Retinoids such as acitretin
Dapsone
Thalidomide
Methotrexate
Mycophenolate mofetil

8. LICHEN PLANOPILARIS

- Follicular variant of lichen planus that results in a scarring alopecia (Fig. 9-5)

8.1. Background
- More common in females than males
- More common in Caucasians

8.2. Clinical Presentation
- In the early stages of classic lichen planopilaris (LPP), patients complain of increased hair loss, scalp pruritus, and tenderness.
- Patchy alopecia of the frontal and vertex scalp with perifollicular erythema and follicular hyperkeratosis is most common, progressing eventually into scarred plaques with surrounding active inflammation.
- Up to 50% of patients will exhibit lichen planus-type lesions elsewhere on the skin at some point in the disease process.
- The frontal fibrosing variant demonstrates the above clinical features but stays limited to the anterior and temporal hairlines and is most common in postmenopausal Caucasian women.
  - Loss of eyebrows is common.

8.3. Evaluation
- Diagnosis requires histologic confirmation.
  - A punch biopsy should be taken at the edge of the alopecic plaque where the inflammation is most prominent.

8.4. Treatment
- Treatment of LPP can be difficult, and subtle disease progression may occur in the absence of clinical signs of inflammation.[8]
  - See Table 9-5 for treatment options.

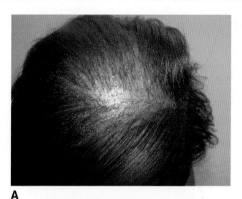

A

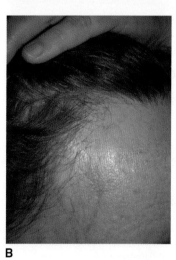

B

Figure 9-5. A: Lichen planopilaris, classic. **B:** Lichen planopilaris, frontal fibrosing variant. (**A,** courtesy of Susan J. Bayliss, MD; **B,** courtesy of Susan J. Bayliss, MD.)

Table 9-5	Treatment of Lichen Planopilaris and Frontal Fibrosing Alopecia

High-potency topical corticosteroids
• Clobetasol propionate 0.05% solution or ointment b.i.d.
• Fluocinonide 0.05% solution b.i.d.
Triamcinolone acetonide 3–5 mg/mL injections q 4–6 wk
Hydroxychloroquine 200 mg b.i.d. (6.5 mg/kg/d)
Minocycline 100 mg b.i.d.
Topical minoxidil 2%–5% b.i.d.
Pioglitazone hydrochloride
Acitretin

9. DISSECTING CELLULITIS

- Chronic and relapsing suppurative disease of the scalp (Fig. 9-6)
  - Evolves to scarring alopecia
- Commonly presents in young black males in 20s to 30s

9.1. Background

- Pathogenesis involves follicular hyperkeratosis with retention of keratin, predisposing to bacterial superinfection and follicular rupture. Keratin debris in the dermis leads to a foreign body–type reaction and eventual scarring.
- Dissecting cellulitis is considered part of the "follicular occlusion tetrad" along with hidradenitis suppurativa, acne conglobata, and pilonidal cysts.[4]

9.2. Clinical Presentation

- Fluctuant nodules and plaques with draining sinus tracts that eventually progress to scarring and hair loss
- Can be painful or asymptomatic

9.3. Evaluation

- Diagnosis is based on clinical history and exam.

9.4. Treatment

- First-line treatment is oral isotretinoin 1 mg/kg daily for 6 to 12 months.[8]
  - Can be used in conjunction with intralesional injections of triamcinolone acetonide (10 to 40 mg/mL)
- Other treatments include oral antibiotics such as doxycycline hyclate 100 mg b.i.d.

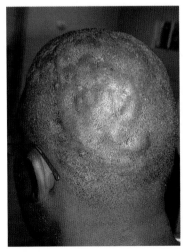

Figure 9-6. Dissecting cellulitis. (Courtesy of Susan J. Bayliss, MD.)

10. FOLLICULITIS DECALVANS

• Highly inflammatory form of scarring alopecia most commonly seen in young to middle-aged adults

10.1. Background

• *Staphylococcus aureus* and an abnormal host immune response are thought to be driving factors in the pathogenesis of this disorder.[9]

10.2. Clinical Presentation

• Begins as a painful and purulent folliculitis most prominent on vertex and occipital scalp that progresses to boggy scarred plaques of alopecia.
  • Tufting of hairs within scars as well as hemorrhagic crusts and erosions may be seen.

10.3. Evaluation

• Bacterial culture swab of the scalp or an intact pustule is recommended to rule out staph infection.
• Punch biopsy at the hair-bearing periphery of an active area shows a neutrophilic inflammatory infiltrate.

10.4. Treatment

• Treatment is directed at eradicating *S. aureus* infection and controlling inflammation.
  • Rifampicin 300 mg b.i.d. along with clindamycin 300 mg b.i.d. × 10 to 12 weeks has been reported to be successful.
  • Long-term doxycycline (100 mg b.i.d.) may be needed to suppress disease activity.
  • PO antibiotics can be used in conjunction with class I or II topical corticosteroids such as clobetasol 0.05% solution b.i.d. or intralesional triamcinolone acetonide 10 mg/mL injections q 4–6 w.

11. SECONDARY SCARRING ALOPECIAS

• Deep burns
• Radiation dermatitis
• Cutaneous sarcoidosis
• Cutaneous malignancies, both primary and metastatic
• Infections, including bacterial and fungal

12. HYPERTRICHOSIS

• Excessive hair growth that may be generalized or local. It may also be inherited or acquired. The excess hair may be lanugo, vellus, or terminal. Lanugo hair is the fine, nonpigmented downy hair that is normally shed in utero or in neonatal period.

Table 9-6	Common Causes of Hypertrichosis

Congenital forms:

Porphyrias (can be acquired as in pseudoporphyria)
- Sun-exposed areas

Universal hypertrichosis
- Rare, autosomal dominant

Congenital hypertrichosis lanuginosa
- Rare, autosomal dominant

Becker nevus
- Congenital hamartoma of upper trunk, usually in males
- Hyperpigmented patch that develops hypertrichosis after puberty

Acquired forms:

Acquired hypertrichosis lanuginosa
- Paraneoplastic disorder associated with lung, colon, and breast cancer
- May be accompanied by fissured tongue

Drug induced:
- Phenytoin
- Cyclosporine
- Minoxidil
- Diazoxide
- Streptomycin
- Glucocorticosteroids
- Psoralens
- Interferon alpha
- EGFR inhibitors

Malnutrition (anorexia nervosa)
Repeated friction, trauma, or inflammation (e.g., under a cast)
Posttraumatic brain injury

- Congenital forms of hypertrichosis are very rare. More commonly seen are acquired variants, often as side effects of medications (Table 9-6).

13. HIRSUTISM

- Excess growth of terminal hair in a male pattern in female patients
- Indicative of androgen excess and affects approximately 5% of women of reproductive age.[10]

13.1. Background

- The source of the excess androgens is most often ovarian or adrenal; however, female patients may have features of hirsutism in the absence of significant hormonal imbalance, that is, constitutional hirsutism.
  - SAHA syndrome (seborrhea, acne, hirsutism, alopecia) may be an isolated clinical finding.
- See Table 9-7 for a list of causes of hirsutism.

13.2. Clinical Presentation

- Hirsutism may be accompanied by other signs of virilization such as acne, male pattern AGA, oligo- or amenorrhea, and increased muscle mass.

Table 9-7	Causes of Hirsutism

Ovarian causes:
- Polycystic ovarian syndrome
- Ovarian tumors
- Ovarian hyperthecosis

Adrenal causes:
- Congenital adrenal hyperplasia
- Adrenal tumors
- Hypercortisolism (Cushing syndrome)

Iatrogenic:
- Anabolic steroids (danazol)
- Glucocorticoids
- Oral contraceptives with progesterone

Hyperprolactinemia
Acromegaly
Severe insulin resistance

- An adrenal cause of hirsutism should be considered in any female pt presenting with terminal hair growth in a central distribution—anterior neck to upper pubic area.
- An ovarian cause of hirsutism usually presents with lateral distribution of hair growth (sides of face, neck, and on breasts) and may be accompanied by menstrual abnormalities and obesity.

13.3. Evaluation
- A thorough clinical history should be taken, taking into account the patient's age, ethnicity, medications, family history of hirsutism, and menstrual cycles.
- Physical exam should look for signs of virilization, peripheral hyperandrogenism, and insulin resistance.
- Basic laboratory evaluation should include total and free testosterone as well as DHEA-S, prolactin, and Δ-4-androstenedione.
  - DHEA-S is a marker of adrenal gland androgens.
  - Δ-4-androstenedione is indicative of an ovarian source of androgens.
- If significant abnormalities are found, referral to an endocrinologist or gynecologic endocrinologist should be considered.

14. NAIL DISORDERS

- The nails often give many diagnostic clues about a patient's underlying health status, including inflammatory, traumatic, environmental, neoplastic, drug-induced, and psychiatric disease[11,12] (Table 9-8).
- Involvement of all or most of the fingernails and/or toenails indicates a systemic cause of dystrophy, while involvement of one or two nails usually suggests exogenous source of injury, neoplasm, or local infection.

Table 9-8	Common Nail Signs		
Nail disorder	**Physical finding**	**Causes and associated diseases**	**Image**
Beau lines	Transverse depression of nail plate due to temporary decrease in mitosis in nail matrix	*Multiple nails:* may be due to severe systemic illness, drug, high fever, viral infection *Single nail:* trauma to matrix or paronychia	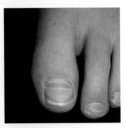
Onychomadesis	Proximal shedding of nail	*Multiple nails:* usually due to systemic illness, high fever *Single nail:* most often traumatic or paronychia	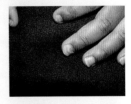
Pitting	Multiple punctate depressions of nail plate	Psoriasis: irregular pitting often in association with oil spots and onycholysis Pitting also can be seen in AA	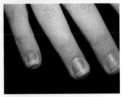
Onychorrhexis	Nail brittleness and fragility in longitudinal direction	May be due to severe nail dryness and often is normal finding in older patients Can be seen with lichen planus	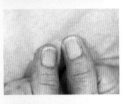
Leukonychia	White discoloration of nail due to either nail bed abnormalities *(apparent leukonychia)* or nail plate abnormalities *(true leukonychia)*	*Terry nails:* apparent leukonychia of proximal 2/3 of nail associated with liver cirrhosis *Half and half nails:* proximal half of nail is white, common in hemodialysis patients *Muehrcke lines:* transverse white bands often seen with cirrhosis or due to chemotherapy	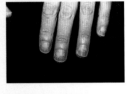

continued on following page

Nail disorder	Physical finding	Causes and associated diseases	Image
Trachyonychia (20-nail dystrophy)	Rough, sandpapered appearance of all 20 nails	Most commonly associated with AA, also seen with lichen planus, psoriasis, or eczema	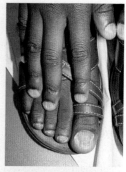
Onycholysis	Detachment of distal nail plate	Trauma, psoriasis, onychomycosis, tumors (solitary affected nail), or drug induced • Tetracyclines (often after exposure to UV light) • Fluoroquinolones • Psoralens • NSAIDs	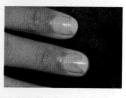
Subungual hyperkeratosis	Accumulation of keratin debris under nail causing detachment and thickening of nail	Onychomycosis, psoriasis, trauma	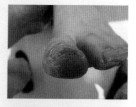
Paronychia	Erythema, swelling, and pain of nail folds, usually absent cuticle	Acute paronychia: often one nail affected, due to bacterial infection Chronic paronychia: often one or more nails due to chronic irritation from manicures, exposure to water, often with yeast colonization Other causes: EGFR inhibitors, retinoids, indinavir	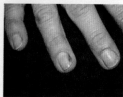

Nail disorder	Physical finding	Causes and associated diseases	Image
Green nail syndrome	Green-brown discoloration of nail due to pyocyanin pigment produced by *Pseudomonas aeruginosa* infection Often with onycholysis and paronychia	Predisposing factors include prolonged exposure to water, trauma, health care work. Treatment includes 4% thymol iodide in absolute alcohol applied to nail b.i.d. and dilute acetic acid soaks	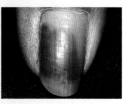
Longitudinal melanonychia	Brown-black pigmented streak on nail, common in dark-skinned patients	*Multiple streaks:* may be due to medications or systemic disease *Single streak:* may be due to subungual nevus or melanocyte hyperplasia, need to rule out subungual melanoma	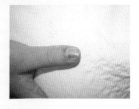
Subungual malignant melanoma	May present as brown-black longitudinal streak, often irregular, or subungual pigmented ulcer, or amelanotic lesion resembling a pyogenic granuloma	*Hutchinson sign:* extension of pigmentation onto periungual skin, suggestive of melanoma when seen with longitudinal melanonychia	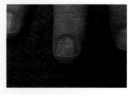

Onychorrhexis image from Mohr WK. *Psychiatric-mental health nursing.* 8th ed. Philadelphia, PA: Wolters Kluwer Health; 2013; Green Nail Syndrome image from: Goodheart HP, Gonzalez ME. *Goodheart's photoguide to common pediatric and adult skin disorders.* 4th ed. Philadelphia, PA: Wolters Kluwer Health; 2016.
Images courtesy of David Sheinbein, MD, Susan Bayliss, MD, and M. Laurin Council, MD.

REFERENCES

1. Sawaya ME, Price VH. Different levels of 5alpha-reductase type I and II, aromatase, and androgen receptor in hair follicles of women and men with androgenetic alopecia. *J Invest Dermatol* 1997;109:296–300.
2. Arias-Santiago S, et al. Male androgenetic alopecia. In: Preedy VR, ed. *Handbook of hair in health and disease*. The Netherlands: Wageningen Academic Publishers; 2012:98–116.
3. Lucky AW, Piacquadio DJ, Ditre CM, et al. A randomized, placebo-controlled trial of 5% and 2% topical minoxidil solutions in the treatment of female pattern hair loss. *J Am Acad Dermatol* 2004;50(4):541–553.
4. Sperling LC, Sinclair RD, El Shabrawi-Caelen L. Alopecias. In: Bolognia J, et al., eds. *Dermatology*. 3rd ed. Philadelphia, PA: Elsevier Saunders; 2012:1093–1109.
5. Trueb RM. Diffuse hair loss. In: Blume-Peytavi U, et al. *Hair growth and disorders*. Leipzig, Germany: Springer; 2008:259–272.
6. Ravindran AV, da Silva TL, Ravindran LN, et al. Obsessive-compulsive spectrum disorders: a reviewed of the evidence-based treatments. *Can J Psychiatry* 2009;54:331–343.
7. Gathers RC, Lim HW. Central centrifugal cicatricial alopecia: past, present, and future. *J Am Acad Dermatol* 2009;60(4):660–668.
8. Harries MJ, Sinclair RD, et al. Management of primary cicatricial alopecias: options for treatment. *Br J Dermatol* 2008;159(1):1–22.
9. Otberg N, Kang H, Alzolibani AA, Shapiro J. Folliculitis decalvans. *Dermatol Ther* 2008;21:238–244.
10. Camacho-Martinez FM. Hypertrichosis and hirsutism. In: Bolognia J, et al., eds. *Dermatology*. 3rd ed. Philadelphia, PA: Elsevier Saunders; 2012:1115–1127.
11. Piraccini BM. *Nail disorders: a practical guide to diagnosis and management*. Italy: Springer; 2014.
12. Tosti A, Piraccini BM. Nail disorders. In: Bolognia J, et al., eds. *Dermatology*. 3rd ed. Philadelphia, PA: Elsevier Saunders; 2012:1129–1144.

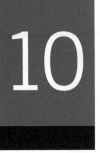

10 Cutaneous Manifestations of Systemic Disease

Urvi Patel, MD and Amy Musiek, MD

It is important to not think of the skin as an isolated organ. Many systemic disorders have an associated skin involvement including autoimmune connective tissue disease and sarcoidosis, where cutaneous signs can aid in diagnosis. There are also primary skin conditions with secondary systemic involvement such as autoimmune blistering disease. Examples of these and further evaluation and management are reviewed here.

1. LUPUS

1.1. Background[1,2]
- Multisystem autoimmune disorder, characterized by presence of multiple antibodies.
- Skin involvement can be seen in up to 85% of patients with lupus; cutaneous signs make up four of the major criteria of systemic lupus erythematosus (SLE).
- Cutaneous lupus can be subdivided into three categories: acute, subacute, and chronic. Chronic cutaneous lupus contains multiple subtypes, including discoid lupus, that have different clinical manifestations.

1.2. Clinical Presentation
- Acute cutaneous lupus erythematosus (ACLE)
  - Bilateral malar erythema, classically sparing the nasolabial folds following sun exposure
  - May also occur as a generalized photosensitive eruption, often involving the extensor forearms and dorsal hands
  - Is a manifestation of SLE
- Subacute cutaneous lupus erythematosus (SCLE) (Fig. 10-1)
  - Annular pink, scaly plaques, typically photodistributed on the upper chest and back.
  - Drug-induced variant: known drug triggers include hydrochlorothiazide, terbinafine, calcium channel blockers, nonsteroidal anti-inflammatory drugs (e.g., naproxen), griseofulvin, and antihistamines.
  - Neonatal lupus is a form of SCLE in neonates that can occur in mothers with anti-SSA antibodies. The eruption is similar to that of SCLE, with a predilection for the scalp and periorbital areas. Internal organ involvement can be seen with congenital heart block (with a mortality of 20% if untreated), hepatobiliary disease, and thrombocytopenia.

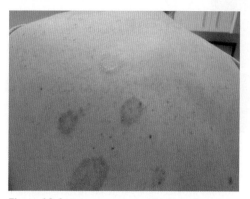

Figure 10-1. Subacute cutaneous lupus erythematosus. Nonscarring, erythematous, scaly, annular plaques on the back.

- Chronic lupus erythematous
  - Discoid lupus erythematosus (DLE) (Fig. 10-2): indurated, erythematous thin papules and plaques with adherent scale on the face, scalp, and/or ears. Lesions heal with scarring, and 25% of patients can have oral involvement. There is increased risk of developing squamous cell carcinoma in scars or chronically inflamed lesions.

1.3. Evaluation

- Skin biopsy can help differentiate cutaneous lupus from other skin disorders.
- Each subtype of lupus has a varying risk of developing systemic lupus.
- Blood tests
  - Acute lupus erythematosus
    - Antinuclear antibody (ANA), double-stranded DNA (dsDNA), Sjogren syndrome–related antigen A and B (SS-A and SS-B), Smith antibody, U1 small nuclear ribonucleoprotein (U1RNP), histone antibodies, complete blood

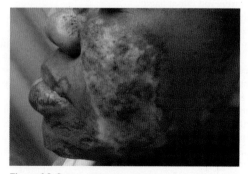

Figure 10-2. Discoid lupus erythematosus. Erythematous to hyperpigmented plaques with central scarring and atrophy.

count (CBC), complete metabolic panel (CMP), urinalysis (UA), and complement levels
- Subacute cutaneous lupus erythematosus
  - ANA, SS-A, and SS-B.
  - 18% to 50% of patient will possess the criteria for SLE.[3]
- Discoid lupus erythematosus
  - ANA often negative
  - 5% to 15% risk of developing SLE

1.4. Treatment[4]

- Lifestyle: strict photoprotection and smoking cessation.
- First-line agents: topical or intralesional steroids, class 1 steroid often required.
- Antimalarial agents are standard of care when systemic therapy is needed.
  - First line: hydroxychloroquine at 200 mg twice a day for most patients.
  - Alternative: chloroquine.
  - Quinacrine may be added to either of the above agents.
- Antimalarial-resistant lupus
  - Methotrexate
  - Thalidomide
  - Mycophenolate mofetil
  - Dapsone

2. DERMATOMYOSITIS

2.1. Background[5]

- Autoimmune inflammatory myopathy with cutaneous findings and systemic involvement, currently with unknown pathogenesis.
- Skin manifestations and pathogenic autoantibodies can help differentiate dermatomyositis (DM) from other autoimmune disorders as well as different subtypes of DM.

2.2. Clinical Presentation

- Classic dermatomyositis (Fig. 10-3)
  - Gottron papules: violaceous papules overlying the dorsal interphalangeal or metacarpophalangeal, elbow, or knee joints
  - Linear extensor erythema: erythema running along the extensor tendons on the hands
  - Heliotrope rash: violaceous erythema and edema involving the periorbital region and eyelids
  - Shawl sign: pink poikiloderma across the upper back
  - V-distributed erythema: photodistributed pink and erythematous patches on the mid- to upper chest
  - Holster sign: erythematous patches on the hips
  - Mechanic's hands: erythematous, scaly, hyperkeratotic papules and plaques on the palms and lateral surfaces with fissuring
  - Periungual telangiectasias and "ragged" cuticles
  - Calcinosis cutis

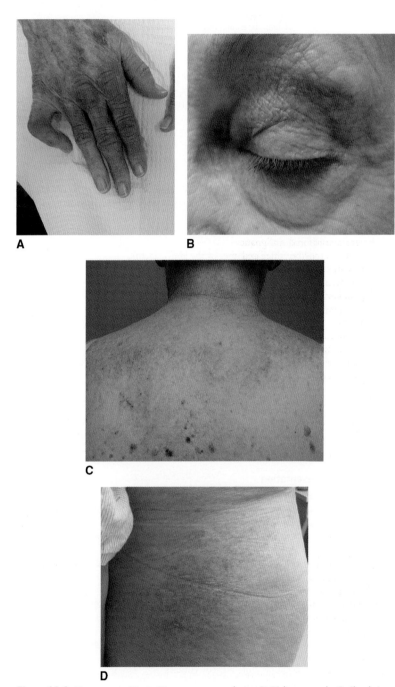

Figure 10-3. Dermatomyositis. **A:** Linear extensor erythema. **B:** Heliotrope rash. **C:** Shawl sign. **D:** Holster sign.

- Antisynthetase syndrome[6]
  - Mechanic's hands: most characteristic finding of antisynthetase syndrome
  - Other cutaneous features: Gottron papules and Raynaud phenomenon.
  - Extracutaneous findings: interstitial lung disease (ILD), arthritis, myositis, and fever
  - Associated antibodies: to aminoacyl-transfer ribonucleic acid (tRNA) synthetases, including Jo-1, OJ, KJ, PL-7, and PL-12
- Amyopathic dermatomyositis
  - Typical skin findings noted above, without the findings of muscle involvement within 6 months after onset of skin findings.
  - Associated antibodies: transcriptional intermediary factor 1-γ antibody (TIFI-γ; 80% of patients) and clinically amyopathic dermatomyositis-40 (CADM-140) antibodies (10% to 15% of patients). Those with CADM-140 antibodies have a risk of severe, progressive ILD that can lead to death from respiratory failure.
- Dermatomyositis and malignancy[7,8]
  - In adults, there is an increased risk (5% to 7%) of developing a malignancy.
  - Most common malignancies: ovarian, lung, pancreatic, stomach, and colorectal carcinomas.
  - Can present anywhere from 2 years preceding to 3 years after presentation of DM.
  - Poorer prognostic factors include older age, male, cutaneous ulceration, and dysphagia.
  - Associated antibodies: TIF1-γ (formerly known as p-155).
- Extracutaneous involvement
  - Musculoskeletal: symmetric, proximal muscle weakness initially, but can progress to all muscle groups
  - Pulmonary: ILD, pulmonary hypertension, and pneumothorax
  - Gastrointestinal: dysphagia secondary to pharyngeal muscle involvement, esophageal reflux, and dysmotility
  - Cardiac: arrhythmias and conduction defects
- Drug induced[9]
  - Hydroxyurea and statins are the most common culprits.

2.3. Evaluation[5]

- Skin biopsy can help point toward a diagnosis of DM.
- Muscle involvement: serum creatinine kinase and aldolase, EMG, MRI, and muscle biopsy.
- Serology testing
  - ANA positive <10% of the time
  - Other myositis antibodies (as above) may be helpful, but they are not always widely available.
- Refer for pulmonary function testing to evaluate for ILD.
- Physical exam and history, age-appropriate malignancy screening, and computed tomography scan (CT scan) of the chest, abdomen, and pelvis in patient at risk for malignancy.

2.4. Treatment[5]

- Muscle disease is more responsive to treatment than is cutaneous disease.
- Initial (acute) therapy: corticosteroids.

- Steroid-sparing agents
  - First line: hydroxychloroquine—helpful for cutaneous disease, questionable efficacy for muscle disease
  - Second line: methotrexate, azathioprine, mycophenolate mofetil, intravenous immunoglobulin, rituximab

3. SARCOIDOSIS

3.1. Background[10]

- A chronic, granulomatous multisystem disorder with unclear etiology.
- Cutaneous disease is present in at least 20% of patients and can be the initial sign in one-third of these patients.
- Ninety to ninety-five percent of patient with skin disease will have pulmonary involvement.
- Cutaneous manifestations can vary greatly.

3.2. Clinical Presentation

- Classically red-brown to violaceous indurated papules and plaques (Fig. 10-4).
- Lupus pernio
  - Violaceous papules and plaques favoring the nose, ears, and cheeks. The classic presentation is a beaded appearance around the nasal rim.
  - Association with chronic sarcoidosis of the lungs (~75% of patients) and of the upper respiratory tract (~50% of patients).
  - Can heal with scarring.
- Papular sarcoidosis
  - Skin-colored papules typically on the face, specifically on the eyelid and nasolabial folds, that heals without scarring
  - Favorable disease prognosis
- Darier-Roussy
  - Skin-colored, subcutaneous, firm, mobile nodules on the extremities; usually painless (differentiating it from erythema nodosum)

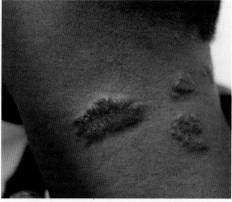

Figure 10-4. Sarcoid. Hyperpigmented, dermal plaques.

- Lofgren syndrome
  - Acute form of sarcoidosis that includes erythema nodosum, polyarthralgias, and bilateral hilar lymphadenopathy
- Scar sarcoidosis
  - Infiltration of sarcoidal granulomas in previous surgical sites, tattoos, piercings, and other sites of trauma
- Higher incidence in African Americans and women.
- African Americans have more severe disease.
- Japanese patients are more likely to have cardiac and ocular involvement.

3.3. Evaluation

- Skin biopsy should show noncaseating granulomas with no or sparse surrounding inflammation.
- Labs: CMP, serum calcium, 1,25 dihydroxyvitamin D, and angiotensin-converting enzyme level (may decline with therapy, but does not have prognostic value).
- Chest x-ray or high-resolution CT scan of the chest to determine nodal and parenchymal involvement.
- Pulmonary function testing and carbon monoxide diffusion capacity.
- Electrocardiogram to evaluate cardiac involvement.

3.4. Treatment

- Topical and intralesional steroids for limited cutaneous involvement
- Systemic steroids for widespread or disfiguring involvement
- Hydroxychloroquine, methotrexate, tetracyclines, and TNF-alpha inhibitors for maintenance

4. SCLERODERMA AND RELATED DISORDERS

4.1. Background

- Scleroderma describes fibrosis of the dermis and subcutaneous tissue. Scleroderma can be classified as either localized cutaneous disease or cutaneous with systemic disease.
- Morphea is also known as localized scleroderma. It is generally self-limiting and typically appears as solitary and linear plaques.[11]
- Systemic sclerosis includes both limited scleroderma (CREST) and progressive systemic sclerosis.[12]
- Lichen sclerosus et atrophicus (LSA) is another inflammatory skin disorder that affects superficial dermis and mucosa leading to atrophic scarring.[13]

4.2. Clinical Presentation

- Morphea[11]
  - Begins as erythematous to violaceous plaques that evolve into white, sclerotic plaques and will resolve as hyperpigmented atrophic plaques
- Scleroderma[12]
  - Limited scleroderma (CREST)
    ○ Calcinosis cutis, Raynaud phenomenon, esophageal dysmotility, sclerodactyly, telangiectasia
  - Progressive systemic sclerosis
    ○ Hallmarks are sclerodactyly and digital pitting scars.

- o Other features include taut and waxy skin, calcinosis cutis, nail fold capillary changes, mat-like telangiectasias, Raynaud phenomenon, and salt and pepper dyspigmentation.
- o Morbidity and mortality are from pulmonary, renal, cardiac, and gastrointestinal involvement.
- The physician should differentiate between morphea and systemic sclerosis. Systemic involvement, sclerodactyly, nail fold changes, and Raynaud phenomenon are not seen in morphea but are seen in systemic sclerosis.
- Lichen sclerosus et atrophicus[13] (LSA)
  - Erythematous patches that evolve into atrophic white plaques. Lesions are more commonly located in the anogenital area and can have significant pruritus.
  - This can be complicated by fissuring, fusion of labia minora to majora, introital narrowing, phimosis, dyspareunia, and dysuria.
  - Increased risk of developing squamous cell carcinoma in anogenital lesions.
  - Women with genital LSA should have alternate evaluations with dermatology and gynecology.

4.3. Evaluation
- These are clinical diagnoses, where skin biopsies can be supportive but not diagnostic among this group of disorders.
- No further evaluation for LSA and morphea.
- Systemic sclerosis[12]
  - ANA, anticentromere antibody (CREST), and antitopoisomerase I (aka Scl-70) antibodies
  - Pulmonary involvement: chest x-ray, pulmonary function testing, and high-resolution CT
  - Gastrointestinal involvement: esophagogram, esophagoduodenoscopy, and small bowel series

4.4. Treatment
- Morphea[14]
  - First line: topical steroids and topical calcineurin inhibitors
  - Refractory disease: phototherapy and methotrexate
  - Physical therapy in the case of contractures
- Scleroderma[12]
  - No agent reverses the process. Disease-modifying agents that have been used with mixed success include methotrexate and cyclophosphamide. In the most severe cases, stem cell transplantation has also been used in clinical trials, but currently is not the standard of care.
  - Proton pump inhibitors and/or H_2 blocker for GERD symptoms. Esophageal strictures may need esophageal dilation. Metoclopramide and erythromycin can promote upper GI motility. Octreotide is useful to lower GI motility.
  - Angiotensin-converting enzyme inhibitors to prevent scleroderma renal crisis.
  - Prostacyclin analogs, bosentan, and sildenafil have been used for pulmonary hypertension.
  - Treatment of digital ulceration includes proper wound care and treatment of bacterial superinfections.
- Lichen sclerosus at atrophicus[13]
  - First line: topical steroids and topical calcineurin inhibitors
  - Second line: phototherapy

5. BULLOUS DISORDERS

5.1. Background

- A heterogeneous group of acquired disorders consisting of bullous cutaneous findings secondary to autoantibodies to antigens in the epidermis and basement membrane
- Pemphigus vulgaris (PV) and pemphigus foliaceus (PF)[15]
  - Due to IgG autoantibodies to proteins important in cell to cell adhesion
    PF: Desmoglein 1
    PV: Desmoglein 3
- Bullous pemphigoid (BP)[16]
  - Most common immunobullous disorder, typically affecting the elderly (Fig. 10-5)
  - Antibodies to bullous pemphigus (BP) antigen 230 (aka BPAg1) and BP antigen 180 (BPAg2) located in the basement membrane

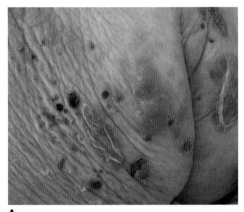

A

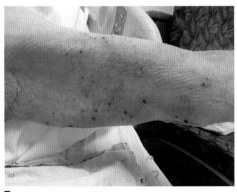

B

Figure 10-5. Bullous pemphigoid. **A:** Erythematous, urticarial plaque with tense vesicles. **B:** Tense bullae on erythematous background.

- Dermatitis herpetiformis (DH)[17]
  - Autoimmune disorder due to IgA antibodies to epidermal transglutaminase (also known as tissue transglutaminase 3)

5.2. Clinical Presentation

- Pemphigus vulgaris and foliaceus[15]
  - Skin findings consist of flaccid blisters and erosions in both types.
  - Mucosal involvement is only seen in PV and presents as painful erosions.
- Bullous pemphigoid[16]
  - Tense vesicles and bullae on erythematous, urticarial, or eczematous plaques
  - Association with neurologic disorders, specifically Parkinson disease, dementia, psychiatric disorders, stroke, and multiple sclerosis
- Dermatitis herpetiformis[17]
  - Grouped erythematous papules and vesicles commonly on bilateral extensor surfaces, scalp, and buttocks. Lesions are very pruritic and are replaced with erosions and excoriations. These erosions can be the initial presentation.
  - All patients with DH have celiac disease, which can be clinically silent.
  - Associated disorders include type 1 diabetes mellitus and Hashimoto thyroiditis.
  - Patients have a higher risk of non-Hodgkin lymphoma, particularly enteropathy-associated T-cell lymphoma.

5.3. Evaluation

- Skin biopsy for H&E and for direct immunofluorescence (DIF)
  - A biopsy for DIF should be perilesional (contain normal skin).
- PV and PF[15]
  - ELISA for desmogleins 1 and 3.
- BP[16]
  - Indirect immunofluorescence
  - ELISA for BP180 and BP230
- DH[17]
  - Total IgA level.
  - Antitissue transglutaminase (tTG2), IgA, and IgG.
  - Antiepidermal transglutaminase (tTG3), IgA, and IgG.
  - Antiendomysial IgA and IgG.
  - Check for associated disorders, that is, thyroid function testing, blood glucose tolerance, and CBC.

5.4. Treatment

- Pemphigus vulgaris and foliaceus[18]
  - First line: rituximab and oral corticosteroids
  - Second line: intravenous immunoglobulin, azathioprine, and mycophenolate mofetil
- Bullous pemphigoid[16]
  - First line: topical and oral steroids
  - Second line: mycophenolate mofetil, azathioprine, and methotrexate

• Dermatitis herpetiformis[19]
  • First line: adherence to gluten-free diet and dapsone

6. NUTRITIONAL DEFICIENCIES[20]

• Most nutritional deficiencies have cutaneous manifestations, and some are pathognomonic for specific deficiencies (Table 10-1).

Table 10-1	Nutritional Deficiencies		
Deficiency	**Clinical manifestation**	**Treatment**	**Misc.**
Vitamin A	Aka phrynoderma; keratotic, follicular papules typically extremities and buttocks	Vitamin A 50,000–200,000 IU/d depending on age and clinical severity	Can have night blindness, keratomalacia, and stunted growth
Vitamin K	Purpura and ecchymoses	Phytonadione Newborn: 0.5–1.0 mg Children: 2 mg Adults: 5–10 mg Fresh frozen plasma in cases of acute hemorrhage	Will have elevated prothrombin time and INR
Vitamin B_1 (thiamine)	Aka beriberi; glossitis and skin breakdown	Thiamine 100 mg TID IV × several days, then switch to 100 mg/d.	
Vitamin B_2 (riboflavin)	Aka oral-ocular-genital syndrome; angular stomatitis (macerated papules and fissuring at corners of the mouth), cheilitis (erythema and fissuring of lips), glossitis, crusted and erythematous patches and plaques in the inguinal folds extending to vulva/scrotum and inner thighs, photophobia and conjunctivitis	Riboflavin: Infants and Children: 1.0–2.0 mg/d Adults: 10–20 mg/d	

continued on following page

Deficiency	Clinical manifestation	Treatment	Misc.
Vitamin B_3 (niacin or nicotinic acid)	Aka pellagra; photodistributed erythematous and hyperpigmented plaques on face, chest, neck, and dorsal hands	Nicotinamide (aka nicotinic acid) 500 mg daily for several weeks	Classic tetrad: dermatitis, dementia, diarrhea, death
Vitamin B_6 (pyridoxine)	Seborrheic dermatitis periorificially including face and perineum, angular cheilitis, glossitis with ulceration	Pyridoxine 100 mg daily	
Vitamin B_{12} (cobalamin)	Glossitis with fissuring, hyperpigmentation	Cyanocobalamin 1 mg weekly × 1 months, then monthly if persistent	
Vitamin C	Aka scurvy; ecchymoses and follicular petechiae and hyperkeratosis; corkscrew hairs (Fig. 10-6)	Ascorbic acid 100 mg to 300 mg/d	
Folic acid (vitamin B_9)	Cheilitis, glossitis with mucosal erosions, and hyperpigmentation	Folic acid 1–5 mg daily	
Biotin (vitamin B_7)	Erythema and crusting in seborrheic and periorificial distribution, alopecia	Biotin 150 µg daily	
Iron	Pallor, koilonychia, glossitis, angular cheilitis, alopecia	Elemental iron: 100–200 mg of elemental iron daily	
Zinc	Eczematous plaques that can become eroded and macerated periorificially, alopecia, diarrhea	Elemental zinc: Inherited: 3 mg/kg daily Acquired in children: 0.5–1 mg/kg/d Acquired in adults: 15–30 mg/d	Can be an acquired or inherited deficiency, latter of which is known as acrodermatitis enteropathica
Marasmus	Dry, wrinkled, and loose skin; aged facial appearance due to loss of buccal fat pads, alopecia	Slow replacement of protein and calories	Total nutrient deficiency
Kwashiorkor	Desquamation and erosions	Aggressive nutritional replacement	Hypoproteinemia

[a]Vitamin D and E deficiencies do not have cutaneous manifestations.
From Schaefer SM, Hivnor CM. Nutritional diseases. In: Bolognia J, et al., eds. *Dermatology*. 3rd ed. Philadelphia, PA: Elsevier Saunders; 2012:737–751.

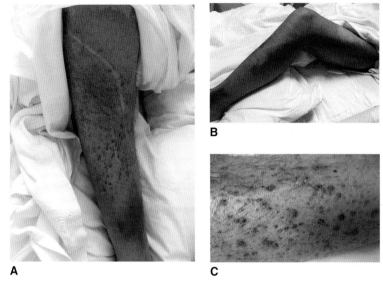

Figure 10-6. Scurvy. **A:** Petechiae. **B:** Extensive ecchymoses. **C:** Perifollicular petechiae with corkscrew hairs.

REFERENCES

1. Rothfield N, Sontheimer RD, Bernstein M. Lupus erythematosus: systemic and cutaneous manifestations. *Clin Dermatol* 2006;24(5):348–362.
2. Lee LA, Werth BP. Lupus Erythematosus. In: Bolognia JL, ed. *Dermatology*. 3rd ed. China: Elserview Saunders; 2012:615–629.
3. Grönhagen CM, Fored CM, Granath F, et al. Cutaneous lupus erythematosus and the association with systemic lupus erythematosus: a population-based cohort of 1088 patients in Sweden. *Br J Dermatol* 2011;164(6):1335–1341.
4. Kuhn A, Ruland V, Bonsmann G. Cutaneous lupus erythematosus: update of therapeutic options part I. *J Am Acad Dermatol* 2011;65(6):e179–e193.
5. Kovacs SO, Kovacs SC. Dermatomyositis. *J Am Acad Dermatol* 1998;39:899–920.
6. Katzap E, Barilla-LaBarca ML, Marder G. Antisynthetase syndrome. *Curr Rheumatol Rep* 2011;13(3):175–181.
7. Hill CL, Zhang Y, Sigurgeirsson B, et al. Frequency of specific cancer types in dermatomyositis and polymyositis: a population-based study. *Lancet* 2001;357(9250):96–100.
8. Wang J, Guo G, Chen G, et al. Meta-analysis of the association of dermatomyositis and polymyositis with cancer. *Br J Dermatol* 2013;169(4):838–847.
9. Seidler AM, Gottlieb AB. Dermatomyositis induced by drug therapy: a review of case reports. *J Am Acad Dermatol* 2008;59(5):872–880.
10. Haimovic A, Sanchez M, Judson MA, et al. Sarcoidosis: a comprehensive review and update for the dermatologist: part I. Cutaneous disease. *J Am Acad Dermatol* 2012;66(5):699.e1–e18.
11. Fett N, Werth VP. Update on morphea: part I. Epidemiology, clinical presentation, and pathogenesis. *J Am Acad Dermatol* 2011;64(2):217–228.

12. Chung L, Lin J, Furst DE, et al. Systemic and localized scleroderma. *Clin Dermatol* 2006;24(5):374–392.
13. Meffert JJ, Davis BM, Grimwood RE. Lichen sclerosus. *J Am Acad Dermatol* 1995;32(3):393–416.
14. Fett N, Werth VP. Update on morphea: part II. Outcome measures and treatment. *J Am Acad Dermatol* 2011;64(2):231–242.
15. Ruocco V, Ruocco E, Lo Schiavo A, et al. Pemphigus: etiology, pathogenesis, and inducing or triggering factors: facts and controversies. *Clin Dermatol* 2013;31(4):374–381.
16. Di Zenzo G, Della Torre R, Zambruno G, et al. Bullous pemphigoid: from the clinic to the bench. *Clin Dermatol* 2012;30(1):3–16.
17. Bolotin D, Petronic-Rosic V. Dermatitis herpetiformis. Part I. Epidemiology, pathogenesis, and clinical presentation. *J Am Acad Dermatol* 2011;64(6):1017–1024.
18. Cianchini G, Lupi F, Masini C, et al. Therapy with rituximab for autoimmune pemphigus: results from a single-center observational study on 42 cases with long-term follow-up. *J Am Acad Dermatol* 2012;67(4):617–622.
19. Bolotin D, Petronic-Rosic V. Dermatitis herpetiformis. Part II. Diagnosis, management, and prognosis. *J Am Acad Dermatol* 2011;64(6):1027–1033.
20. Jen M, Yan AC. Syndromes associated with nutritional deficiency and excess. *Clin Dermatol* 2010;28(6):669–685.

11 Dermatologic Surgery

Christopher R. Urban, MD and Eva A. Hurst, MD

Cutaneous surgery is an important part of dermatology and necessary for the treatment of benign and malignant neoplasms. Understanding key principles of dermatologic surgery is important for both primary care physicians and dermatologists.

1. PREOPERATIVE ASSESSMENT

- It is important to begin with a careful preoperative patient evaluation.
- In addition to a comprehensive review of past medical and surgical history, special attention should be paid to several areas.

1.1. Anticoagulant Use

- Patients must be questioned about cardiovascular disease and hypercoagulability, blood-thinning medications, and the presence of implantable cardiac devices (pacemakers and defibrillators).
- It is important to know if the patient has any history of cardiovascular disease including myocardial infarctions, strokes, transient ischemic attacks, atrial fibrillation, and cardiac or vascular stents; this is crucial for making decisions about having patients either continue or discontinue anticoagulants and medications that increase the risk of bleeding.
  - In patients without cardiovascular disease or the conditions listed above, it is common to ask them to hold preventative aspirin as well as vitamin E, multivitamins, fish oil, and omega-3 fatty acid supplements 14 days before a surgical excision.
  - Reversible platelet inhibitors such as NSAIDs require only 2 days of discontinuation prior to a procedure.
  - Preventative blood thinners are typically not discontinued for small procedures such as biopsies.
  - In patients who have a history of cardiovascular disease or hypercoagulability of any type, it is important to emphasize that they need to continue their regular anticoagulants such as aspirin, warfarin, and clopidogrel because the risk of serious life-threatening events outweighs the benefit of minimizing minor bleeding complications.[1]
- Patients should also be queried regarding bleeding disorders or thrombocytopenia.
  - Guidelines set forth by the American Society of Clinical Oncology state that major invasive procedures may safely be performed with platelet counts of 40,000 to 50,000.[2]
  - Platelet transfusion should be considered for patients with platelets under 30,000 for excisions, although small biopsies can likely be performed with care in patients with even lower levels when utilizing aggressive hemostasis.

1.2. Implantable Cardiac Devices

- In patients without implanted electrical devices, it is safe to use electrocoagulation to stop normal bleeding.
- The concern with using electrosurgery in patients with implanted electrical devices is that the current from the electrical device may be detected and interpreted as cardiac electrical activity. Although in practice it is unlikely, this could theoretically alter pacemaker function or stimulate the firing of a defibrillator.
- In patients with a pacemaker but no defibrillator, it is safe to use unipolar electrocoagulation or electrodessication in short bursts of less than a few seconds at the lowest effective settings as long as the treatment area is not directly over the cardiac device.
- In patients who have a defibrillator, the safest option is to use heat cautery only, although a recent study suggests bipolar electrocautery devices are safe.[3]

1.3. Infection Precautions

- Patients should be questioned about a history of shingles or herpes.
  - Many studies have described the effectiveness of valacyclovir prophylaxis following laser resurfacing and chemical peels.[4] If the patient reports a positive history of shingles or herpes at the surgical site, a prophylactic course of valacyclovir 500 mg twice per day for a week, starting the day of surgery, may be prescribed to reduce the risk of a flare or recurrence.
- Most wounds in dermatologic surgery are created on normal skin using clean or sterile technique and are considered clean wounds. The infection rate is very low, and prophylactic antibiotics are typically not necessary.
- Wounds on the oral cavity, axilla, and perineum are considered clean-contaminated, and the infection rate approaches 10%.
- Other risk factors include diabetes, immunocompromised states secondary to immune deficiency or medications, smoking, and malnutrition.
- Patients who have had joint replacement surgery with insertion of artificial joints within the past 6 months should be given prophylactic oral antibiotics preoperatively.
  - Other risk factors for prosthetic joint infection include inflammatory arthropathies such as systemic lupus or rheumatoid arthritis, hemophilia, and prior joint infection.
  - A typical treatment covering common skin pathogens is cephalexin 2 grams at least 60 minutes before surgery. Clindamycin 600 mg can be used in patients with a penicillin allergy.[5]
- Bacterial endocarditis prophylaxis may be considered for patients at high risk who have prosthetic cardiac valves, previous bacterial endocarditis, complex congenital heart disease, and surgical pulmonary shunts.
  - A similar 1-hour preoperative dose with cephalexin or clindamycin can be given.

1.4. Anesthetic Concerns

- Female patients should be asked if they are pregnant or breast-feeding.
  - During pregnancy, lidocaine is a category B medication and is considered safe, but epinephrine is category C, which means pregnancy risk has not been ruled out.
    - If a procedure such as the excision of a malignant melanoma is necessary and cannot be delayed until after delivery, surgeons may safely use plain lidocaine for anesthesia.

- During breast-feeding, lidocaine can be detected in breast milk, and if procedures are necessary, the best option may be to pump and dispose of the breast milk for 24 hours after treatment. Epinephrine is safe during breast-feeding.
- Finally, it is important to ask and document whether the patient has an allergy or adverse reaction to the local anesthetic, typically 1% lidocaine with epinephrine 1:100,000.
  - Other options for local anesthesia for minor procedures such as biopsy include diphenhydramine hydrochloride (Benadryl) 12.5 mg/mL, intradermal injection of normal saline, or cryoanesthesia with ice.[6]

1.5. Informed Consent

- All risks of the procedure should be clearly explained to patients before any cutaneous surgery.
- For most surgeries, this may include, but is not limited to, pain, swelling, erythema, infection, bleeding, surgical dehiscence, scarring, hyperpigmentation or hypopigmentation, and incomplete response.
- The health care provider who will be performing the procedure should review the relevant risks and give the patient time to ask any questions or express concerns before written consent is obtained.

1.6. Surgical Preparation

- Surgical preparation begins with careful positioning of the patient.
  - The goal is to maximize patient comfort while providing the surgeon with easy access to the surgical site.
  - Typically, patients are situated in the supine position on their backs to maximize comfort unless lesions are located on the back or posterior legs.
  - Rolled up towels placed under the knees and behind the head can be helpful to relieve pressure.
  - For even minor biopsies, it is recommended that the patient be reclined to minimize the risk of vasovagal reaction.

1.7. Antiseptics

- Antiseptics have a broad spectrum and are important for infection control.
  - For minor procedures such as punch and shave biopsies, isopropyl alcohol preparation and clean nonsterile gloves can be used.
  - Invasive procedures such as surgical excisions and repairs of defects after Mohs micrographic surgery should be cleaned with either povidone-iodine or chlorhexidine scrub.
    - Both of these agents have good coverage of Gram-positive and Gram-negative bacteria plus viruses.
    - Chlorhexidine gluconate leads to ototoxicity and keratitis, so it is necessary to avoid contact with eyes and the external auditory canal.
    - Iodine is safe to use around the eyes and ears but must be allowed to dry to become effective.
      - Side effects of iodine include skin irritant and allergic contact dermatitis.
  - Sterile towels should also be placed around the field, and patients should be reminded to keep their hands away from the sterile field.[7]

1.8. Anesthesia

- Most cutaneous surgical procedures can be done under local anesthesia.
- These agents act by blocking the sodium and potassium channels of nerve cells to prevent depolarization.
  - Unmyelinated C-type nerve fibers conduct pain and temperature signals and are most effectively blocked by local anesthesia.
  - Pressure sensations are transmitted by myelinated A-type fibers that are less effectively blocked by local anesthesia.
    - For this reason, patients commonly report being able to feel pressure but no pain during procedures.
- While small procedures such as biopsies can easily be performed using injected plain 1% lidocaine, the most commonly used local anesthetic in cutaneous surgery is lidocaine 1% with 1:100,000 epinephrine.
- Most local anesthetics lead to vasodilation and increased bleeding at the surgical site.
- Epinephrine is a vasoconstrictor and is added to reduce surgical site bleeding, prolong the effectiveness of local anesthetics, and reduce systemic toxicity to local anesthetics by decreasing systemic absorption.
  - Although the anesthetic effects of lidocaine occur within minutes, the full vasoconstrictive effect of epinephrine takes approximately 15 minutes.
  - Use of epinephrine is contraindicated in untreated hyperthyroidism and pheochromocytoma.
  - It should be used cautiously in hypertensive patients because it can lead to increases in blood pressure.
  - Although a true allergy to epinephrine is uncommon, patients often describe physiologic symptoms of epinephrine sensitivity including mild tremors and racing heart rate or palpitations.
- The combination of lidocaine 1% with 1:100,000 epinephrine has a very low pH and is painful during injection.
  - The pain can be mitigated by adding sodium bicarbonate to neutralize the solution; however, this must be freshly prepared because the basic pH reduces the water solubility and shelf life of the anesthetic.
- Other techniques for reducing pain and burning during injection include injecting slowly, warming the solution to room temperature before injection, using a small-gauge needle (30 g), and placing subsequent needle sticks in areas that are already numb.
- Lidocaine is an amide anesthetic and is metabolized by liver enzymes.
  - In patients with liver disease, it may be preferable to use an ester anesthetic.
- In patients with reported anesthesia allergies, careful history must be taken to elucidate the actual cause and determine reasonable alternatives.[6]
  - Occasionally, the help of an allergist must be employed.

2. PROCEDURAL TECHNIQUES

- There are several commonly performed procedures in cutaneous surgery.

2.1. Shave Biopsy

- A shave biopsy involves removal of a relatively shallow piece of skin with a 15-blade scalpel or a flexible blade such as the DermaBlade (see Chapter 1, Figure 1-2).

- Suturing is not performed, and the area is allowed to heal by second intention.
- This is an effective procedure for accurately diagnosing benign and malignant neoplasms and less commonly skin rashes.
- This technique is most appropriate for raised lesions including papules and plaques.
- An accurate prebiopsy differential diagnosis will be helpful for providing the pathologist with an adequate tissue sample for making the correct diagnosis.
  - A relatively superficial tissue sample is usually satisfactory for diagnosis of a basal cell carcinoma.
  - To make the diagnosis of a squamous cell carcinoma, a deeper biopsy is necessary because the pathologist needs to visualize the dermal-epidermal junction and some of the papillary and upper reticular dermis.
    - This allows visualization and differentiation of in situ versus invasive squamous cell carcinoma.
  - With experience, when performing the procedure in the correct upper dermal tissue plane, there should be a slight feeling of reduced resistance, and the resulting defect should have spots of pinpoint bleeding indicating a depth of the upper cutaneous vascular plexus.
- Shave biopsies extending deep into the dermis often lead to atrophic or indented scarring.
- A concern about performing shave biopsies for diagnosis of pigmented lesions is that the biopsy could transect the deeper component of a melanoma.
  - When this happens, only a provisional Breslow depth thickness can be assigned. This affects prognosis and treatment because deeper melanomas are staged differently and may require further testing and treatments such as sentinel lymph node biopsies.
  - Despite this risk, recent studies have suggested that the deep shave biopsy is a safe and effective technique for diagnosis of melanocytic lesions in experienced hands.[8]
- Many rashes, particularly those that are elevated, can be diagnosed with shave biopsy including eczema and psoriasis.
  - Broad shave biopsies are considered the preferred biopsy technique to diagnose mycosis fungoides and cutaneous T-cell lymphoma.
- Once the shave biopsy is taken, hemostasis can be acquired either with electrodessication or with aluminum chloride (Drysol).
  - It is important to note that this solution often contains alcohol and may be flammable.
  - If bleeding continues after application of the solution, it must be completely cleaned off before subsequent use of heat or electric cautery to avoid risk of fire.
- Shave biopsies heal by second intention and wound care consists of petrolatum and a daily bandage change until healed.
  - Typical shave biopsies heal in about a week.

2.2. Punch Biopsy

- Punch biopsies are an important technique in the diagnosis of neoplasms and rashes that are macules and patches and can be used for papules and plaques (see Chapter 1, Figure 1-3).
- Typically, rashes are best diagnosed with punch biopsies so the pathologist has the ability to look at the epidermis, entire dermis, and upper subcutaneous fat.
- This is helpful for the diagnosis of vasculitis, panniculitis, drug hypersensitivities, and alopecia.

- A punch excision can be performed to completely remove a pigmented lesion down to the subcutaneous fat and with a small rim of normal tissue.
- Punch biopsies are helpful for assessing whether a neoplasm such as a basal cell carcinoma has recurred within or underneath a scar from prior treatment.
- The technique of a punch biopsy first involves choosing the correct size.
  - Most rashes are diagnosed with a four-millimeter punch tool.
  - Punch excision to remove a neoplasm is done with the smallest sized punch tool necessary to completely remove the lesion.
    - By applying pressure with one edge of the punch biopsy tool and pushing the skin toward that edge, it is possible to fit a slightly larger lesion into a smaller punch.
- Once the lesion or area of rash to be biopsied is within the punch, firm downward pressure while rotating the punch biopsy tool in one direction will cut through the epidermis and dermis and into the subcutaneous fat.
- Once dermal release is achieved and the punch biopsy tool is retracted, the circular plug of tissue will typically rise above the surrounding skin.
  - This elevation can be increased by placing downward pressure on the surrounding skin.
  - After gently lifting one edge of the plug of tissue with forceps, the plug of tissue can be easily cut free from its attachment to the subcutaneous fat with surgical scissors.
  - Care must be taken not to crush the tissue with the forceps during this process, or the cellular and tissue architecture will be distorted and crush artifact will be present on histology.
- Sutures are typically used to close the punch biopsy.
  - When using punch biopsy tools 5 mm or less in size, it is common for only epidermal sutures to be placed.
  - When punch biopsies of 6 mm or greater are performed, the defect may be closed in a layered manner with an absorbable deep suture plus epidermal sutures.
- Placing surgical scar lines in the natural relaxed skin tension lines results in improved cosmetic outcomes.
  - By slightly stretching the skin perpendicular to the relaxed skin tension lines, the punch biopsy defect will become a slight oval shape with the long axis in the direction of the relaxed skin tension lines and allow the scar to be in the appropriate orientation.

2.3. Snip Removal

- For some pedunculated lesions such as skin tags, warts, seborrheic keratoses, and dermatosis papulosa nigra, snip excision with curved or straight iris surgical scissors is the preferred technique.
- The sharpest part of the scissor blades is typically located centrally along the scissor blades instead of right at the tips.
- Pedunculated lesions may have a vascular connection at the pedicle and may bleed after removal.
  - Hemostasis can be achieved with either aluminum chloride or electrodessication.
  - It is often useful to inject local anesthetic such as lidocaine with epinephrine into skin tags with a substantial pedicle.
    - This reduces pain during removal and allows for electrodessication if control of bleeding is necessary.
- Wound care consists of petrolatum and a bandage.

2.4. Excision

- Standard excision is performed for diagnosis and treatment of skin neoplasms and pigmented lesions (Fig. 11-1).
- It is used to treat symptomatic benign lesions such as epidermoid cysts and skin malignancies such as basal cell carcinomas, squamous cell carcinomas, and melanoma.
- Different skin cancers require different surgical margins.
  - For basal cell and squamous cell carcinomas, complete pathologic removal is recommended. To achieve that end, once the lesion is anesthetized, it may be helpful to use a three- or four-millimeter curette to scrape the lesion and better define the borders. Afterward, the safety margins may be measured.
    - If this technique is performed on elderly patients with fragile skin, it is important to note that even gentle pressure from the curette can tear skin and lead to an overestimate of the true borders of the malignancy.
  - For standard excision of basal cell carcinoma, a clinical margin of approximately 3 to 4 mm is commonly used in order to achieve pathologic clearance.
  - For well-differentiated squamous cell carcinoma, a margin of 5 mm is usually sufficient.

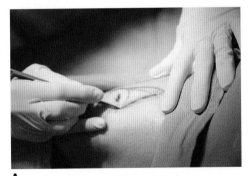

A

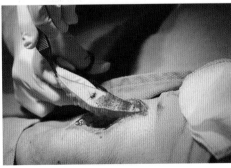

B

Figure 11-1. Elliptical excision. **A:** Margins and cones of redundant tissue are marked and incised. **B:** Specimen is excised to the appropriate tissue depth.

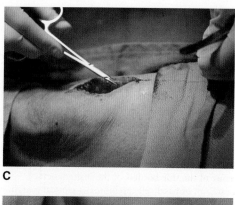

C

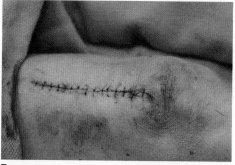

D

Figure 11-1. (*Continued*) **C:** Buried absorbable sutures reapproximate wound edges. **D:** Simple interrupted sutures reapproximate the epidermis. (Courtesy of M. Laurin Council, MD.)

- In tumors with a diameter larger than two centimeters or with moderate to poor differentiation, a larger margin ranging from 6 to 10 mm is often necessary.[9]
- Margins for excisions of melanomas are set forth by the American Joint Committee on Cancer and include 5-mm margins for melanoma in situ and 1-cm clinical margins for thin melanomas.[10]
- Excisions are designed with an elliptical or fusiform shape approximately three times as long as the defect is wide to allow for linear closure with minimal puckering at the ends.
- Scars should be oriented along relaxed skin tension lines when possible.
- For most body areas, a 15-blade scalpel is the most appropriate tool for performing excisions.
  - Exceptions to this include the use of a smaller 15c blade for more precise control around the eyelids and a larger 10 blade for excisions on thick skin such as the back.
- Cutting the skin with the scalpel blade at a 90-degree angle is common for standard excisions, though for thick skin of the back sometimes it is beneficial to "bevel out" slightly and take a few millimeter wider margins under the epidermis.

- This helps ensure that you take satisfactory margins in the deeper tissue and may help in approximating the epidermis during suturing.
- Different types of malignancies also require different depths of excision.
  - Treatment of basal cell carcinomas and squamous cell carcinomas typically require excising down to the level of the mid-to-deep subcutaneous fat.
  - Treatment of melanoma in situ requires excising down to the deep subcutaneous fat.
  - Treatment of invasive melanoma requires excision down through the subcutaneous fat to the fascia overlying muscles.

2.5. Surgical Repairs

- Repairing postexcision defects requires several steps including undermining, hemostasis, and suturing.
- Undermining is necessary for allowing the edges of the defect to slide over the exposed tissue.
- It results in a plate-like scar under the skin that reduces stretch of the scar and improves cosmetic outcomes.
- The recommended depth of undermining depends on the location.
  - On the cheeks, the proper level is the upper subcutaneous fat to ensure that nerves and vessels, which run in deeper tissue planes, are protected.
  - On the scalp, the ideal plane is below the galea because this is a relatively bloodless area to work.
  - On the trunk and extremities, undermining is often performed in the deep subcutaneous fat or fascia.
- Blunt-ended surgical scissors are typically used for undermining to reduce risk of damage to nerves and vessels.
  - On the back, it may be safe to carefully use the 10 blade to quickly undermine since there are minimal important structures at risk for damage.
- Hemostasis with electrocoagulation or heat cautery is typically done after undermining to control bleeding from small severed vessels.
- Once undermining is complete and hemostasis achieved, suturing is performed to close the defect and complete the repair.
- The first step in suturing is to place deep dermal sutures with absorbable materials, typically Monocryl (poliglecaprone 25) or Vicryl (polyglactin 910).
- Size of the suture depends on the location, with 5-0 suture typically used for the face/neck, 4-0 for the scalp and extremities, and 3-0 for thicker areas under tension such as the back.
- The deep dermal sutures should both bring the dermal edges of the wound together in good approximation and also contribute to eversion of the wound edges.
- Once the deep layer of sutures are completed, the epidermal sutures can be placed either as simple interrupted sutures or a running suture.
- Either nonabsorbable sutures (polypropylene or nylon) or absorbable sutures (fast absorbing gut) can be utilized.
- Simple interrupted sutures are more time consuming to place but are very good at approximating the wound edges and useful for wounds under tension.
- Running top stitches are both quick to perform and also useful for approximating and everting the wound edges.
- On cosmetically sensitive areas where "track marking" from top sutures is a concern and the wound is under low tension, a running subcuticular suture may be placed.
- Nonabsorbable sutures should be removed in 1 week for facial locations and in 10 to 14 days for extremities and trunk.

2.6. Mohs Micrographic Surgery

- It is important to understand the advantages and benefits of Mohs micrographic surgery in the treatment of cutaneous neoplasms such as basal cell carcinoma and squamous cell carcinoma.
- Mohs surgery, named for Dr. Frederic Mohs, is based on the principle that these cutaneous malignancies are contiguous tumors without skip areas.
- The treatment offers the highest cure rates and lowest recurrence rates for certain tumors because the technique allows visual confirmation of clear peripheral and deep margins.
- While traditional permanent tissue processing takes days before the slides can be analyzed, with the Mohs technique, fresh tissue is frozen, cut, stained, and ready for microscopic analysis in approximately 1 hour.
- If positive margins are found, additional tissue is removed in a second "stage," and the process is repeated.
- This allows the surgeon to take numerous "stages" as needed to clear the tumor on the day of surgery and ensures that the tumor is fully removed before the defect is repaired.
- The process is considered tissue sparing because conservatively sized pieces of tissue can be excised with each stage.
- The other significant difference is the way the tissue is cut.
  - In permanent processing, tissue is cut vertically. This is similar to how a loaf of bread is sliced. In a loaf of raisin bread, individual slices may show raisins in cross section, but the majority of the margins are not being visualized.
  - For Mohs micrographic surgery, the tissue is cut horizontally. This can be conceptualized by visualizing the lesion as a pie with the bulk of the tumor making up the pie filling and the surrounding deeper peripheral tissues as the crust.
  - The stage is taken by cutting with a 45-degree bevel so that the tissue can be laid flat on glass microscope slides.
  - This allows for microscopic examination of one hundred percent of the margins with the peripheral epidermis around the edges and the deep margins in the middle.
- This technique is especially beneficial for treatment of lesions on cosmetically and functionally important areas such as the face and hands because minimal margins can be taken for tumor clearance.
- It is also beneficial for high-risk tumors with aggressive histologic appearance and recurrent tumors because the rate of recurrence with standard excision or other treatment modalities is much higher than with the Mohs micrographic surgery technique.

2.7. Cryosurgery

- Cryosurgery involves applying an extremely cold agent either through a spray or directly via a cotton-tipped applicator.
- The most commonly used agent is liquid nitrogen, which has a boiling point of 196°C (320°F).
- Benign lesions such as verruca, condyloma, seborrheic keratoses, and prurigo nodules and premalignant lesions such as actinic keratoses may be treated with cryotherapy.
- The mechanism of action of cryosurgery initially involves the transfer of heat away from the skin to the cryogen.

- This leads to cell freeze and both the formation of intracellular and extracellular ice crystals.
- A fast freeze leads to more intracellular ice crystal formation and increased tissue damage.
- Cell injury also occurs during the thawing phase because of the occurrence of vascular stasis.
  - A rapid freeze followed by a slow thaw maximizes tissue damage.
- Blister formation may occur due to separation of the basement membrane.
- Inflammation is the final stage and leads to redness and swelling.
- Different cell types have different susceptibilities to cryotherapy.
  - The most sensitive are melanocytes, which are damaged at –4 to –7°C.
    - For this reason, hypopigmentation is a common side effect of cryosurgery and should always be discussed before treatment, especially in patients with darker skin pigmentation (Fitzpatrick types 4 and 5).
  - Keratinocytes are damaged at –20 to –30°C.
    - The benign and premalignant lesions listed above typically fall into this category, and treatment times range from approximately 5 to 10 seconds of constant liquid nitrogen spray for one or two cycles.
    - One study reported that two cycles of liquid nitrogen were more effective at treating verruca on the feet, but one cycle was equivalent and better tolerated for treating verruca on the hands.[11]
  - Fibroblasts of the dermis are usually damaged at –30 to –35°C.
- Treatment of malignant tumors such as basal cell carcinomas and squamous cell carcinomas has been described but requires measurement of core tissue temperature of –50°C.[12]

2.8. Electrodesiccation and Curettage

- This is a treatment option for benign and malignant cutaneous neoplasms.
- In electrodessication, a high-voltage electric current is generated at the metal tip of the device.
- By directly applying this metal tip to the lesion, heat is delivered and the tissue is rapidly dried leading to superficial destruction.
- Once the tissue has been heated and dried, a curette can be used to scrape off the upper portions of the lesion.
- Benign seborrheic keratoses can be treated in as few as one cycle of electrodessication and curettage, resulting in a smooth base of superficially eroded skin that should heal with minimal scarring.
- When treating malignancies such as basal cell carcinoma, the curette is first used to scrape off the tumor.
  - This is effective because the tumor cells do not hold together like normal tissue. With firm pressure from the semisharp curette edge, the tumor scrapes off, while the underlying normal tissue remains intact.
- Once the tumor is removed with the curette, the base and a few millimeter margin are treated with electrodessication.
- Three passes of curettage and electrodessication are typically performed for the treatment of malignancies.[13]
- Electrodessication and curettage are typically utilized for the treatment of small (<1 cm) malignancies on the trunk and extremities.

- Facial areas are typically avoided due to the risk of atrophic or hypopigmented scarring.
- The main types of cancers treated are low-risk superficial or nodular basal cell carcinomas and occasionally squamous cell carcinoma in situ.
- It is not an effective treatment for invasive squamous cell carcinoma or melanoma.
- Lesions are allowed to heal by second intention with petrolatum and a bandage.

3. WOUND DRESSINGS

- The main functions of wound dressings are to provide pressure for hemostasis, to maintain a moist environment that promotes healing, and to provide protection from mechanical trauma and infection.
- A moist healing environment leads to more rapid re-epithelialization.
  - It is important to prevent a wound from drying out and forming an eschar.
- Small procedures such as shave and punch biopsies can be dressed with petrolatum and a bandage.
- For surgical excisions and larger procedures, the typical postsurgical wound dressing consists of a generous amount of petrolatum covered by folded clean cotton gauze held tightly in place with paper tape.
  - Petrolatum is recommended instead of over-the-counter antibiotic ointments such as Neosporin or Polysporin because a significant proportion of the population either has or will develop an allergic contact dermatitis to these products.
  - Studies have shown equivalent healing using petrolatum compared to topical over-the-counter antibiotic preparations, with lower risk of allergic contact dermatitis.[14]
- There are other occlusive dressings that include films, foams, hydrogels, alginates, and hydrocolloids. These are all semipermeable but have different advantages.
  - Films are translucent and provide a barrier to outside bacteria but may lead to an accumulation of exudate.
  - Foams are very absorbent and comfortable but cannot be used on dry wounds and are opaque.
  - Hydrogels are soothing, cooling, and moisturizing but may have a higher risk of infection.
  - Alginates are the most highly absorbent but require a secondary dressing and may have an undesirable appearance and odor.
  - Hydrocolloids are useful for chronic ulcers and burns but risk leading to maceration of surrounding skin.[15,16]

4. WOUND HEALING

- Breakdown of the epidermal barrier occurs following injury, burns, and surgical procedures.
- These processes activate mechanisms to allow for repair and healing.
- Wound healing occurs in phases consisting of the inflammatory phase, proliferative phase, and the remodeling phase.
  - The acute inflammatory phase takes place 1 to 2 days after surgery and is characterized by cellular and vascular responses.
    - Damage to endothelial cells, blood vessels, and collagen leads to platelet activation and release of growth factors as well as platelet plug formation for initiation of hemostasis.

- o Neutrophils are the first leukocytes to migrate to the site of injury. They function to eliminate bacteria and break down proteins in the wound bed.
- o Macrophages are critical for repair and wound healing. They eliminate pathogens and tissue debris, destroy remaining neutrophils, and induce new blood vessel growth.
- o Many chemical mediators are also important for the inflammatory phase including histamine, serotonin, and prostaglandins.
- The proliferative phase reestablishes a barrier through reepithelialization and blood flow through angiogenesis.
  - o Fibroblasts migrate into the wound between 2 and 3 days and produce the dermal matrix.
  - o Myofibroblasts contribute to wound contraction.
- In the remodeling phase, collagen is synthesized and present.
  - o Initially, type III collagen is the major component, but over time type I collagen predominates.
  - o After 1 month, the wound tensile strength approaches 40% of original strength.
  - o By 1 year, it reaches its maximum strength, which is only 80% of the original.[15,17]

5. SURGICAL COMPLICATIONS

- Common surgical complications include bleeding, hematoma, dehiscence, and infection.
- Bleeding usually occurs in the first 24 hours following a procedure.
  - As the vasoconstrictive effect of the epinephrine wears off, there is increased small-vessel bleeding and the blood clots that form initially may move or be displaced.
  - The bleeding risk is reduced with a tight pressure dressing held in place for 24 to 48 hours.
  - While a small quantity of bleeding is tolerable, if the bleeding soaks through the bandage, the patient should attempt to hold firm pressure for at least 20 minutes.
  - Applying pressure with an ice pack may also help.
  - If the bleeding continues, the patient should seek evaluation for possible exploration of the wound.[1,18]
- If bleeding occurs under the skin and accumulates, a hematoma forms (Fig. 11-2).
  - Initially, the collection is soft, and if patients present early enough, the hematoma can be easily evacuated or drained. Antibiotics should be administered following drainage.

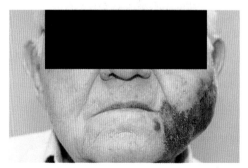

Figure 11-2. Hematoma. (Courtesy of M. Laurin Council, MD.)

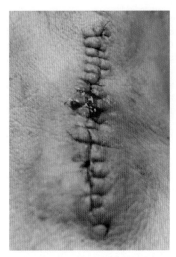

Figure 11-3. Infection. (Courtesy of M. Laurin Council, MD.)

- If the hematoma goes undetected and untreated for several days, it will organize and harden.
- At this point, if it is not compromising the integrity of the surgical closure, it is often best to allow the body to resorb the hematoma, which will take several weeks.
- The risk of infection may be increased with the presence of a resorbing hematoma so the administration of oral antibiotics and close clinical follow-up is beneficial.
- Surgical site infection usually occurs around postoperative day five (Fig. 11-3).
  - Increased pain, redness, and drainage or pus are common signs of infection.
  - Antibiotics should be started based on the most likely causative organisms. The wound should be cultured to identify the organism and determine sensitivities.
  - Cephalexin has good coverage of normal skin pathogens and is often started while the cultures are pending.
  - In cases where there is concern for Gram-negative infection such as Pseudomonas, ciprofloxacin may be used.[5]
  - Sometimes it is challenging to determine whether a surgical site is infected or if there is an allergic contact dermatitis reaction.
    - Usually, allergic contact dermatitis will be itchy rather than painful and redness will be present around the surrounding areas where antibiotic ointment or adhesives have been applied.
- Dehiscence is when the wound edges separate. This most commonly occurs at the time of suture removal but may also occur before or after (Fig. 11-4).
  - Risk factors for dehiscence include excessive wound tension, infection, and wound edge necrosis.
  - Areas of dehiscence will heal from the bottom up by second intention and may later require scar revision.[18]

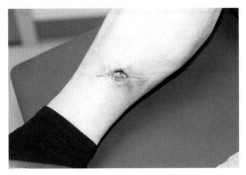

Figure 11-4. Dehiscence. (Courtesy of M. Laurin Council, MD.)

REFERENCES

1. Hurst EA, Yu SS, Grekin RC, et al. Bleeding complications in dermatologic surgery. *Semin Cutan Med Surg* 2007;26(4):189–195.
2. Schiffer CA, Anderson KC, Bennett CL, et al. Platelet transfusion for patients with cancer: clinical practice guidelines of the American Society of Clinical Oncology. *J Clin Oncol* 2001;19(5):1519–1538.
3. Weyer C, Siegle RJ, Eng GG. Investigation of hyfrecators and their in vitro interference with implantable cardiac devices. *Dermatol Surg* 2012;38(11):1843–1848.
4. Beeson WH, Rachel JD. Valacyclovir prophylaxis for herpes simplex virus infection or infection recurrence following laser skin resurfacing. *Dermatol Surg* 2002;28(4):331–336.
5. Hurst EA, Grekin RC, Yu SS, et al. Infectious complications and antibiotic use in dermatologic surgery. *Semin Cutan Med Surg* 2007;26(1):47–53.
6. Koay J, Orengo I. Application of local anesthetics in dermatologic surgery. *Dermatol Surg* 2002;28(2):143–148.
7. Rogues A. Infection control practices and infectious complications in dermatologic surgery. *J Hosp Infect* 2007;65(3):258–263.
8. Mendese G, Maloney M, Bordeaux, J. To scoop of not to scoop: The diagnostic and therapeutic utility of the scoop-shave biopsy for pigmented lesions. *Dermatol Surg* 2014;40(10):1077–1083.
9. Brodland DG, Zitelli JA. Surgical margins for excision of primary cutaneous squamous cell carcinoma. *J Am Acad Dermatol* 1992;27(2 Pt 1):241–248.
10. American Joint Committee on Cancer. https://cancerstaging.org
11. Berth-Jones J, Bourke J, Eglitis H, et al. Value of a second freeze-thaw cycle in cryotherapy of common warts. *Br J Dermatol* 1994;131(6):883–886.
12. Kokoszka A, Scheinfeld N. Evidence-based review of the use of cryosurgery in treatment of basal cell carcinoma. *Dermatol Surg* 2003;29(6):566–571.
13. Rodriguez-Vigil T, Vázquez-López F, Perez-Oliva N. Recurrence rates of primary basal cell carcinoma in facial risk areas treated with curettage and electrodesiccation. *J Am Acad Dermatol* 2007;56(1):91–95.
14. Saco M, Howe N, Nathoo R, et al. Topical antibiotic prophylaxis for prevention of surgical wound infections from dermatologic procedures: a systematic review and meta-analysis. *J Dermatolog Treat* 2015;26(2):151–158.
15. Menaker GM, Mehlis AL, Kasprowiczs. Dressings. In: Bolognia J, et al., eds. *Dermatology.* 3rd ed. Philadelphia, PA: Elsevier Saunders; 2012:2365–2379.

16. Thomas S. Hydrocolloid dressings in the management of acute wounds: a review of the literature. *Int Wound J* 2008;5(5):602–613.
17. Sun BK, Siprashvili Z, Khavari PA. Advances in skin grafting and treatment of cutaneous wounds. *Science* 2014;346(6212):941–945.
18. Alam M, Ibrahim O, Nodzenski M, et al. Adverse events associated with mohs micrographic surgery: multicenter prospective cohort study of 20,821 cases at 23 centers. *JAMA Dermatol* 2013;149(12):1378–1385.

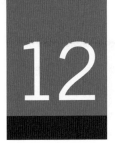

12 Pediatric Dermatology

Monique Gupta Kumar, MD, MPhil, Kara Sternhell-Blackwell, MD, and Susan J. Bayliss, MD

Skin disorders are one of the most common problems in pediatrics. While there is overlap with adult dermatology, there are often unique disease processes in this age group. Conservative treatment is often recommended.

NEONATAL AND INFANTILE DERMATOLOGY

1. NEONATAL ACNE (CEPHALIC PUSTULOSIS)

1.1. Clinical Presentation
- Small pustules and papules on the face (resembles miliaria rubra) (Fig. 12-1). Comedones are absent.
- Transient. Generally develops at 2 to 3 weeks of age and resolves within 6 months.
- May represent an inflammatory reaction to *Malassezia* species.

1.2. Treatment
- No treatment is usually necessary; wash face with baby soap. In severe cases, consider ketoconazole cream.

2. APLASIA CUTIS CONGENITA

2.1. Clinical Presentation
- Absence of skin with scar formation in a localized area, most commonly on the scalp (Fig. 12-2).
- Defects are present from birth.
- Larger or multiple lesions may be associated with other congenital anomalies or genetic syndromes.

2.2. Evaluation
- MRI should be considered before biopsy.

2.3. Treatment
- Small defects often heal on their own, leaving scar tissue and alopetic patch. Larger defects may require skin grafting or other surgical intervention.

3. ERYTHEMA TOXICUM NEONATORUM

3.1. Clinical Presentation
- Scattered yellowish, erythematous papules and pustules may occur anywhere on the body, except palms and soles (Fig. 12-3).

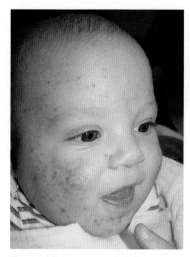

Figure 12-1. Acne neonatorum. (From Dusenbery SM, White A. *The Washington Manual of Pediatrics.* Philadelphia, PA: Lippincott Williams & Wilkins; 2009.)

• More common in full-term infants. Generally appears in the first 24 to 48 hours of life and resolves within 1 week.

3.2. Evaluation

• Diagnosis is clinical. Can be confirmed by the presence of eosinophils on a smear of the pustule.

3.3. Treatment

• Self-limited condition. No treatment needed.

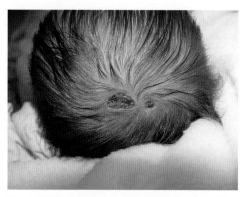

Figure 12-2. Aplasia cutis congenita. (From Dusenbery SM, White A. *The Washington Manual of Pediatrics.* Philadelphia, PA: Lippincott Williams & Wilkins; 2009.)

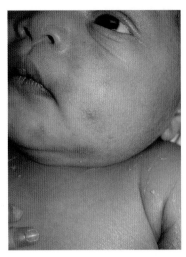

Figure 12-3. Erythema toxicum neonatorum. (From Dusenbery SM, White A. *The Washington Manual of Pediatrics.* Philadelphia, PA: Lippincott Williams & Wilkins; 2009.)

4. MILIA

4.1. Clinical Presentation

• 1- to 2-mm pearly white, firm papules found most commonly on the face (Fig. 12-4) but may occur anywhere. Represent tiny inclusion cysts
• May be present at birth
• Rarely associated with certain syndromes such as epidermolysis bullosa, orofaciodigital syndrome type 1, and Basan syndrome

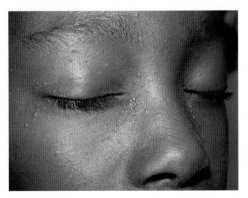

Figure 12-4. Milia. (From Dusenbery SM, White A. *The Washington Manual of Pediatrics.* Philadelphia, PA: Lippincott Williams & Wilkins; 2009.)

4.2. Treatment

• Usually resolve without treatment by 2 to 6 months of age. If persistent, lesions can be punctured and expressed.

5. MILIARIA

• General term describing obstruction of the eccrine ducts at different levels, often secondary to heat and humidity

5.1. Clinical Presentation

• Miliaria crystallina: 1- to 2-mm clear vesicles without erythema in intertriginous areas, neck, and chest. Obstruction is in the most superficial level of the stratum corneum.
• Miliaria rubra ("heat rash"): erythematous papules in the same distribution that result from obstruction deeper in the epidermis, with resulting erythema.

5.2. Treatment

• Treatment involves correcting overheating conditions.

6. NEVUS SEBACEUS

• Nevus sebaceus is an organoid hamartoma of sebaceous and apocrine glands that is present at birth. It is caused by a postzygotic somatic gene mutation in *HRAS* or *KRAS*.[1]

6.1. Clinical Presentation

• Alopetic, yellow-colored plaque tends to have a bumpy surface (Fig. 12-5).
• Usually present from birth on the scalp or elsewhere on head and neck. Lesion becomes less prominent after the newborn period but later becomes more papular or verrucous around puberty, when hormone levels increase.

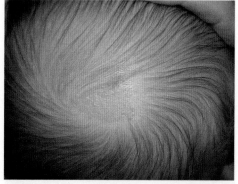

Figure 12-5. Nevus sebaceus. (From Dusenbery SM, White A. *The Washington Manual of Pediatrics.* Philadelphia, PA: Lippincott Williams & Wilkins; 2009.)

6.2. Treatment

- Treatment is surgical excision or observation.
  - Surgery is often deferred until puberty when the lesion begins to grow.
  - Plaque can be followed by clinical observation until excision because there is a low risk of developing neoplastic growths within the lesion.[2]
    - Most neoplasms within the nevus sebaceus are benign and include syringocyst-adenoma papilliferum and trichoblastoma.
    - Rarely, malignant tumors can be identified such as basal cell carcinoma and squamous cell carcinoma.

7. SUBCUTANEOUS FAT NECROSIS

7.1. Clinical Presentation

- Localized indurated erythematous plaques or subcutaneous nodules on buttocks, thighs, trunk, face, and/or arms. Lesions may be fluctuant (Fig. 12-6).

7.2. Evaluation

- Subcutaneous fat necrosis (SCFN) is usually diagnosed clinically. Diagnosis can be confirmed by skin biopsy.

7.3. Treatment

- Patches appear at 1 to 6 weeks of life and generally resolve without treatment in 2 to 6 months. Fluctuant nodules require drainage.
- Uncommonly, can be associated with significant hypercalcemia as well as localized calcification. Infants should be monitored for hypercalcemia for at least 6 months after appearance of extensive lesions.

8. TRANSIENT NEONATAL PUSTULAR MELANOSIS

8.1. Clinical Presentation

- Present at birth. More common in dark-skinned infants.

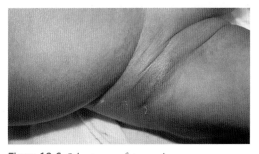

Figure 12-6. Subcutaneous fat necrosis.

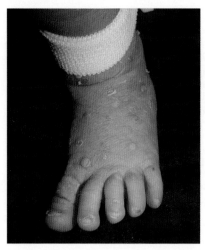

Figure 12-7. Transient neonatal pustular melanosis. (From Dusenbery SM, White A. *The Washington Manual of Pediatrics*. Philadelphia, PA: Lippincott Williams & Wilkins; 2009.)

• Pustular lesions rupture easily with a collarette of scale and leave hyperpigmented macules on the neck, chin, forehead, lower back, and shins (Fig. 12-7), which fades over 6 to 12 months.

8.2. Treatment

• Self-limited. Pustules resolve within days, but hyperpigmentation may take months to resolve. No treatment needed.

PIGMENTED LESIONS

9. CAFÉ AU LAIT MACULES

9.1. Clinical Presentation

• Light brown macules (Fig. 12-8) can occur anywhere on the body, ranging from small (<0.5 mm) to large, including segmental patches.

9.2. Evaluation

• May occur in isolation or with a syndrome.
  • Neurofibromatosis 1: The presence of six or more macules >0.5 cm in diameter in prepubertal children or >1.5 cm in postpubertal, as well as inguinal or axillary freckling.
  • Large, very irregular truncal patches may be associated with McCune-Albright syndrome.

9.3. Treatment

• Treatment is generally not required. Laser therapy with Q-switched lasers can be attempted but is not permanent.

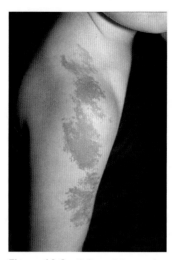

Figure 12-8. Café au lait macules. (From Dusenbery SM, White A. *The Washington Manual of Pediatrics.* Philadelphia, PA: Lippincott Williams & Wilkins; 2009.)

10. CONGENITAL DERMAL MELANOCYTOSIS (MONGOLIAN SPOT)

10.1. Clinical Presentation

- Blue-gray poorly circumscribed macules most commonly in lumbosacral area but can be seen anywhere (Fig. 12-9).
- More common in pigmented skin; present at birth.

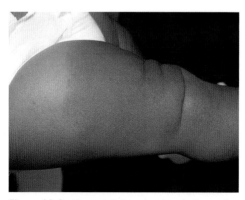

Figure 12-9. Congenital dermal melanosis (mongolian spots). (From Dusenbery SM, White A. *The Washington Manual of Pediatrics.* Philadelphia, PA: Lippincott Williams & Wilkins; 2009.)

- Lumbosacral lesions tend to lighten in childhood; however, lesions in other locations usually persist.

11. CONGENITAL MELANOCYTIC NEVI

11.1. Clinical Presentation

- Present at birth or become evident in the first year of life.
- Brown pigmented macules or plaques may have dark brown or black papules or other irregular pigmentation within the lesions (Fig. 12-10). Lesions can have hypertrichosis. Larger lesions may have ulceration, a cobblestoned surface, nodules, and/or satellite lesions.
- They are found in 1% to 3% of newborn babies.
- These nevi enlarge in proportion to the child's growth and are classified based on their projected final adult size, with the following categories:
  - Small CMN: <1.5 cm in diameter (projected adult size)
  - Medium CMN: 1.5 to 20 cm in diameter (projected adult size)
  - Large or giant CMN: >20 cm in diameter (projected adult size)
  - Giant congenital melanocytic nevi (CMN) can cover a large portion of the body (e.g., in a "bathing trunk" or "cape" distribution) and are rare, found in fewer than 1 in 20,000 newborn infants.

11.2. Evaluation

- The small increased risk of melanoma development within lesions makes close follow-up important. This risk is <1% over a lifetime for small and medium CMN and is extraordinarily low before puberty. Risk of melanoma is greatest (~5%) in giant CMN, over a lifetime.
- Children with giant and/or numerous (e.g., >20) CMN also have an increased number of melanocytes around their brain, which is referred to as neurocutaneous melanocytosis.
- Magnetic resonance imaging with contrast of the brain and spine may be performed in large CMN with >20 satellite lesions, giant CMN, or CMN over posterior axis, to rule out neurocutaneous melanosis.

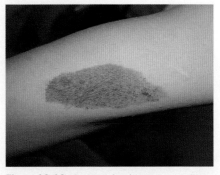

Figure 12-10. Congenital melanocytic nevi. (From Dusenbery SM, White A. *The Washington Manual of Pediatrics.* Philadelphia, PA: Lippincott Williams & Wilkins; 2009.)

11.3. Treatment

- CMN are managed on an individual basis depending on their location, size, appearance, and evolution over time. Factors that may prompt surgical excision of a congenital nevus include cosmetic concerns, difficulty in monitoring the lesion, and worrisome changes in its appearance.

12. SPITZ NEVUS

12.1. Clinical Presentation

- Dome topped tan-pink papule appears over a few months and is a subtype of melanocytic nevus. Common in first two decades of life. Usual locations for pediatric Spitz nevi include head, neck, and extremities.

12.2. Evaluation

- Biopsy confirms diagnosis.

12.3. Treatment

- The management of pediatric Spitz nevi has no clear consensus. Surgical excision may be considered.

VASCULAR LESIONS

13. CAPILLARY MALFORMATION (PORT-WINE STAIN)

13.1. Clinical Presentation

- Pink, red, or purple blanchable small to large patch caused by capillary malformations (Fig. 12-11). This is due to a somatic mutation in GNAQ.[3]

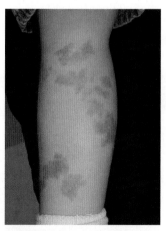

Figure 12-11. Capillary malformation (port-wine stain). (From Dusenbery SM, White A. *The Washington Manual of Pediatrics.* Philadelphia, PA: Lippincott Williams & Wilkins; 2009.)

13.2. Evaluation

• Lesions in hemifacial (involving upper quarter and cheek) distribution on the face should be evaluated for associated glaucoma and/or Sturge-Weber syndrome. Lesions persist and generally become darker and thicker with age.

13.3. Treatment

• Therapy is serial pulsed-dye laser treatment.

14. CUTIS MARMORATA TELANGIECTATICA CONGENITA

14.1. Clinical Presentation

• Fixed, blanchable purple, reticular pattern most commonly on unilateral extremity. Focal areas with atrophy and/or ulceration. Considered a vascular malformation
• Does not disappear with rewarming (unlike cutis marmorata)
• May be associated with body asymmetry
• May improve with age but rarely disappears completely

14.2. Treatment

• No treatment is usually needed, and can improve with time. Poorly responsive to pulsed-dye laser treatment.

15. INFANTILE HEMANGIOMA

• Most common vascular tumor of infancy

15.1. Clinical Presentation

• Superficial: bright red vascular plaques or nodules
• Deep: bluish purple nodules, sometimes with overlying telangiectatic markings (Fig. 12-12)

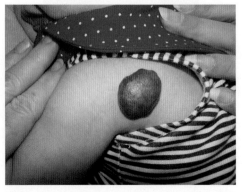

Figure 12-12. Hemangioma. (From Dusenbery SM, White A. *The Washington Manual of Pediatrics*. Philadelphia, PA: Lippincott Williams & Wilkins; 2009.)

15.2. Course
- Lesions usually are not present at birth, or a precursor lesion may be present.
  - Appear as faint vascular markings initially and then enlarge and develop characteristic appearance over 2 to 4 months.
  - Between 6 and 12 months, infantile hemangioma (IH) stabilizes in size and appearance and then slowly involutes by 5 to 10 years of age. Many leave behind residual markings or fibrous tissue.

15.3. Complications and Associations
- Ulceration: may occur in any hemangioma but is more common on the lip and in the diaper area.
- Depending on the location and size, the IH may cause disfigurement or may interfere with vision or breathing.
- Disseminated neonatal hemangiomatosis: multiple scattered small hemangiomas. Can be accompanied by internal involvement in the liver, brain, or gastrointestinal tract.
- PHACES syndrome: **p**osterior fossa malformations, **h**emangiomas, **a**rterial anomalies, **c**oarctation of the aorta, **e**ye anomalies, and **s**ternal cleft
- Segmental facial hemangiomas: may be associated with PHACES syndrome or severe GI bleeding.
- Chin and neck hemangiomas: may be associated with tracheal involvement
- Sacral hemangiomas: may be associated with tethered cord or spinal dysraphism
- LUMBAR syndrome: **l**ower body segmental IHs with **u**rogenital anomalies, **u**lceration, **m**yelopathy, **b**ony deformities, **a**norectal malformations, **a**rterial anomalies, and **r**enal anomalies.

15.4. Evaluation
- Early evaluation is imperative if treatment is needed. Evaluation depends on type and presentation of hemangioma.
  - If periocular, ophthalmologic evaluation is warranted.
  - If concerned for PHACES syndrome, workup includes MRI/MRA of brain and neck, echocardiogram, and ophthalmology evaluation. Patients should be referred to a physician familiar with vascular lesions.
  - For multifocal hemangiomas (>5), obtain ultrasound of liver.

15.5. Treatment
- For most uncomplicated hemangiomas, active nonintervention is the best management option. If large, ulcerated, or disfiguring, the treatment of choice is topical and/or oral beta blockers.[4] Other options include intralesional/oral steroids, pulsed-dye laser, and surgical removal.

16. NEVUS SIMPLEX

16.1. Clinical Presentation
- Pink macular patches (Fig. 12-13), generally on the eyelids, glabella, or nape of neck.
- Lesions on the eyelids usually improve at 1 year and fade by 3 years.
  - Those on the nape of the neck tend to persist.
  - No treatment is needed.

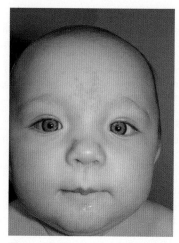

Figure 12-13. Nevus simplex (angel's kiss). (From Dusenbery SM, White A. *The Washington Manual of Pediatrics.* Philadelphia, PA: Lippincott Williams & Wilkins; 2009.)

DERMATITIS

17. ATOPIC DERMATITIS

17.1. Clinical Presentation

* Characterized by pruritic, erythematous papules and plaques.
* Secondary changes include lichenification, postinflammatory hyperpigmentation, or hypopigmentation.

17.2. Epidemiology

* There is a strong association with personal or family history of asthma and allergic rhinitis.
* Most eczema improves by 10 years of age, but severe atopic dermatitis (AD) can persist into adulthood.
* Severe, recalcitrant eczematous dermatitis may be associated with immunodeficiencies, including hyper-IgE syndrome, Wiskott-Aldrich syndrome, and severe combined immunodeficiency syndrome.
* Often associated with mutations in the *filaggrin* gene.[5]
* Children with eczema are prone to viral superinfection (e.g., herpes simplex virus [HSV], molluscum contagiosum, coxsackie) and colonization with *Staphylococcus aureus.*[6]

17.3. Subtypes

* Infantile
  * From 2 months to 2 years
  * Commonly involves cheeks (Fig. 12-14A), scalp, trunk, and extensor surfaces of the extremities

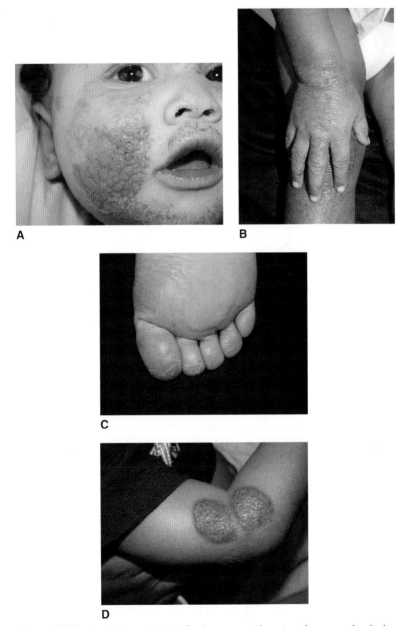

Figure 12-14. Atopic dermatitis. **A:** Infantile eczema with oozing plaques on the cheeks. **B:** Childhood eczema-lichenified plaques with excoriations. **C:** Juvenile plantar dermatosis (foot eczema). **D:** Nummular eczema. (From Dusenbery SM, White A. *The Washington Manual of Pediatrics*. Philadelphia, PA: Lippincott Williams & Wilkins; 2009.)

- Childhood
  - From 2 years to adolescence
  - Commonly involves flexural surfaces, including antecubital, popliteal fossae, neck, wrists, and feet (Fig. 12-14B, C)
- Adolescent/Adult
  - Flexural surfaces; may be limited to hands and/or face
- Nummular
  - Coin-shaped erythematous, oozing plaques that may have papules or vesicles at the periphery
  - Often occur on hands, arms, or legs (Fig. 12-14D)
- Dyshidrotic
  - Bilateral hand and/or foot dermatitis
  - Intensely pruritic with small vesicles along sides of fingers and toes

17.4. Treatment

- General skin care
  - Limit bathing to once daily in lukewarm water. Plain water is best. Use mild soaps (e.g., Dove, Aveeno) only in small amounts and in the area necessary.
  - Apply moisturizers immediately after bathing. Ointments (e.g., petroleum jelly [Vaseline] or Aquaphor) are more effective than are lotions.
- Education of patients, including emphasizing the chronicity of disease and the need for consistent application of prescribed treatment, can improve compliance and outcomes.
- Topical steroids[7]
  - Classification
  - Low strength (e.g., hydrocortisone 1% or 2.5% ointment): can be used for mild to moderate disease.
  - Mid strength (e.g., triamcinolone 0.1% ointment): can be used for limited amounts of time on more severe, localized areas of disease. These agents can cause atrophy if used chronically.
  - High strength (e.g., fluocinonide or clobetasol ointment) for palmar and plantar dermatitis or lichenified plaques.
  - Avoid using topical steroids on the face and intertriginous areas. Risks of topical steroids include skin atrophy, striae, and hypopigmentation.
- Immunomodulators
  - Topical tacrolimus (0.03% or 0.1%) or topical pimecrolimus (1%) may be useful in limited areas such as the face, where topical steroids may cause undesirable side effects with prolonged use.
  - These agents are recommended in children over age 2 years.
- Antihistamines
  - Oral diphenhydramine, hydroxyzine, or cetirizine may cause sedation, restricting their use to night time, to help with sleeping.
- Systemic steroids
  - Used in short bursts for severe exacerbations.
  - Regular or long-term use is not recommended.
- Antibiotics
  - *S. aureus* is the most common cause of bacterial superinfection. Dilute bleach baths can decrease colonization (1/4 cup for tub of water). Oral antibiotics may be necessary depending on the severity of infection. Methicillin-resistant *S. aureus* is becoming more prevalent. Cultures to determine antibiotic susceptibility may be helpful.
- If eczema is still refractory, systemic therapy with cyclosporine and methotrexate may be considered.[8]

18. CONTACT DERMATITIS (ALLERGIC)

18.1. Clinical Presentation

- Erythematous papules and vesicles with oozing and crusting. Pruritus may be intense. This is a type IV (delayed/cell-mediated) hypersensitivity reaction.
- Common causes include poison ivy/oak, nickel, cosmetics and fragrances, topical medications, chemicals in diaper wipes, tape, or adhesives (Fig. 12-15A, B). The distribution often gives clues to the causative agent (e.g., exposed areas for poison ivy, umbilicus for nickel, eyelids and face for nail polish or other cosmetics, buttocks and posterior thigh for toilet seat).

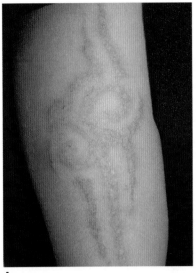

A

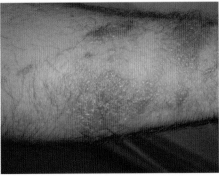

B

Figure 12-15. Contact dermatitis. **A:** Henna tattoo allergy. **B:** Poison ivy. (From Dusenbery SM, White A. *The Washington Manual of Pediatrics*. Philadelphia, PA: Lippincott Williams & Wilkins; 2009.)

• May be accompanied by eczematous dermatitis at sites far from initial exposure (hypersensitivity reaction).

18.2. Evaluation

• If condition is recurrent and no causative agent can be identified, skin patch testing may be indicated.

18.3. Treatment

• Contact with the offending allergen should be avoided. Topical midpotency and high-potency steroids decrease inflammation. In severe eruptions, systemic steroids may be needed (2 to 3 week taper).

19. DIAPER DERMATITIS

• Many potential causes of diaper dermatitis, with the most common being irritant. Other causes: seborrheic dermatitis, candidiasis, psoriasis, zinc deficiency, and Langerhans cell histiocytosis.

19.1. Clinical Presentation

• Irritant dermatitis: erythematous patches with maceration occur in diaper area, sparing the creases due to the moist environment. In more severe cases, papules, erosions, and ulcerations may be present.

19.2. Evaluation

• Diagnosis is straightforward and uncomplicated. However, if the dermatitis is refractory to treatment, widespread, or unusual, additional studies (such as measurement of zinc levels or biopsy) may be warranted.

19.3. Treatment

• Treatment includes frequent diaper changes, avoidance of diaper wipes, low-strength topical steroids and/or topical antifungals, and use of barrier creams.

20. SEBORRHEIC DERMATITIS

20.1. Clinical Presentation

• Characterized by erythematous patches covered by thick, yellow scale on the vertex of the head and intertriginous areas.
• "Cradle cap" occurs on the scalp of infants (Fig. 12-16). Other commonly affected sites in babies include diaper area, axillae, and other creases. Dermatitis may be complicated by Candida or bacteria, with postinflammatory hypopigmentation.
  • It is most common at 2 to 10 weeks and may last for 8 to 12 months.

20.2. Treatment

• Treatment in infants is hydrocortisone 0.5% to 1% cream or ointment.
• Scale may be removed with a soft brush while shampooing. Salicylic acid preparations should be avoided as they cause salicylism through absorption.
• Avoid "medicated shampoos" as this will aggravate eczema if this is a complicating factor.

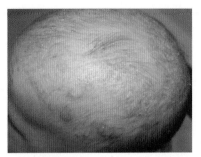

Figure 12-16. Seborrheic dermatitis. (From Dusenbery SM, White A. *The Washington Manual of Pediatrics*. Philadelphia, PA: Lippincott Williams & Wilkins; 2009.)

INFECTIOUS DISEASES

21. TINEA

• Fungal infections in children commonly occur on the scalp (tinea capitis) (Fig. 12-17A, B), face (tinea faciei), and body (tinea corporis) (Fig. 12-18).

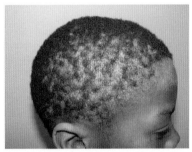

A

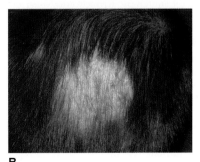

B

Figure 12-17. A,B: Tinea capitis. (From Dusenbery SM, White A. *The Washington Manual of Pediatrics*. Philadelphia, PA: Lippincott Williams & Wilkins; 2009.)

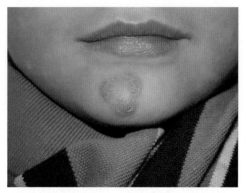

Figure 12-18. Tinea corporis. (From Dusenbery SM, White A. *The Washington Manual of Pediatrics.* Philadelphia, PA: Lippincott Williams & Wilkins; 2009.)

- Most often caused by *Microsporum* and *Trichophyton* species.
- Transmitted by contact with affected individuals, cats, or dogs.

21.1. Clinical Presentation

- Scalp infections are characterized by scaling and patchy hair loss. They may be confused with seborrheic dermatitis if there is minimal hair loss and inflammation. A kerion is a sharply demarcated, tender, inflammatory pustular plaque.
- Tinea corporis is characterized by annular, scaly plaques or plaque with central clearing and erythematous scaly border.

21.2. Evaluation

- Diagnosis may be made by clinical appearance, potassium hydroxide (KOH) slide "prep" showing branching hyphae, or fungal culture.

21.3. Treatment

- Scalp infections: topical antifungals are ineffective when used alone; requires systemic antifungal treatment (griseofulvin for 6 to 8 weeks minimum or terbinafine for 2 to 4 weeks, depending on fungal species), plus antifungal shampoo (selenium sulfide 2.5% or ketoconazole 1% to 2%), 2 to 3 times per week
- Skin infections: topical antifungals (e.g., miconazole, clotrimazole, terbinafine) b.i.d. for 3 to 4 weeks or until scaling clears

22. VERRUCAE

- Verrucae are caused by human papillomavirus infection of skin keratinocytes.

22.1. Clinical Presentation

- Verruca vulgaris
  - Round papules with an irregular, papillomatous surface that disrupts skin lines (Fig. 12-19A)

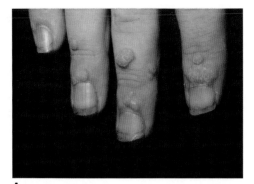

A

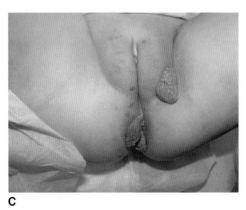

B

C

Figure 12-19. Warts. **A:** Verrucae vulgaris. **B:** Flat warts. **C:** Genital warts (condylomata acuminata). (From Dusenbery SM, White A. *The Washington Manual of Pediatrics*. Philadelphia, PA: Lippincott Williams & Wilkins; 2009.)

- Common on the hands but may occur anywhere
- Verruca plantaris
  - Flat hyperkeratotic papules on plantar feet. Thrombosed capillaries may appear as black dots.
  - Painful with pressure of walking.
- Verruca plana
  - Skin-colored slightly raised, flat-topped papules (Fig. 12-19B).
  - They often occur in groups on the legs and face.

22.2. Treatment

- Most warts resolve spontaneously within 2 years. Therapeutic methods include:
  - Topical keratolytics (e.g., salicylic acid) or cryotherapy available over the counter; however, they may be slow to work.
  - Liquid nitrogen cryotherapy performed every 2 to 4 weeks in office.
- Flat warts on legs: patients should avoid shaving because microtrauma can lead to new lesions.
- Refractory lesions: more intensive intervention, including pairing, Candida antigen injections, topical immunotherapy, laser therapy, or surgical removal, may be considered.
- Anogenital warts (Fig. 12-19C): use imiquimod. Therapy is usually 6 to 12 months, applied 2 to 3 times per week. May be caused by autoinoculation of common warts or vertical transmission during childbirth. Screening for sexual abuse in a child ages 2 to 14 years if warranted.

23. MOLLUSCUM CONTAGIOSUM

- Caused by a poxvirus; transmitted by swimming, bathing, or other close contact with an infected person

23.1. Clinical Presentation

- Skin-colored pearly papules with central umbilication. If inflamed, they may become red, tender, pustular, and increase in size (Fig. 12-20).

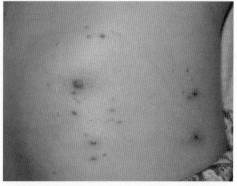

Figure 12-20. Molluscum contagiosum. (From Dusenbery SM, White A. *The Washington Manual of Pediatrics.* Philadelphia, PA: Lippincott Williams & Wilkins; 2009.)

23.2. Treatment

- Generally self-limited, and the condition often resolves in 12 months.
- For extensive or persistent lesions, curettage or topical cantharidin (blistering agent) may be effective. Imiquimod is not effective.

MISCELLANEOUS

24. ACNE VULGARIS

- The etiology of acne is multifactorial. Causes include follicular plugging, increased sebum production, *Propionibacterium acnes* overgrowth, and inflammation.

24.1. Clinical Presentation (Types)

- Comedonal: open comedones (blackheads) and closed comedones (whiteheads) (Fig. 12-21A)

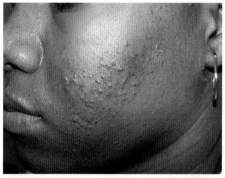

A

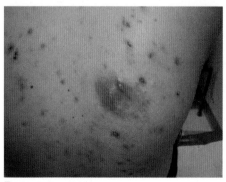

B

Figure 12-21. Acne vulgaris. **A:** Comedonal acne. **B:** Cystic acne. (From Dusenbery SM, White A. *The Washington Manual of Pediatrics.* Philadelphia, PA: Lippincott Williams & Wilkins; 2009.)

- Inflammatory: erythematous, inflammatory papules and pustules in addition to comedones
- Cystic: nodules and cysts on face, chest, and back (Fig. 12-21B)

24.2. Treatment

- General skin care: washing of face with soap or acne wash 2 times per day. Avoid scrubbing and excessive washing.
- Comedonal acne[9]
  - Benzoyl peroxide 2.5%, 5%, and 10% preparations. Benzoyl peroxide products should not be used at the same time as a topical retinoid.
  - Topical retinoids come in a variety of strengths: adapalene 0.1% (least potent) and 0.3%; tretinoin 0.025%, 0.05%, and 0.1% creams and gels; and tazarotene 0.05% and 0.1% cream (most potent). Start with the least potent for patients with dry or sensitive skin and work up as tolerated.
  - Benzoyl peroxide and retinoids can be irritating. Advise patients to use only a pea-sized amount on the face. Use every other day initially if redness/drying occurs, and then increase to daily as tolerance develops.
  - Products combining a topical antibiotic (clindamycin 1%, erythromycin) and benzoyl peroxide OR topical antibiotic and retinoid are available to simplify regimens.
- Inflammatory acne[9]
  - Add oral antibiotic (doxycycline, minocycline, tetracycline) to topical regimen for comedonal acne. Per guidelines, oral antibiotics should be continued for 3 to 6 months to assess efficacy.
  - Advise patients to avoid excessive sun exposure and to use sunscreen to avoid photosensitivity, and take antibiotics with a large glass of water to minimize esophagitis.
- Cystic/nodular or scarring acne
  - Systemic retinoid therapy (isotretinoin)
  - Requires monitoring of lipid profile, aspartate aminotransferase, alanine aminotransferase, and strict contraception in females because the agent is teratogenic.
- For females, consider an endocrine workup if there are virilizing signs or irregular menses to look for androgen excess disorder (polycystic ovary syndrome).

25. ERYTHEMA MULTIFORME

25.1. Clinical Presentation

- Characterized by erythematous papules or plaques that evolve into target lesions with dusky centers. Oral lesions may be present (Fig. 12-22).
- Most common precipitants are HSV infection, drug, or mycoplasma.

25.2. Treatment

- Oral systemic steroids may be helpful if given early, for 7 to 10 days.
- Prophylactic acyclovir may be useful to prevent recurrent HSV-related disease.
- Antihistamines provide symptomatic relief.

See Chapter 5 for additional discussion of reactive viral exanthems.

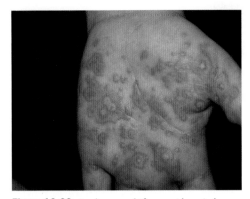

Figure 12-22. Erythema multiforme with typical target lesions. (From Dusenbery SM, White A. *The Washington Manual of Pediatrics*. Philadelphia, PA: Lippincott Williams & Wilkins; 2009.)

REFERENCES

1. Groesser L, Herschberger E, Ruetten A, et al. Postzygotic HRAS and KRAS mutations cause nevus sebaceous and Schimmelpenning syndrome. *Nat Genet* 2012;44(7):783–787.
2. Idriss MH, Elston DM. Secondary neoplasms associated with nevus sebaceous of Jadassohn: a study of 707 cases. *J Am Acad Dermatol* 2014;70(2):332–337.
3. Shirley MD, Tang H, Gallione CJ, et al. Sturge-Weber syndrome and port-wine stains caused by somatic mutation in GNAQ. *N Engl J Med* 2013;386(21):1971–1979.
4. Léauté-Labrèze C, Dumas de la Roque E, Hubiche T, et al. Propranolol for severe hemangiomas of infancy. *N Engl J Med* 2008;358(24):2649–2651.
5. Palmer CN, Irvine AD, Terron-Kwiatkowski A, et al. Common loss-of-function variants of the epidermal barrier protein filaggrin are a major predisposing factor for atopic dermatitis. *Nat Genet* 2006;38(4):441–446.
6. Eichenfield LF, Tom WL, Chamlin SL, et al. Guidelines of care for the management of atopic dermatitis: section 1. Diagnosis and assessment of atopic dermatitis. *J Am Acad Dermatol* 2014;70(2):338–351.
7. Eichenfield LF, Tom WL, Berger TG, et al. Guidelines of care for the management of atopic dermatitis: section 2. Management and treatment of atopic dermatitis with topical therapies. *J Am Acad Dermatol* 2014;71(1):116–132.
8. Sidbury R, Davis DM, Cohen DE, et al. Guidelines of care for the management of atopic dermatitis: section 3. Management and treatment with phototherapy and systemic agents. *J Am Acad Dermatol* 2014;71(2):327–349.
9. Eichenfield LF, Krakowski AC, Piggot C, et al. Evidence-based recommendations for the diagnosis and treatment of pediatric acne. *Pediatrics* 2013;131(suppl 3):S163–S186.

13 Geriatric Dermatology

Kathleen Nemer, MD and David M. Sheinbein, MD

Diseases of elderly adults are becoming increasingly important as life expectancy increases worldwide. To promote healthy aging, it is important to understand and recognize the skin changes associated with aging. Structural and physiologic skin changes, coupled with a lifetime's worth of environmental insults, make the elderly especially susceptible to dermatologic disorders.[1]

As the skin ages, cellular turnover slows, with progressive loss of cells in the epidermis, dermis, and extracellular matrix.[2,3] Histologically, the rete pegs, which help to hold the epidermis to the dermis, are retracted,[4] leading to skin that is wrinkled, lax, and easier to tear.[5,6] Years of sun exposure predispose the elderly to benign skin conditions (**solar lentigo, rosacea**) as well as malignant skin conditions (**actinic keratosis, basal cell carcinoma, squamous cell carcinoma, lentigo maligna, malignant melanoma**).

Reduced stratum corneum lipid biosynthesis impairs permeability barrier function,[7] increasing the likelihood of **xerosis, pruritus, and seborrheic dermatitis**. There is decreased cutaneous blood flow and remodeling of microvasculature,[8,9] increasing the risk for vascular abnormalities such as **actinic (solar) purpura, stasis dermatitis, chronic leg ulcers**, and **pressure ulcers** (Fig. 13-1). Thermoregulation is also weakened due to a decreased number of sweat glands and diminished subcutaneous fat,[5] increasing the elderly's sensitivity to moisture, heat, and cold (**skin maceration, intertrigo, erythema ab igne**).

A parallel blunting of normal immune function in the elderly produces higher levels of autoimmune skin disorders such as **bullous pemphigoid** and **pemphigus vulgaris**. Immunologic senescence also increases the potential for reactivation of latent viruses such as **herpes zoster (shingles)**.

With age come skin growths that are often unwanted and unsightly, such as the exceedingly common **seborrheic keratosis**. Endearingly termed "wisdom spots," these benign skin thickenings are hereditary and increase proportionally with age. They are often confused with skin cancer and as such are a frequent cause for referral to the outpatient dermatology clinic.

The etiology of allergic responses in the elderly can be challenging to diagnose. Patients often present with itchy, inflamed skin. The prevalence of polypharmacy in the elderly increases their risk for drug reactions and **urticaria**. Although elderly individuals have increased cumulative exposures to allergens,[10] normal immune senescence leads to diminished clinical manifestations, making diagnosis more difficult. Overall, it seems that the incidence of **allergic contact dermatitis** decreases with age; however, some allergens such as fragrance demonstrate increased sensitization rates in the elderly.[11] The presence of ulcerated skin also increases sensitization rates, for example, in patients with chronic leg ulcers.[12]

When treating the elderly patient, the physician must take into consideration the patient's physical ability to comply with the recommended therapy as well as

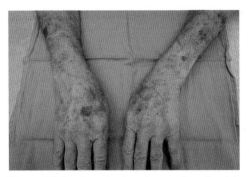

Figure 13-1. Purpuric, irregular macules of actinic (solar) purpura with prominent veins, skin wrinkling, and hemosiderin staining.

socioeconomic factors that impact compliance. Older patients often present with multiple comorbidities and the potential for cognitive dysfunction and/or impaired vision, hearing, and/or mobility. One medical problem can lead to a cascade of others. For example, a diabetic elderly patient is at risk for sensory, motor, and autonomic neuropathy, leading to limited sensation, decreased mobility of the lower extremities, and foot trauma. Immunosuppression in diabetics places them at higher risk for chronic fungal infection (**tinea pedis**, **onychomycosis**). Incidental foot trauma, coupled with fungal pathogens, creates a portal of entry for bacterial invasion of subcutaneous tissues (**cellulitis**).[13]

When treating elderly patients, it is important to consider extrinsic factors necessary for compliance. Some patients may not have adequate housing, nutrition, or the financial resources necessary for adequate compliance. For those who do have housing in long-term care facilities, there is increased risk for transmission of contagious infestations such as **scabies**. Scabies can cause a generalized eruption resembling erythroderma (generalized scaling and erythema over an extensive part of the body) in the elderly, the institutionalized, and those with immunosuppression or neurologic dysfunction. The inability to scratch in these patients can lead to **crusted or Norwegian scabies**, a more severe form of scabies with a higher mite burden.

Polypharmacy in the elderly increases the risk for medication confusion, while skin fragility increases safety concerns with overuse of topical medications prescribed. Given these factors, simple regimens for the shortest course possible are preferable in elderly patients. Extra effort may be necessary on the clinician's part to write down medication instructions for patients and caregivers so that they are accurately followed.

Many of the dermatologic conditions afflicting the elderly are seen in a wide range of ages. These entities are listed by chapter in Table 13-1 with a short clinical description of "*what to look for*" when distinguishing between them. Further details can be found within the appropriate chapter. The remaining common skin ailments in the elderly are discussed, with an emphasis on general skin care for dry, itchy skin, as these are intertwined as two of the most common skin complaints seen in the outpatient elderly patient.

Table 13-1	Common Elderly Dermatoses

Disorder	*Look for...*	Page
Inflammatory disorders		
Rosacea	Facial flushing, localized erythema, telangiectasias, erythematous papules and pustules on the nose, cheeks, brow, and chin; rhinophyma is more common in men.	
Allergic contact dermatitis	Red, itchy, burning rash in the distribution of allergen exposure. Look for well-demarcated borders and geometric shapes. Eyelid edema is seen when the allergen is innocently transferred from finger to lid. In nursing home patients, consider rubber catheters and body lotions as potential culprits. Patch testing may be necessary to identify the offending allergen.	
Seborrheic dermatitis	Loose, bran-like, or greasy white scales often with background erythema. Characteristic sites: scalp (dandruff), eyebrows, eyelids, nasolabial folds, within and behind ears, sternum, umbilicus, groin (scrotum, labia minora), and perianal area. This is a common, chronic entity in the elderly and can be quite severe in HIV and Parkinson disease.	
Infections and infestations		
Tinea pedis	Pruritic plaques on the dorsum of the foot; advancing edge with prominent erythema and scale. Plantar surface with powdery, white scale in a "moccasin" distribution. Interdigital web space scaling and white maceration (fourth web space most common).	
Intertrigo	Erythema or erosions of opposing skin surfaces: axillae, groin, perineum, inframammary creases, and abdominal folds. Patients are often obese and/or diabetic. In obese patients, look for inflammation in neck creases, popliteal or antecubital fossae, thigh and groin folds, and under pendulous breasts. Satellite papules suggest *Candida*.	
Herpes zoster (shingles)	1 to 3 d prodrome of burning pain/paresthesias followed by an eruption of grouped papules and vesicles on an erythematous base. Usually confined to a distinct dermatome and not crossing midline. Postherpetic neuralgia can be quite painful and is more common in those over 70 years old.	

Disorder	*Look for...*	Page
Cellulitis	Rapidly progressive areas of skin edema, redness, warmth, tenderness, and lymphangitic streaking. Fever, malaise, and chills are common in immunosuppressed individuals. Tinea pedis and diabetes are risk factors.	
Scabies	Look for burrows: fine, thread-like, serpiginous lines with a terminal tiny black speck (the mite) with surrounding small erythematous papules and vesicles in the interdigital web spaces of the hands, flexor wrists, elbows, areolae, axillae, umbilicus, genitals, and buttocks. Spares the head and neck. Pruritus is intense, especially at night. Pruritic lesions on the areola in women and penis and scrotum in men are highly suggestive of scabies. Scabies is very contagious. Inquire about symptoms in family members and caretakers.	
Crusted/ Norwegian scabies	Thick, crusted plaques may be localized but are more often generalized involving the scalp, face, trunk, extremities, and periungual areas. Patients may present with generalized erythema and scaling. Typical burrows may be absent. The diagnosis is frequently missed, and transmission continues to those in physical contact with the individual. Always consider this diagnosis in any elderly, institutionalized, or immunocompromised patient with pruritus.	

Reactive disorders and drug eruptions

Stasis dermatitis	Bilateral erythema, hyperpigmentation, and scaling on the ankle and distal lower legs. Often, there is edema, varicosities, and atrophic patches indicative of venous insufficiency. Advanced disease may have a woody induration due to chronic adipose tissue ischemia (lipodermatosclerosis), characterized by an "inverted champagne bottle" due to fibrosis in the distal leg and edema in the proximal leg. Stasis dermatitis is often confused with cellulitis. Unlike cellulitis, stasis dermatitis is usually *scaly* and *bilateral*.	
Urticaria (hives)	Well-circumscribed, erythematous, edematous papules, patches, or plaques, often with a pale center. No single lesion lasts >24 h. May occur anywhere on the body but most often on the trunk.	

continued on following page

Disorder	Look for...	Page
Morbilliform drug eruption	Blanchable red macules and papules arising on the trunk and spreading symmetrically to the proximal extremities. Areas of pressure may be more severely affected. Pruritus is common. Superficial desquamation (scaling) occurs as the rash resolves. Onset is usually within 7 to 14 d of initiating a medication.	

Benign skin lesions

Seborrheic keratoses	Tan, brown, black, waxy, "stuck-on" appearing papules with a well-defined border. Pigmentation may vary within a single lesion. They occur anywhere except the palms, soles, and mucous membranes. **No malignant potential** but can be itchy and annoying; irritated by clothing (bra straps, underwear elastic) and jewelry (necklaces). Patients often scratch them off only to have them grow back.	
Solar lentigo	Tan to dark brown irregular macules on areas of sun exposure including the face, upper chest, shoulders, dorsal arms, and hands. Caused by chronic sun exposure. Present in 90% of Caucasians over 60 years old. A solar lentigo that looks different from the others or is enlarging or darkening should be biopsied to rule out lentigo maligna.	

Malignant skin lesions

Basal cell carcinoma	Nonhealing, pearly papule with a rolled border and telangiectasias on sun-exposed skin (face, trunk). Can bleed and ulcerate. Increased risk in fair-skinned patients	
Actinic keratosis	Erythematous, raised, rough papules with associated scale; their "gritty" texture makes them easier felt than seen.	
Squamous cell carcinoma	Nonhealing, red papule, plaque, or nodule on sun-exposed skin (face, scalp, trunk, extremities). Over time, the tumor often develops a depressed center. Increased risk in fair-skinned and solid organ transplant patients	
Lentigo maligna	Irregularly bordered, hyperpigmented (tan-brown) flat patch usually on the face of an elderly person. Predilection for the nose and cheeks. Looks like a "stain" on the skin of a fair-skinned person with a history of significant sun exposure.	

Disorder	*Look for...*	Page
Malignant melanoma	**Asymmetry:** draw a line through the lesion and the two sides do not match. **Border:** irregular, notched, or scalloped borders. **Color:** different shades of brown, tan, black, red, or white. **Diameter:** >6 mm is concerning (size of a #2 pencil eraser). **Evolution:** changing in size, shape, or color; pain, pruritus, or bleeding. Caucasian men: most common location is the back. Caucasian women: most common location is the back and legs.	

Disorders of the hair and nails

Onychomycosis	Thickened, yellowed fingernails or toenails (latter more common). Associated subungual debris and onycholysis (lifting of the nail plate from the nail bed at its distal end, resembling a half-moon). Commonly associated with concurrent tinea pedis.	

Cutaneous manifestations of systemic disease

Bullous pemphigoid	Large, tense bullae on an erythematous base filled with serous or blood-tinged fluid. Most often seen on the forearms, lower abdomen, and thighs of elderly individuals over 60 years old. Pruritus is very common and may precede bullae. Bullae are *tense* compared to the flaccid bullae of pemphigus vulgaris and are rarely seen on the mucosa.	
Pemphigus vulgaris	Flaccid bullae that break easily, leaving denuded erosions and risk for bacterial infection; frequently begins with oral lesions; blister spreads apart with application of pressure; first onset is in individuals 50–60 years old.	
Lichen sclerosus et atrophicus	Flat, ivory white, shiny scar-like plaques with a violaceous border. Most commonly found on the vulva and perianal skin in women and glans and prepuce of the penis in men but can be extragenital. Severely pruritic. Squamous cell carcinoma can arise in genital lesions. Complications related to genital scarring include dyspareunia, urinary obstruction, ulceration, painful erection, and phimosis. When on the genitals, the lesions may have purpura, and elderly abuse must be ruled out.	

continued on following page

Disorder	*Look for...*	Page
Geriatric dermatology		
Actinic purpura	See below.	
Erythema ab igne	See below.	
Leg ulcers	See below.	
Skin maceration	See below.	
Xerosis/Pruritus	See below.	
The Washington Manual of Outpatient Internal Medicine[14]		
Pressure ulcers	Erythema, shallow erosion, or ulceration over a bony prominence or pressure point (sacrum, heels, occiput, elbows). More prevalent in patients who are bed or wheel-chair bound	pp. 716–718

1. ACTINIC PURPURA

1.1. Background

- Actinic purpura, also known as solar or senile purpura, is a benign form of purpura found almost exclusively in the elderly. Years of ultraviolet radiation induces atrophy of the dermis, rendering dermal blood vessels vulnerable to minor trauma. While the trauma itself often goes unrecognized, it causes noticeable leakage of red blood cells into the dermis.

1.2. Clinical Presentation (Fig. 13-2)

- Asymptomatic violaceous macules and patches with irregular borders and sharp margins on the dorsal hands and extensor forearms. Ecchymoses may vary in deepness of color depending on their age and can persist for several weeks. They are most pronounced in fair-skinned individuals. Other signs of actinic damage are often present.

1.3. Evaluation

- This is a clinical diagnosis. Of note, patients usually do not give a history of trauma and are often taking medications that exacerbate the condition (warfarin, clopidogrel, aspirin).

1.4. Treatment

- Minimize trauma to the skin.
- Protect the forearms from the sun with sunscreen and from trauma with a double layer of clothing. Long athletic socks with the feet cut off at the ankle can provide a protective layer for the arms when around the house/long-term care facility.

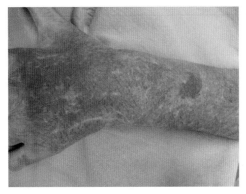

Figure 13-2. Hemosiderin deposition with a sharp demarcation between normal and abnormal skin. The linear white scars suggest dermal atrophy.

2. ERYTHEMA AB IGNE

2.1. Background

• Erythema ab igne, derived from Latin for "redness from fire," is characterized by hyperpigmentation caused by long-term exposure to heat. The elderly are especially susceptible given prolonged exposure to hot water bottles, heating pads, or electric blankets. Sitting near a wood stove or fireplace as well as using a laptop computer on the lap are also risk factors. The disorder is seen more commonly in women.

2.2. Clinical Presentation

• Reticular (net-like) or mottled patches of pink, purple, red, and eventually brown (from melanin deposition) in areas of heat exposure. Telangiectasia and other poikilodermatous changes (hypopigmentation, hyperpigmentation, or atrophy) can appear in long-standing cases. Burns do not occur, but pruritus or mild burning paresthesias can be present. The resultant pigmentation changes can be permanent.

2.3. Evaluation

• This is a clinical diagnosis. When erythema ab igne is suspected, ask the patient specific questions regarding direct heat exposure (e.g., heating pad, hot water bottle, exposure to radiant heat from a radiator, stove, or fireplace). Do not confuse with livedo reticularis and cutis marmorata, which are more erythematous and vascular appearing, have no associated hyperpigmentation, and are not related to heat exposure (more likely to be related to cold exposure).

2.4. Treatment

• Eliminate the source of the chronic heat exposure. In mild cases, the hyperpigmentation may remit. Elderly individuals, especially those with dementia, warrant an environmental safety assessment.

3. LEG ULCERS

3.1. Background

- 90% of leg ulcers result from venous insufficiency, 5% result from arterial disease, and 5% are due to miscellaneous causes including diabetic microangiopathy, pyoderma gangrenosum, malignancies, vasculitis, and infections.[14]
- Venous ulcers are caused by incompetent one-way venous valves, leading to insufficient venous blood return, leg venous hypertension, aberrant tissue perfusion, and ischemia. Risk increases with age, a history of thrombosis, phlebitis, obesity, or leg injury such as fracture.
- Arterial ulcers are caused by inadequate blood supply to the skin from progressive atherosclerosis (peripheral vascular disease) or arterial embolization. Risk increases with diabetes mellitus, smoking, hyperlipidemia, obesity, rheumatoid arthritis, coronary artery disease, hypertension, hyperhomocysteinemia, male sex, and a sedentary lifestyle.

3.2. Clinical Presentation

- Venous ulcers
  - Shallow, irregular borders; yellow, fibrinous exudate.
  - Most common on the medial malleolus in areas of preceding stasis dermatitis. May become circumferential over time.
  - Associated features include leg and ankle edema, varicose veins, yellow-brown pigmentation secondary to hemosiderin deposition, eczematous changes with scaling and crusting (stasis dermatitis), and lymphedema.
  - Pulses are normal.
  - Ulcers are not painful.
- Arterial ulcers
  - Sharply defined, punched out ulcer with a pale base over bony prominences with surrounding smooth, shiny skin.
  - Most common on the lateral malleolus, tips of the toes, and heel.
  - Associated features include cyanosis, pallor, cool extremities, and loss of hair.
  - Pulses are diminished and capillary refill is delayed (more than 3 to 4 seconds).
  - Ulcers are painful and patients often give a history of claudication. Pain is relieved by dependency of the extremity (e.g., dangling the affected limb off the edge of the bed).

3.3. Evaluation

- Ulcers presenting with the distinct characteristics of either venous or arterial disease can be diagnosed clinically. Skin biopsy is often useful in the diagnosis of enigmatic ulcers; however, consideration must be given to the long healing time of biopsy sites on the lower leg, where ulcers are most common.
- In cases of doubt, the best tests to distinguish between arterial and venous disease are ankle-brachial index (ABI) to evaluate for arterial disease and duplex ultrasound to evaluate for venous insufficiency. The correct diagnosis is significant because the management differs for each. For example, compression stockings are a mainstay of treatment for venous disease but worsen arterial disease.
- Ankle-brachial index values:
  - Normal ABI: 1.0 to 1.3
  - Noncompressible calcified vessel: >1.3
  - Positive peripheral arterial disease: <0.9
- A vascular surgeon should evaluate any patient with a decrease in ABI.

3.4. Treatment[15,16]

- Venous ulcers
  - Treatment aims to improve venous return with **leg elevation** and **compression stockings** (e.g., Jobst stockings). Compression stockings should be tailored to fit the patient and the degree of venous insufficiency. Recommended pressure gradients are as follows:
    - **15 to 20 mm Hg**: mild varicose veins and minor leg swelling
    - **20 to 30 mm Hg**: moderate edema and moderate to severe varicosities
    - **30 to 40 mm Hg**: chronic venous insufficiency, severe edema, DVT and postthrombotic syndrome, venous ulceration, lymphedema, and orthostatic hypotension
  - Wet-to-dry dressings provide excellent mechanical debridement for 2 to 3 days, but longer use can interfere with wound healing. Keep wounds clean, covered, and moist with occlusive dressings. Cleanse with saline. Unna wraps are effective in severe cases.
  - Choice of wound dressing should be based on the amount of exudate, the depth of the ulceration, and the presence of slough.
  - Flat, shallow wounds with a low to medium amount of exudate do well with the following:
    - **Semipermeable films** (Tegaderm, OpSite Plus)
    - **Hydrocolloids** (DuoDERM, Tegasorb)
    - **Hydrogels** (IntraSite, Nu-Gel)
    - **Foam** (Allevyn brands)
  - Cavities and undermining wounds with a high amount of exudate do well with the following:
    - **Alginates** (Tegagen, Sorbsan, AlgiSite)
  - Ulcers with extensive necrotic tissue should be debrided. Treat secondarily infected wounds with systemic antibiotics and antimicrobial dressings:
    - **Iodosorb**
    - **Silver-impregnated dressings** (Acticoat, Aquacel Ag, Arglaes)
  - Associated stasis dermatitis may benefit from mid- to high-potency topical corticosteroids applied twice daily. Protect the ulcer with Vaseline petroleum jelly prior to application of corticosteroid.
  - Ulcers recalcitrant to medical treatment may need surgical intervention including punch grafts, split-thickness grafts, epidermal or dermal engineered grafts, and ablation of the superficial venous system (VNUS procedure).
- Arterial ulcers
  - Treatment aims to improve arterial blood flow with wound care, revascularization, and risk factor modification.
  - Arterial ulcers can be treated similarly to venous ulcers (above) with the exception of compression stockings, which *worsen* ischemic ulcers. Arterial ulcers tend to have slough but less exudate; thus, hydrogel dressings (IntraSite, Nu-Gel, Curasol) that rehydrate wounds and promote autolytic debridement are most efficacious.
  - Risk factor modifications:
    - Strict blood sugar control and meticulous foot care in diabetics
    - Tobacco cessation
    - Antiplatelet therapy with aspirin or clopidogrel
    - Antihypertensive therapy
    - Lipid-lowering therapy: goal LDL cholesterol <100 mg/dL and in very high-risk patients <70 mg/dL
    - Encourage exercise as tolerated

- Amputation can be avoided with revascularization procedures: angioplasty, stenting, catheter-based plaque excision, or open lower extremity bypass.
- Nonhealing ulcerations, gangrene, rest pain, and worsening claudication are indications for surgical consideration.

4. SKIN MACERATION

4.1. Background

- Maceration is defined as the softening and breaking down of skin resulting from prolonged exposure to moisture.[17] Excess moisture may be secondary to urinary or fecal incontinence, excessive sweating, occlusive dressings, or produced by a wound bed. In obese individuals, lesions may occur between skin folds. Macerated, moist skin can lead to pressure ulcers. For a detailed discussion of pressure ulcers, see *The Washington Manual of Outpatient Internal Medicine,* pages 716–718.[18]

4.2. Clinical Presentation

- Erythematous, abraded, or excoriated skin; there can be blisters and white or silver patches. Can affect any area constantly in contact with moisture.

4.3. Evaluation

- Elderly who are bedbound or incontinent of urine/feces are at risk of developing lesions on the buttocks or sacrum. These areas should be checked regularly by caregivers for both skin maceration and pressure ulcers.

4.4. Treatment[19]

- Eliminate the cause of moisture:
  - Toileting program for incontinence
  - Condom catheter
  - Indwelling catheter (if condom catheter not adequate)
  - Fecal incontinence collector
- Protect the skin from moisture:
  - Clean gently with a mild, nondrying soap (Dove, Oil of Olay, or Cetaphil) after each incontinent episode.
  - Apply a moisture barrier (Vaseline, Proshield, Smooth and Cool, Calmoseptine, or zinc oxide).
  - For irritated perianal skin, it is useful to apply an over-the-counter low-potency steroid (1% hydrocortisone cream) mixed with a low-potency antifungal (clotrimazole cream [Canesten or Lotrimin]).
  - Use disposable briefs that wick moisture from the skin; use linen incontinence pads when disposable briefs worsen perineal dermatitis.

5. XEROSIS/PRURITUS

5.1. Background

- Dry, itchy skin is a frequent ailment in the elderly. Skin thinning, coupled with decreased permeability barrier function, leads to persistently dry skin.[7] Dryness (xerosis) is the number one cause of itchy skin (pruritus). Other causes of pruritus in the elderly are listed in Table 13-2. When a common cause of pruritus cannot be identified, other avenues must be explored. Pruritus without a rash may be caused by several disparate underlying systemic diseases, listed in Table 13-3. A thorough workup should be undertaken if any such disease is suspected.

Table 13-2	Pruritus in the Elderly

Autoimmune blistering diseases

Acquired epidermolysis bullosa
Bullous pemphigoid
Dermatitis herpetiformis
Pemphigus vulgaris

Autoimmune connective tissue diseases

Dermatomyositis
Sjögren syndrome
Systemic sclerosis

Cutaneous lymphomas

Mycosis fungoides and its variants
Sézary syndrome

Erythematous papulosquamous diseases

Darier disease
Grover disease
Hailey-Hailey disease
Lichen planus
Palmoplantar pustulosis
Pityriasis rubra pilaris
Polymorphic light eruption
Psoriasis

Inflammatory diseases

Allergic contact dermatitis
Atopic dermatitis (eczema)
Dyshidrotic eczema
Urticaria

Other benign skin conditions

Lichen sclerosus et atrophicus
Seborrheic dermatitis
Seborrheic keratosis

Skin infections and infestations

Cutaneous larva migrans
Folliculitis
Herpes simplex
Herpes zoster
Insect bites and arthropod reactions
Intertrigo
Lice (pediculosis)
Scabies
Tinea

Xerosis (dry skin)

Table 13-3	Systemic Diseases with Associated Pruritus

Endocrine diseases

Hyperthyroidism
Hypothyroidism
Hyperparathyroidism
Diabetes

Hematologic diseases

Polycythemia vera (pruritus follows contact with heat, especially hot water)
Hodgkin lymphoma
Non-Hodgkin lymphoma
Leukemias
Myeloma multiplex
Iron deficiency
Systemic mastocytosis
Hypereosinophilic syndrome
Myelodysplastic syndromes

Infectious diseases

HIV infection/AIDS
Infestations (see above)

Kidney disease

Chronic kidney disease

Liver diseases (look for jaundice)

Primary biliary cirrhosis
Primary sclerosing cholangitis
Extrahepatic cholestasis
Hepatitis B and C

Malnutrition

Vitamin deficiencies (iron, vitamin A, vitamin D, zinc, B vitamins)

Neurologic diseases

Postherpetic itch
Notalgia paresthetica
Brain injury/tumor (frequently unilateral pruritus)
Sclerosis multiplex
Small fiber neuropathy

Other malignancies

Solid tumors (paraneoplastic pruritus)
Carcinoid syndrome
Cutaneous lymphomas (mycosis fungoides, Sézary syndrome)

Psychogenic diseases

Obsessive-compulsive disorder (OCD)
Anxiety
Neurotic excoriations
Delusions of parasitosis

- Medication-induced pruritus should be entertained in those individuals with intractable itching after the more usual causes have been excluded. Common drugs associated with pruritus in the elderly include the following:[20–22]
  - **Narcotics** (opioids)
  - **Antihypertensives** (calcium channel blockers, beta adrenergic blockers, angiotensin-converting enzyme inhibitors, angiotensin II antagonists [sartans])
  - **Statins**
  - **Antidiabetic drugs** (biguanides, sulfonylurea derivatives)
  - **Antibiotics**
  - **Antiepileptics**
  - **Antimalarials** (hydroxychloroquine)
  - **Psychotropic drugs** (tricyclic antidepressants, selective serotonin reuptake inhibitors, neuroleptics)
  - **Chemotherapeutics**
  - **Nonsteroidal anti-inflammatory drugs** (NSAIDs)
  - **Corticosteroids**
  - **Sex hormones**
  - **Antithyroid agents**
  - **B vitamins** (cyanocobalamin, niacin, thiamine)

5.2. Clinical Presentation

- Dull, rough, flaky, dry, cracked skin. There can be fine bran-like scales that flake off easily. Can present as large patches of dryness or smaller, nummular lesions. Repeated scratching can result in lichenification (thickened skin), excoriations, infection, and traumatic purpura.
- Xerosis usually worsens in the wintertime, exacerbated by low humidity, frequent bathing, and harsh soaps. Severe xerosis may present as asteatotic eczema, also known as *eczema craquelé* or *winter itch*. The skin is rough and dry with fine scale and interconnected fissures resembling cracked porcelain. Asteatotic eczema classically involves the lower legs but may involve the upper arms, anterior thighs, and lower back.[23]

5.3. Evaluation

- The physical examination should include a search for any other skin manifestations. While pruritus is most often related to xerosis, care should be taken to palpate for thyroid, liver, or lymph node abnormalities, especially if systemic disease is suspected.
- Suggested baseline evaluations for pruritus of unknown etiology are listed in Table 13-4.

5.4. Treatment

- Xerosis and pruritus in the elderly can create substantial suffering and often prove difficult to treat. Treatment focuses on general skin care with avoidance of provocative factors and frequent topical moisturization.
- Bathing
  - Take short baths or showers (<5 minutes).
  - Avoid hot water (use tepid water), especially in the wintertime.
  - Avoid bath oils, which can lead to falls from slippery feet.

Table 13-4	Suggested Evaluations for Pruritus of Unknown Etiology

Complete blood count with differential
Basic metabolic panel
Iron studies (iron, ferritin)
Thyroid-stimulating hormone
Liver function tests
Human immunodeficiency virus test
Chest x-ray
Vitamin levels

- Apply an emollient (ointment is best) within 3 minutes of bathing for maximal effect.
- Invest in a humidifier.
- Soaps
  - Use mild, nondrying soaps such as Dove, Oil of Olay, Cetaphil, Tone, or Purpose.
  - Use of washcloths and loofahs is discouraged as they can harbor bacteria.
  - Limit soap to axilla and groin.
- After bathing
  - Pat dry and apply thick moisturizers while the skin is still wet.
  - Ointments such as Vaseline and Aquaphor are the most lubricating and occlusive, making them the most potent. The downside is that they can be greasy and thus more difficult to apply.
  - Creams are less lubricating than ointments but more lubricating than gels, lotions, and solutions. They also are more likely to have additives that may irritate the skin (lanolin, aloe vera, and parabens). Thus, if a patient complains of burning or stinging with a cream, try switching to the comparable ointment. Recommended creams include Aveeno, Eucerin, Cerave, Curel, Cetaphil, Vanicream, or Lubriderm.
  - Apply ointments/creams multiple times daily.
  - Occlusion with plastic wrap or gloves after application of emollients increases their potency.
- Antipruritics
  - Camphor 1% to 3% and menthol (Sarna) provide a cooling sensation and should be stored in the refrigerator for maximal effect.
  - Topical anesthetics (benzocaine), antihistamines (diphenhydramine), and neomycin are best avoided because of the high rate of contact dermatitis.
  - Systemic antihistamines (H1-receptor antagonists) are helpful for sedative effect (cetirizine, loratadine, hydroxyzine, doxepin).
  - In recalcitrant cases, low-dose mirtazapine (7.5 mg qhs) or gabapentin (300 mg qhs) can be used for pruritus and carefully titrated up if tolerated and effective.
- Corticosteroids
  - Mild to midpotency topical steroids may be used on inflamed pruritic skin.
  - As with emollients, occlusion increases potency. Given the potential for skin thinning, steroid occlusion should be reserved for severe, resistant lesions and for a limited amount of time (such as in the evening while watching television).

- Midpotency topical corticosteroids (classes 3 to 4):
  - Triamcinolone cream or ointment: apply twice daily
  - Mometasone cream or ointment: apply twice daily
  - Fluocinolone cream or ointment: apply twice daily
- Low-potency topical corticosteroids for thinner skin (e.g., face, groin) (classes 6 to 7):
  - Desonide cream, lotion, or ointment: apply twice daily
  - Hydrocortisone 1% (OTC) or 2.5% cream or ointment: apply twice daily
- In sum:
- Patients can minimize the effect of xerosis by increasing the ambient humidity in their living environment, modifying their bathing technique, and using emollients multiple times daily to replace the lipid components of their skin.

REFERENCES

1. Farage MA, Miller KW, Berardesca E, et al. Clinical implications of aging skin: cutaneous disorders in the elderly. *Am J Clin Dermatol* 2009;10(2):73–86.
2. Kligman AM. Perspectives and problems in cutaneous gerontology. *J Invest Dermatol* 1979;73(1):39–46.
3. Branchet MC, Boisnic S, Frances C, et al. Skin thickness changes in normal aging skin. *Gerontology* 1990;36(1):28–35.
4. Waller JM, Maibach HI. Age and skin structure and function, a quantitative approach (I): blood flow, pH, thickness, and ultrasound echogenicity. *Skin Res Technol* 2005;11(4):221–235.
5. Gilchrest BA. Skin aging and photoaging: an overview. *J Am Acad Dermatol* 1989;21(3 Pt 2):610–613.
6. Tindall JP, Smith JG. Skin Lesions of the aged and their association with internal changes. *JAMA* 1963;186:1039–1042.
7. Elias PM, Ghadially R. The aged epidermal permeability barrier: basis for functional abnormalities. *Clin Geriatr Med* 2002;18(1):103–120, vii.
8. Chang E, Yang J, Nagavarapu U, et al. Aging and survival of cutaneous microvasculature. *J Invest Dermatol* 2002;118(5):752–758.
9. Tsuchida Y. The effect of aging and arteriosclerosis on human skin blood flow. *J Dermatol Sci* 1993;5(3):175–181.
10. Na CR, Wang S, Kirsner RS, et al. Elderly adults and skin disorders: common problems for nondermatologists. *South Med J* 2012;105(11):600–606.
11. Buckley DA, Rycroft RJ, White IR, et al. The frequency of fragrance allergy in patch-tested patients increases with their age. *Br J Dermatol* 2003;149(5):986–989.
12. Saap L, Fahim S, Arsenault E, et al. Contact sensitivity in patients with leg ulcerations: a North American study. *Arch Dermatol* 2004;140(10):1241–1246.
13. Al Hasan M, Fitzgerald SM, Saoudian M, et al. Dermatology for the practicing allergist: Tinea pedis and its complications. *Clin Mol Allergy* 2004;2(1):5.
14. Rosman I, Lloyd B, Jassim O. Dermatology. In: De Fer TM, Brisco MA, Muller RS, eds. *The Washington Manual of Outpatient Internal Medicine*. 1st ed. Philadelphia, PA: Lippincott Williams & Wilkins; 2010:831–861.
15. Hafner A, Sprecher E. Ulcers. In: Bolognia JL, Jorizzo JL, Schaffer JV, eds. *Dermatology*. 3rd ed. Philadelphia, PA: Elsevier Saunders; 2012:1729–1746.
16. Menaker GM, Mehlis SL, Kasprowicz S. Dressings. In: Bolognia JL, Jorizzo JL, Schaffer JV, eds. *Dermatology*. 3rd ed. Philadelphia, PA: Elsevier Saunders; 2012:2365–2379.
17. Anderson KN. *Mosby's Medical Nursing and Allied Health Dictionary*. St. Louis, MO: Mosby-Year Book; 1998.

18. Khalid S, Carr DB. Geriatrics. In: De Fer TM, Brisco MA, Muller RS, eds. *The Washington Manual of Outpatient Internal Medicine*. 1st ed. Philadelphia, PA: Lippincott Williams & Wilkins; 2010:699–722.

19. Reuben DB, Herr KA, Pacala JT, et al. *Geriatrics at your fingertips*. 13th ed. New York: American Geriatrics Society; 2011.

20. Reich A, Ständer S, Szepietowski JC. Drug-induced pruritus: a review. *Acta Derm Venereol* 2009;89(3):236–244.

21. Reich A, Ständer S, Szepietowski JC. Pruritus in the elderly. *Clin Dermatol* 2011;29(1):15–23.

22. Tripathi S, Kim B. The Science of Chronic Itch: a current review of the pathophysiology & clinical presentations of chronic pruritus to help you manage your itchy patients. *Rheumatologist* 2014;8(12):32–42.

23. Piérard GE, Quatresooz P. What do you mean by eczema craquelé? *Dermatology* 2007;215(1):3–4.

14 Sun Safety

Rachel L. Braden, MD and Kimberly L. Brady, MD

Exposure to ultraviolet (UV) light is the most important modifiable risk factor for skin cancer. Regular use of broad-spectrum sunscreen can reduce the risk of sunburn, prevent skin cancer, and decrease skin aging. Clothing provides some protection from UV radiation; the amount of protection depends on the weave of the fabric, dye color, fabric material, and dryness. Tanning bed use has been associated with a substantial increased risk for both melanoma and nonmelanoma skin cancer. All patients should be counseled to avoid excessive UV exposure, including indoor tanning.

1. SUNSCREENS

- A primer on UV radiation
  - UV light is the portion of the electromagnetic spectrum that encompasses the wavelengths 100 to 400 nm. The UV spectrum is divided into three bands: UVC (100 to 280 nm), UVB (280 to 320 nm), and UVA (320 to 400 nm). The ozone layer blocks all UVC and 90% of UVB rays produced by the sun; subsequently, the vast majority of the UV radiation that reaches the earth's surface is UVA.[1,2]
  - UV penetration into the skin varies with wavelength, with longer wavelengths penetrating deeper into the skin. UVB causes cross-linking of deoxyribonucleic acid (DNA), leading to pyrimidine dimer formation and pyrimidine-pyrimidone 6,4-photoproducts. UVA induces generation of reactive oxygen species leading to DNA strand breaks.[1]
  - Short-term effects of UV radiation on the skin include sunburn and tanning. UVB induces an inflammatory response that generates the prototypical erythema and blistering of a sunburn. Immediate tanning occurs secondary to UVA-induced oxidation and redistribution of the existing melanin. Delayed tanning peaks 3 days after UV exposure and is due to increased melanin synthesis and increased numbers of melanocytes.[1]
  - Long-term effects of chronic sun exposure include photoaging and photocarcinogenesis. The chronic inflammation induced by repetitive exposure to excessive UV radiation results in skin wrinkling, irregular skin pigmentation, and thickening of the skin that leads to a leathery appearance. The DNA damage induced by UV radiation is known to be important in the pathogenesis of skin cancer.[1,2]
- The UV index
  - The UV radiation level varies with latitude, altitude, time of day, and time of year. UV levels are higher at lower latitudes (closer to the equator), higher altitudes, during midday, and during summer months. Only a small fraction of UV light is filtered by clouds.[2]
  - The UV index (UVI) was developed as a tool to provide the public with an objective measure of UV radiation levels and raise awareness for the need to use sun protection (Table 14-1).[3]

Table 14-1	The UV Index	
	UV index	**Associated risk**
Low	0–2	No danger to the average person
Moderate	3–5	Little risk of harm from unprotected sun exposure
High	6–7	High risk of harm from unprotected sun exposure
Very High	8–10	Very high risk of harm from unprotected sun exposure
Extreme	11–14	Extreme risk of harm from unprotected sun exposure

The index is color coded to ease public recognition and facilitate inclusion of the index in weather forecasts.

- Rationale for use
  - UV radiation is a known carcinogen.[4] However, complete sun avoidance is neither always possible nor practical.
  - The development of both invasive melanoma and nonmelanoma skin cancers is clearly associated with exposure to UV radiation from the sun.[1–6] Sunburn at any age increases an individual's risk for skin cancer.[1,5]
  - Broad-spectrum sunscreens with at least SPF 15 have been proven to decrease the risk of actinic keratoses and squamous cell cancers.[1,3,7] There is limited evidence to support efficacy for prevention of BCC and melanoma. Regular sunscreen use also can prevent photoaging.[1,7]
- Mechanism of action
  - The active agents in sunscreen form a protective coating on the surface of the stratum corneum that attenuates UV radiation in one of two ways: reflection or absorption.
  - **Physical blockers** or "inorganic" sunscreens, such as zinc oxide or titanium dioxide, form a film of inert metal particles on the skin that reflect both UVA and UVB. Advances in nanotechnology have allowed for the development of micronized inorganic sunscreens, which are less opaque and more cosmetically acceptable.[1]
  - **Chemical absorbers** or "organic" sunscreens function as UV filters, which absorb the energy in UVA, UVB, or both; this energy is converted to a negligible amount of heat. The specific absorption spectrum of each chemical varies, and most sunscreens contain a combination of multiple chemical agents to provide broad-spectrum protection and act as stabilizing agents (Table 14-2).[1,7] Aminobenzoates, cinnamates, salicylates, octocrylene, and ensulizole provide protection against UVB, while benzophenones, avobenzone, ecamsule, and meradimate provide UVA protection.
- Sun protection factor
  - The **sun protection factor (SPF)** is a commonly used measure of efficacy for sunscreens. The SPF is the ratio of the minimal erythema dose (MED) of sunscreen-protected skin to the MED of unprotected skin.[1] It is expressed as a factor reflecting the relative amount of time skin can be exposed to sunlight without developing erythema, such that an SPF of 10 would allow 10 times as much time

Table 14-2	The Absorption Spectrum of Ingredients Commonly Used in Chemical and Physical Sunscreens

	Absorption spectrum	
Chemical absorbers	UVB	UVA
Benzophenones		
Dioxybenzone	×	
Oxybenzone	×	×
Sulisobenzone		×
Cinnamates		
Cinoxate	×	
Octinoxate	×	
Salicylates		
Homosalate	×	
Octisalate	×	
Trolamine salicylate	×	
PABA derivatives		
PABA (para-aminobenzoic acid)	×	
Padimate O	×	
Miscellaneous		
Avobenzone		×
Ecamsule		×
Ensulizole	×	
Meramidate		×
Octocrylene	×	
Physical blockers		
Titanium dioxide	×	×
Zinc oxide	×	×

in the sun with the same resultant erythema as would unprotected skin. This assumes perfect use with a thick application of at least 2 mg/cm^2. In reality, most people do not apply sunscreen according to this recommendation.[3,5]

- The SPF is related to the percentage of blocked erythemal radiation (Fig. 14-1). This relationship is nonlinear, such that a sunscreen with SPF 20 blocks 95% of erythemal radiation, while a sunscreen with SPF 40 blocks 97.5%.[1] Sunscreens with a higher SPF do not remain effective longer than do those with a lower SPF and still must be reapplied frequently.[3,6]

- Because UVB radiation is responsible for the erythema produced during a sunburn, **SPF only measures efficacy against UVB**. There is no standard to measure protection against UVA light, but there are in vitro assays utilizing spectrophotometry to calculate the percentage of UVA rays absorbed by a given chemical, as well as in vivo assays measuring either immediate or delayed skin pigment darkening.

- Safety
  - The first commercial sunscreen was developed in 1928. Sunscreens have been widely used since the 1970s and have an excellent safety profile.

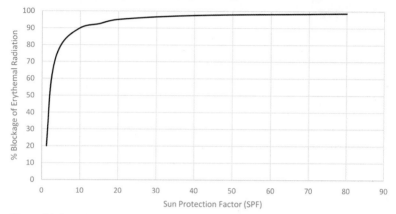

Figure 14-1. The relationship of SPF to the blockage of UVB radiation. This is a nonlinear relationship, and as SPF increases beyond 30, there is minimal added protection.

- The main risks associated with sunscreen use are **minor skin irritation**, which is common, and **allergic contact dermatitis**, which is rare.[1] The most common agents implicated in allergic contact dermatitis include the chemical absorbers oxybenzone, padimate O, and avobenzone. Sunscreens containing only physical blockers are available for patients who develop allergic reactions to one of these agents or for those who have sensitive skin that is prone to irritation.
- UV exposure stimulates vitamin D production in the skin. Casual sun exposure (5 to 15 minutes per day, 2 to 3 times per week) can provide enough vitamin D for most people. **Adequate vitamin D can safely be obtained via dietary sources** without exposure to the risks of UV radiation, and there is no clear evidence that regular sunscreen use causes vitamin D deficiency.[8]
- Regulation
  - Sunscreens are regulated by the Food and Drug Administration (FDA) as over-the-counter medications. In 2012, the FDA changed the labeling requirements for sunscreens. Any sunscreen marketed as **"broad spectrum"** has to pass tests proving efficacy against **both UVA and UVB**.[7]
  - Products that are not broad spectrum or that have SPF < 15 are labeled with a warning to caution that they only prevent sunburn and should not be used for the prevention of skin cancer or early skin aging.
  - Sunscreens can no longer be labeled as "waterproof" or "sweatproof." Sunscreens labeled as **"water resistant" and "very water resistant"** must pass a standardized test to assure they retain their protective effects after prolonged immersion of the skin in water for 40 minutes or 80 minutes, respectively.[7]
  - There is a labeling cap of SPF 50+ on sunscreens in the United States (US), as sunscreens greater than SPF 50 have not been proven to provide increased protection.
- Application
  - Patients, especially those with lighter skin types, should be counseled to use sunscreen on a daily basis.

- Sunscreen used for daily sun protection should be **broad spectrum and have an SPF of at least 15.** All areas of exposed skin should be covered with an adequate layer of sunscreen, including the face.
- **During outdoor activities with exposure to sunlight,** sunscreen should be used that has an **SPF of at least 30.** Sunscreen should be **reapplied every 2 hours,** and more frequently if skin is exposed to water (sweat, swimming). Sunscreen use should not be used with the aim of increasing the duration of sun exposure.

1.1. Sun Protective Clothing
- The UV protection factor
  - UV protection claims for clothing are rated according to the "**Ultraviolet Protection Factor (UPF),**" which is analogous to the SPF rating system for sunscreens. A UPF of 25 means that only 1/25th of UV radiation will pass through the fabric. While SPF only measures a sunscreen's efficacy against UVB radiation, UPF measures efficacy against both UVA and UVB rays.[3,6]
- Rationale for use
  - The UPF of clothing varies depending on several factors, and more protection is provided by tighter weaves, darker dyes, synthetic fabrics, and dry fabrics. Many clothing manufacturers have begun specifically developing and marketing UV-protective clothing. These fabrics have enhanced protection from UV light by virtue of either construction with a dense weave or dyeing with chemicals that function as UV filters.
  - While UV-protective clothing has undergone various standardized tests analyzing UV transmission through fabrics, it important to remember that unlabeled clothing also provides protection from UV light.[3]
  - Hats should have a brim wide enough to shade the entire face (typically >2 inches). The eyes are also vulnerable to UV-induced damage. Sunglasses should be chosen that provide broad-spectrum UV protection.[5]

1.2. Tanning Bed Use
- Risks associated with indoor tanning:
  - Indoor tanning increases the risk for developing both melanoma and nonmelanoma skin cancers. Risks appear to be dose and age dependent, with the youngest and most frequent users at highest risk.[9,10]
  - Any change in skin pigmentation is a sign of overexposure to UV light and resulting DNA damage. A "base tan" from indoor tanning correlates to only an SPF of 1 to 2, and a tan from outdoor tanning correlates to an SPF of 2 to 3.[1]
  - The U.S. Centers for Disease Control and Prevention (CDC) estimates that one in three Caucasian young adult women, the population at highest risk for future skin cancers, engage in indoor tanning each year.[11]
  - The average intensity of UV radiation from indoor tanning devices correlates to a UVI of 13 or 14 (extreme), which is up to five times the amount of UV exposure of natural light. The amount and type of UV radiation emitted varies widely between devices and often exceeds FDA recommended limits.[5]
  - In addition to increasing skin cancer risk, tanning beds carry additional risks including sunburns, damage to the eyes, and skin infections caused by exposure to improperly sanitized devices.
- Regulations
  - In 2009, the World Health Organization (WHO) classified indoor tanning beds as class 1 human carcinogens.[4,11] Many countries, including France, Spain,

Germany, Italy, Norway, and the United Kingdom, have subsequently banned the use of tanning beds for those under age 18. Australia and Brazil recently instituted total bans on indoor tanning for cosmetic purposes.

- In the United States, tanning bed restrictions have thus far been legislated on a state by state basis. As of 2014, 21 states have an age limit on tanning bed use. Some states have instituted limits on tanning bed frequency or tanning time limits.
- The FDA recently reclassified tanning bed devices from class I (low-risk) to class II (moderate-risk) devices.[12] Tanning beds must now carry a visible black box warning explicitly stating that the device should not be used by persons under 18 years of age.

- Alternatives to tanning bed use
  - **Sunless tanning lotions** contain dihydroxyacetone (DHA), a color additive that binds to the stratum corneum and colors the skin to produce a darkened appearance, which does not provide any additional protection against UV radiation. These lotions are **only FDA approved for external application**.
  - **Spray tanning** involves the use of DHA as a misting spray. There are insufficient safety data regarding DHA exposure to mucous membranes, periorbital surfaces, or inhalational exposure; therefore, use of DHA in this fashion is not FDA approved.
  - Pills containing large doses of canthaxanthin or other food color additives have been illegally marketed as "tanning pills" in the US. The dyes deposit in the skin, imparting a darker color. The dyes also deposit in other organs of the body, including the eyes, and retinopathy is a known side effect.
  - Injectable analogs of melanocyte-stimulating hormone, which increase melanogenesis, have been developed and illegally marketed in the last decade. Patients should be counseled that commercially marketed injections claiming to induce melanogenesis are unapproved and may be hazardous to their health.

- Counseling
  - All patients should be counseled regarding the dangers of excessive UV radiation and the importance of sun safety including sun avoidance, sunscreen, and the use of protective clothing.[1,3,5] The U.S. Preventive Services Task Force has specifically recommended that primary care physicians conduct a brief behavioral counseling intervention warning of the dangers of indoor tanning for those at highest risk: patients with fair skin aged 10 to 24 years.[13]
  - Some studies have suggested that counseling focused on the appearance-related side effects of sun exposure is more successful than are cancer prevention-focused messages.

REFERENCES

1. Bolognia JL, Jorizzo JL, Schaffer JV. *Dermatology*. 3rd ed. Philadelphia, PA: Elsevier Saunders; 2012.
2. Lucas R, McMichael M, Smith W, et al.; World Health Organization. *Solar ultraviolet radiation: Global burden of disease from solar ultraviolet radiation*. Geneva, Switzerland, 2006.
3. U.S. Environmental Protection Agency, Office of Air and Radiation. SunWise Program. http://www2.epa.gov/sunwise. Accessed online December 18, 2014.
4. International Agency for Research on Cancer Working Group on the Evaluation of Carcinogenic Risks to Humans, World Health Organization. Radiation. *IARC Monogr Eval Carcinog Risks Hum* 2012;100:7–303.

5. U.S. Department of Health and Human Services. *The surgeon general's call to action to prevent skin cancer.* Washington, DC: U.S. Department of Health and Human Services, Office of the Surgeon General; 2014.

6. Centers for Disease Control and Prevention. Skin cancer: sun safety. http://www.cdc.gov/cancer/skin/basic_info/sun-safety.htm. Accessed online December 18, 2014.

7. U.S. Food and Drug Administration, U.S. Department of Health and Human Services. Labeling and effectiveness testing; sunscreen drug products for over-the-counter human use. Final rule. *Fed Regist* 2011;76:35620–35665.

8. Ross AC, Taylor CL, Yaktine AL, et al.; Institute of Medicine (US). *Dietary reference intakes for calcium and vitamin D.* Washington, DC: National Academies Press (US); 2011.

9. Wehner MR, Shive ML, Chren MM, et al. Indoor tanning and non-melanoma skin cancer: systematic review and meta-analysis. *BMJ* 2012;345:5909.

10. Colantonio S, Bracken MB, Beecker J. The association of indoor tanning and melanoma in adults: systematic review and meta-analysis. *J Am Acad Dermatol* 2014;70:847–857.

11. Centers for Disease Control and Prevention (CDC). Use of indoor tanning devices by adults—United States, 2010. *MMWR Morb Mortal Wkly Rep* 2012;61:323–326.

12. Ernst A, Grimm A, Lim HW. Tanning lamps: health effects and reclassification by the Food and Drug Administration. *J Am Acad Dermatol* 2015;72:175–180.

13. Moyer VA; US Preventive Services Task Force. Behavioral counseling to prevent skin cancer: US Preventive Services Task Force recommendation statement. *Ann Intern Med* 2012;157:59–65.

15 Dermatologic Therapies

Kyle Eash, MD, PhD and Ian Hornstra, MD, PhD

Commonly encountered skin diseases encompass a broad etiologic spectrum including infectious, neoplastic, and autoimmune/inflammatory. Accordingly, a wide variety of classes of therapeutic agents are used in treating dermatologic disease. Given space limitations, only selected therapies that are commonly used, particularly notable, and/ or likely to be less familiar to the generalist practitioner will be discussed here. In particular, the reader should refer to outside sources for complete information on pharmacokinetics, contraindications, side effects, cautions in pregnant or breast-feeding patients, monitoring guidelines, and drug-drug interactions as these are beyond the scope of this chapter.[1-4] The reader is also referred to the sections of this manual on specific disease entities for additional therapeutic information.

The skin forms the body's interface with the external environment, which also makes it easily accessible for treatment with topical or intralesional therapies, modes of drug administration that are somewhat unique to dermatology. Sunscreens are a special category of topically applied compounds and are discussed in Chapter 14. Some disorders can also be treated with light-based therapies including photodynamic therapy, lasers, or phototherapy (see section 4 of this chapter). These modalities provide a concentrated, local therapeutic effect at the site of pathology without significant systemic absorption. Therefore, they often have a favorable side effect profile. Finally, some dermatoses do require systemically acting agents, which are administered via standard oral or parenteral routes.

1. TOPICAL THERAPY OVERVIEW

- Drugs formulated for transdermal administration can target localized skin disease via direct diffusion or the systemic circulation via dermal capillaries. The latter requires that the compound be of low molecular weight and lipophilic and exhibit efficacy at relatively low doses and/or serum concentrations. Because of these constraints, relatively few systemic agents are administered transdermally. Examples include clonidine, testosterone, estrogen, and fentanyl.
- As discussed in Chapter 2, the skin's barrier function is performed by the outermost layer of the epidermis, termed the cornified layer or stratum corneum. It forms a relatively impermeable barrier that prevents water and nutrient loss while effectively blocking entry of most external substances, including pharmaceuticals. The barrier is arranged in a "bricks and mortar" configuration comprising a protein-rich cellular component (keratinocytes or corneocytes) and a lipid-laden extracellular matrix. Topical delivery of drugs is accomplished by small amounts of diffusion through the stratum corneum. Therefore, compounds with the greatest bioavailability will be of low molecular weight and lipophilic.
- The majority of a topically applied drug remains on the skin surface because of poor absorption. This remaining drug is subject to loss from factors such as exfoliation, sweating, washing, rubbing, degradation, etc. Clinicians should be cognizant of this

fact when determining dosing interval and, in the case of superpotent glucocorticoids or topical chemotherapeutics, counseling about the potential for exposure of others (especially neonates) in the home environment.
- The rate of percutaneous absorption of a drug is proportional to the soluble concentration in the vehicle (C) and the partitioning coefficient (k). This partitioning coefficient k describes the ability of the drug to move out of the vehicle and into the stratum corneum. Both variables C and k are highly dependent on the particular vehicle in which the drug is delivered.

1.1. Vehicles
- Formulations include creams, ointments, lotions, gels, solutions, foams, and patches.
- Many specific components in vehicles enhance absorption via positive effects on solubility and/or partitioning. Examples of enhancers include ethanol and propylene glycol. Often, components that increase absorption come at a cost of increased risk of irritant or allergic side effects.
- The properties of the vehicle can have a marked effect on drug potency. Thus, a given pharmaceutical compound can have a wide range of potencies depending on its formulation. This is exemplified in the classification of glucocorticoids wherein the same drug can fall into several different potency classes depending on its concentration and vehicle, for example, cream versus ointment versus gel (Table 15-1).[5,6]
- In practice, ointments are generally more potent than are creams or lotions. Although nominally equipotent alternative formulations have been developed, the occlusion, hydration, and augmented barrier function provided by ointments makes them more clinically effective in most cases.
- Solutions or gels can be used on hair-bearing skin or for a drying effect, while creams, lotions, or foams rub in to the skin easily and may be preferred to greasy ointments by some patients.
- Alcohol-containing formulations should be avoided on fissured or eroded skin because they will cause stinging and pain in these instances.

1.2. Clinical Factors Affecting Drug Absorption
- The thickness and composition of the stratum corneum and thus drug absorption varies by body site and must be taken into account when administering topical therapy. A rough guideline in order from most to least permeable is scrotum/genital region, face/scalp/axillae, trunk/extremities, palms/soles, nails.
- Hydration of the skin via soaking or prolonged occlusion increases barrier permeability and, thus, drug delivery. Occlusion with impermeable or semipermeable material (plastic wrap, medical tape, cloth dressing, or old clothing) is a reliable and easy way to increase drug delivery and therefore efficacy. Aside from increased hydration, occlusion also prevents loss of yet-to-be absorbed drug from the skin surface.
- Skin folds (inguinal, gluteal, inframammary, and axillary regions) are naturally hydrated and occluded regions, and care should be taken to avoid potent formulations with the potential for overdosage and side effects in these areas (e.g., ointments, superpotent topical glucocorticoids).
- Drug absorption is increased in skin disorders that are characterized by impaired skin barrier function. A classic example is atopic dermatitis. In most cases, this is therapeutically advantageous. However, in disorders characterized by severe epidermal dysfunction (e.g., toxic epidermal necrolysis, congenital ichthyosis) or with the increased skin permeability of preterm infants, caution must be taken as uptake will be dramatically increased, possibly resulting in significant serum levels of drug.

Table 15-1	Potency Classification of Selected Topical Glucocorticosteroid Products		
Name	Trade name(s)	Vehicle(s)	Concentration (%)
Class 1 (superpotent)			
Betamethasone dipropionate, augmented	Diprolene	O, L, G	0.05
Clobetasol	Temovate, Clobex, Olux	O, C, L, G, F, Sh, Sol, Sp	0.05
Halobetasol	Ultravate	O, C	0.05
Fluocinonide	Vanos	C	0.1
Flurandrenolide	Cordran	Tape	4 mcg/cm^2
Diflorasone diacetate	Psorcon	O	0.05
Class 2 (potent)			
Betamethasone dipropionate	Diprolene AF, Diprosone	C, O	0.05
Halcinonide	Halog	O, C, Sol	0.1
Fluocinonide	Lidex	O, C, G, Sol	0.05
Desoximetasone	Topicort	O, C	0.25
Desoximetasone	Topicort	G	0.05
Class 3 (upper midstrength)			
Betamethasone dipropionate	Diprosone	C, L	0.05
Betamethasone valerate	Luxiq	F	0.12
Desoximetasone	Topicort LP	C	0.05
Diflorasone diacetate	Psorcon, Florone	C	0.05
Fluticasone propionate	Cutivate	O	0.005
Fluocinonide	Lidex-E	C	0.05
Mometasone furoate	Elocon	O	0.1
Triamcinolone acetonide	Kenalog, Aristocort, Triderm	O, C	0.5
Class 4 (midstrength)			
Clocortolone pivalate	Cloderm	C	0.1
Desoximetasone	Topicort E	C	0.25
Fluocinolone acetonide	Synalar	O	0.025
Flurandrenolide	Cordran	O	0.05
Hydrocortisone valerate	Westcort	O	0.2
Mometasone furoate	Elocon	C, L, Sol	0.1
Triamcinolone acetonide	Kenalog	O, C, Sp	0.1

Name	Trade name(s)	Vehicle(s)	Concentration (%)
Class 5 (lower midstrength)			
Betamethasone dipropionate	Diprosone	L	0.05
Betamethasone valerate	Beta-Val, Betatrex, Valisone	C	0.05
Desonide	DesOwen, Desonate	O, G	0.05
Fluocinolone acetonide	Synalar	C	0.025
Flurandrenolide	Cordran	C, L	0.05
Hydrocortisone butyrate	Locoid	O, C, L, Sol, Sp	0.1
Hydrocortisone valerate	Westcort	C	0.2
Prednicarbate	Dermatop	O, C	0.1
Triamcinolone acetonide	Kenalog	L, O	0.1, 0.025
Class 6 (mild)			
Alclometasone dipropionate	Aclovate	O,C	0.05
Betamethasone valerate	Beta-Val, Valisone	L	0.1
Desonide	DesOwen, Lokara, Verdeso	C, L, F	0.05
Fluocinolone acetonide	Synalar, Capex, Derma-Smoothe	C, Sol, Sh, Oil	0.01
Triamcinolone acetonide	Kenalog, Aristocort	C, L	0.025
Class 7 (least potent)			
Hydrocortisone	Hytone, Cortaid, Cortizone	O, C, L, Sol, Sp	2.5–0.5
Hydrocortisone acetate	Pramosone, Wellcortin	O, C, L, F	2.5–1.0

Abbreviations: O, ointment; C, cream; L, lotion; G, gel; F, foam; Sp, spray; Sol, solution, Sh, shampoo.
Data from Jacob SE, Steele T. Corticosteroid classes: a quick reference guide including patch test substances and cross-reactivity. *J Am Acad Dermatol* 2006;54(4):723–727; Tadicherla S, Ross K, Shenefelt PD, et al. Topical corticosteroids in dermatology. *J Drugs Dermatol* 2009;8(12):1093–1105.

1.3. Quantity of Application

The volume of medication is an important consideration, with respect to both the total volume to be dispensed to the patient for a given treatment area and duration and the amount used per application by the patient or caregiver. Although some formulas are discussed below as rough guidelines, in clinical practice, the actual amounts required can be quite variable.

Table 15-2   Dosing Estimates for Topical Therapy in Adults

Area/region	FTU	Flat hand areas	Single application (grams)	BID application × 1 week (g)
25 × 25 cm, 625 cm^2	2	4	1	14
Face and neck	2.5	5	1.25	17.5
Single arm, excluding hand	3.5	7	1.75	24.5
One hand, both sides	1.5	3	0.75	10.5
Trunk, one side (chest and abdomen or back)	6	12	3	42
Buttocks/groin	2	4	1	14
Single leg and thigh, excluding foot	6	12	3	42
One foot	2	4	1	14
Total body	**42.5**	**85**	**~21**	**~300**

Abbreviations: FTU, fingertip unit; BID, twice daily.
Data from Long CC, Finlay AY. The finger-tip unit—a new practical measure. *Clin Exp Dermatol* 1991;16(6):444–447; Long CC, Mills CM, Finlay AY. A practical guide to topical therapy in children. *Br J Dermatol* 1998;138(2):293–296.

- Medication should be applied in a thin layer not to exceed 0.1 mm in thickness.
- One "fingertip unit" (FTU) is the amount of ointment dispensed in a line from the distal crease to the tip of the index finger, is equivalent to 0.5 g, and can cover the area of two flat hands.
- Practically speaking then, a single application to one hand would require 0.5 g of medication, the face and neck 1.25 g, one arm 1.75 g, one leg 3 g, and either the front or back of the trunk 3 g. Therefore, once-daily application for 10 days' duration requires approximately a 15-g tube for the arm, hand, or face, but at least a 50-g tube for the leg or trunk.
- Total body application can vary from 20 to 100 g depending on patient characteristics, thickness of application, and preparation.
- Several studies have objectively quantified these parameters and provide a useful guide for dispensing and application of topical medications (Table 15-2).[7,8]

2. GLUCOCORTICOSTEROIDS

These are the most commonly prescribed anti-inflammatory medications in dermatology and medicine at large. They have efficacy in a large number of inflammatory dermatoses, but can have significant side effects, especially with long-term (>4 weeks) therapy. Accordingly, they come in a wide variety of formulations and routes of administration.

2.1. Mechanism of Action

These drugs are various modifications of the four-ring cholesterol-based structure of the endogenous hormone cortisol. They bind to the glucocorticoid receptor, a cytosolic hormone receptor, which then translocates to the nucleus and modifies the transcription of a wide variety of genes involved in inflammation. They also interact with other key inflammatory transcription factors. Glucocorticosteroids (CS) can also exert direct effects without receptor binding. The end result is decreased levels of proinflammatory molecules including cytokines and prostaglandins and decreased activation, cell number, and localization of most inflammatory cells including neutrophils, eosinophils, and lymphocytes.

2.2. Hypothalamic-Pituitary-Adrenal (HPA) Axis

The HPA axis controls the production of cortisol by the adrenal glands. Peak secretion of cortisol occurs in the morning. CS suppress the adrenal production of cortisol via negative feedback. Generally, morning dosing is used to minimize HPA suppression. Split (twice daily) dosing can be used to increase efficacy at a cost of increased side effects. A dose of 5 mg/d of prednisone approximates physiologic levels of cortisol. Three weeks or less treatment duration is considered short-term therapy; in these cases, adrenal function is usually sufficiently preserved so that tapering is not required from an adrenal recovery standpoint.

2.3. Pharmacology

CS are readily orally bioavailable, with peak plasma levels 30 to 90 minutes after administration and wide tissue distribution. They are bound to serum proteins, so free levels are increased in the setting of low serum proteins as can be seen in liver or kidney disease. Additionally, some CS (hydrocortisone and prednisolone) require functioning hepatic enzymes for conversion to their active metabolites. Because they are hormonally and transcriptionally mediated, the effects of CS persist for some time after the drug has been metabolized.

2.4. Topical and Intralesional Therapy

Principles of topical therapy are discussed in in section 1 of this chapter.
- **Indications/use.** Include but are not limited to psoriasis, various forms of dermatitis including contact, atopic, stasis, and seborrheic (Chapter 3), urticaria and drug eruptions (Chapter 5), vitiligo (Chapter 6), alopecia areata (Chapter 9), and autoimmune/connective tissue disease including discoid lupus (Chapter 10).[9]
- **Dosing.** Topical CS (TCS) are divided into seven potency classes based on topical vasoconstrictor assays and objective clinical activity (Table 15-1).[5,6]
  - The clinician should choose the potency based on type, severity, extent, and location. Preparations are applied up to twice daily, although daily application may be sufficient.
  - The least potent agent that is expected to achieve a response should be chosen, and the potency and/or frequency of application should be tapered as rapidly as possible while still maintaining a response.
  - *Intralesional* **triamcinolone acetonide** in concentrations ranging from 2 to 40 mg/mL diluted in saline can be administered via 30-gauge needle directly into the dermis, thus bypassing the need for cutaneous absorption and delivering a higher concentration of CS directly to the site of pathology. This therapy is generally administered by a dermatologist and reserved for deeper, thicker, and/or more severe disease processes.
- **Therapeutic considerations**
  - Agents of potency class 3 or greater should generally be avoided in pediatric patients.
  - TCS are very safe in general; serious or important adverse effects are rare and typically involve exceedingly long-term use or gross misapplication of the medication.

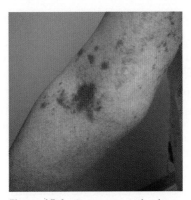

Figure 15-1. Cutaneous atrophy due to topical corticosteroid use. Close-up of the right antecubital fossa shows decreased pigmentation; thin, translucent skin; and prominent blood vessels. (Courtesy Milan J. Anadkat, MD.)

- High-potency formulations should be avoided when treating large areas, as some systemic absorption can occur.
- Common side effects with *short-term* use including mild itching, burning, redness, and stinging that are usually transient. More rarely, true urticaria, irritant contact dermatitis, or allergic contact dermatitis can develop (Chapters 3 and 5). Allergy can develop to vehicle components or the CS molecule itself.
- **Desoximetasone (Topicort)** is in a distinct structural class from other topical steroids. It is sometimes used in cases where TCS allergy is suspected based on the theory that there is a decreased chance of allergic cross-reactivity.
- The most common and important side effect with prolonged (more than 2 to 3 weeks) therapy is **cutaneous atrophy** (Fig. 15-1). Clinically, atrophy is characterized by thin, lax, shiny, wrinkled skin, often with easy bruising (purpura), lightening or darkening of the skin (pigmentary changes/dyspigmentation), prominently visible small blood vessels (telangiectasias), and, in severe cases, ulceration.
- Rebound upon discontinuation of TCS and loss of efficacy to ongoing treatment (tachyphylaxis) are known to occur. A related disorder known as **perioral dermatitis** (Fig. 15-2) occurs on the face after prolonged or potent TCS exposure. Its clinical appearance can have features of acne rosacea and/or atopic dermatitis (Chapter 3). The treatment for perioral dermatitis is discontinuation of TCS and use of a topical calcineurin inhibitor (TCI) and/or tetracycline class antibiotics if needed.
- An infectious etiology, particularly superficial fungal species such as **candida** or **tinea** (Chapter 4), should be considered in eruptions that worsen or recur with TCS therapy.

2.5. Systemic Therapy

- **Indications/use.** Severe dermatitis (Chapter 3), urticaria, drug eruptions (Chapter 5), and a number of systemic diseases with skin manifestations including

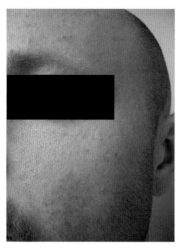

Figure 15-2. Perioral dermatitis. This disorder occurs on the face in the setting of topical steroid use and is characterized by redness, acne-like papules, and eczema-like scaling and flaking. (Courtesy Milan J. Anadkat, MD.)

vasculitis, sarcoidosis, lupus erythematosus, dermatomyositis, scleroderma, and bullous diseases (Chapter 10).

- **Dosing.** Prednisone is readily available and can be easily titrated and tapered. A relatively standard dose would be 40 to 60 mg/d (0.5 to 1 mg/kg) tapered over a 2- to 4-week period, initially in intervals of 20 mg and then in 10 mg, 5 mg, or even lower amounts as the dose is lowered (see HPA above). Generally, cutaneous inflammatory disease does not respond satisfactorily to lower doses or shorter courses of CS, and some diagnoses require prolonged or chronic therapy in the case of bullous or autoimmune disease, respectively.
- **Therapeutic considerations**
  - Short-term therapy for acute dermatoses such as contact dermatitis, drug eruptions, or urticarial is generally safe and well tolerated.
  - Adverse effects with even short-term therapy include mood changes, insomnia, increased appetite and weight gain, fluid retention, hypertension, insulin resistance, and poor wound healing.
  - Systemic fungal infection is a contraindication to therapy. Risk of infection of all types is increased in patients on systemic CS.
  - With prolonged therapy, patients are at risk for a number of serious adverse events that can affect multiple body systems. These side effects are a major limitation on the use of CS and include osteoporosis, osteonecrosis, growth retardation, myopathy, cataracts, glaucoma, peptic ulcer disease, intestinal perforation, hyperglycemia, obesity, hypertension, atherosclerosis, adrenal suppression including adrenal crisis, mood changes, and psychosis.
  - Cutaneous findings in patients on CS therapy are distinctive and include atrophy, purpura, striae, hirsutism, and acne.

- Vitamin D and calcium supplementation at standard doses (1.5 g and 800 to 1,000 U, respectively) is easy to implement and should be recommended to all patients on systemic CS.
- For patients expected to be on >3 months duration of therapy, an assessment of osteoporotic fracture risk should be performed including baseline bone mineral densitometry via DEXA scan. Since the greatest bone loss occurs in the first 6 months of therapy, bisphosphonate therapy should be initiated promptly.

3. RETINOIDS

These compounds are structural and functional analogues of vitamin A. Endogenous retinoids (vitamin A and its derivatives) function in embryonic development and in proliferation, differentiation, and maintenance of various epithelial surfaces. They have a key role in the epidermis and its various appendages; thus, synthetic retinoids, with the exception of ATRA (all *trans* retinoic acid) for a rare subtype of leukemia, are almost exclusively utilized for a number of dermatologic disorders.

3.1. Mechanism of Action

Both endogenous and synthetic retinoid compounds exert a diverse set of effects on epithelial and immune cells in the skin including decreased inflammation, promotion of apoptosis, decreased tumor formation, decreased keratinization, alterations in the extracellular matrix, and decreased sebum production. A complete understanding of the cellular and molecular basis of these effects is lacking, but it is known that retinoids bind RAR and/or RXR nuclear hormone receptors, which then induce a complex transcriptional program that is then responsible, at least in part, for the observed effects.

3.2. Pharmacology and Teratogenicity

- Retinoids are lipophilic compounds. They are orally bioavailable on the order of 25% to 60%, and, although not required, absorption is increased by administration with a fat-containing meal. Topical retinoids have minimal systemic absorption. Systemic retinoids are metabolized in the liver and excreted via biliary and renal routes.
- Retinoids are extremely potent teratogens. There is no known minimal safe level of retinoid compounds during pregnancy. Exposure, especially during the first trimester when organogenesis occurs, may lead to craniofacial, cardiovascular, CNS, and limb anomalies that result in abortion, preterm birth, or perinatal death.
- These drugs are therefore absolutely contraindicated in pregnancy, lactation, and patients attempting to conceive. Topicals range from category C to X, while all systemic retinoids are category X. Patients of childbearing potential should be counseled about these risks, and appropriate contraceptive measures and serial serum pregnancy tests are required before, during, and after therapy. Contraception and documentation of negative pregnancy status is performed for 1 month prior to initiation of therapy, monthly during therapy, and for at least 1 month after therapy.
- The elimination half-life of retinoids is variable, from 1 hour to 120 days. Prolonged elimination is due to the lipophilic nature of the compound and resulting depot storage in adipose tissue. Because of this property, patients on acitretin (but not other retinoids) must undergo contraception for 2 to 3 years after cessation of therapy.

- Although the theoretical systemic exposure and therefore teratogenic risk is much lower, topical retinoids are also avoided during pregnancy and lactation. Similarly, retinoid therapy in the male partner of a female who is pregnant or attempting to become pregnant should be avoided.

3.3. Topical Retinoid Compounds

Topical retinoid compounds in common dermatologic use include **tretinoin (Retin-A)**, **adapalene (Differin)**, and **tazarotene (Tazorac)**. They all act via binding the RAR receptor. They are all available in gel and cream formulations, with some also available in lotion or solution format.

- **Indications/use.** The most common indication for the use of a topical retinoid is inflammatory or comedonal acne vulgaris (Chapter 3). They are first-line treatment for this common disorder. The other indication the general practitioner should be aware of is the use of topical retinoids (including low-potency, over-the-counter, vitamin A cosmeceutical products) for cosmetic benefit in the treatment of photoaging.
- **Dosing.** A small amount of medication should be applied in a thin layer to dry skin nightly or every other night. Maximal efficacy is not evident until 1 to 2 months of therapy.
- **Therapeutic considerations.** Aside from the risk of teratogenicity discussed above, the major side effect of topical retinoids is skin irritation, also known as retinoid dermatitis. Moisturizing lotions and sunscreens can decrease the irritation. Patients should be encouraged to continue treatment through mild irritation because after approximately 1 month, it generally improves as the skin develops tolerance to the medication. For severe irritation, decreased concentration, frequency, and/or duration of application may be necessary.
- **Bexarotene** gel acts via the RXR receptor and is used topically to treat early-stage CTCL (cutaneous T-cell lymphoma; see Chapter 8).

3.4. Systemic Retinoid Drugs

Systemic retinoid drugs include isotretinoin, acitretin, and bexarotene. Isotretinoin binds the RAR receptor, while acitretin only weakly interacts with retinoid receptors, yet exerts significant activation of these receptors and their pathways.

- **Isotretinoin (Accutane)** is the mainstay of treatment for severe, scarring, or recalcitrant acne vulgaris. It is the only agent known to induce long-term remission in the disease. This may be related to the fact that it is the only retinoid that decreases sebum production.
  - **Dosing.** Generally 0.5 to 1.0 mg/kg/d. Both disease flares and the most severe cutaneous side effects are often seen in the first month of therapy; therefore, half-strength doses are often used initially. In practice, patients are usually started at between 20 and 40 mg daily and titrated to a maximal dose of 40 to 80 mg. A total dose of 120 mg/kg is recommended to achieve sustained remission, corresponding to a typical duration of treatment of 4 to 6 months.
  - **Therapeutic considerations.** Isotretinoin is regulated by the government-mandated iPLEDGE program, primarily because of the combination of its teratogenicity and frequent use in young females of childbearing age. Patients, providers, and pharmacies must be enrolled before the medication can be dispensed. The program and its website (www.ipledgeprogram.com) formalize and document the functions of obtaining consent, monitoring pregnancy avoidance measures, and

confirming nonpregnant status via HCG testing. In addition to its teratogenicity and dermatitis side effects, the other common and important side effects of isotretinoin therapy are myalgias and arthralgias and elevations in lipid levels and liver enzymes. All are generally self-limited with discontinuation or dose reduction; chronic hepatitis, liver failure, and pancreatitis are exceedingly rare complications. The laboratory parameters (AST, ALT, total cholesterol, triglycerides) should be monitored at the initiation of and at regular intervals during therapy.

- **Acitretin (Soriatane)** is a treatment option for psoriasis. An additional indication is severe hand eczema. It is particularly effective in the erythrodermic or pustular variants (as opposed to plaque type) of psoriasis. Effective doses are between 25 and 75 mg (~0.5 to 1.0 mg/kg) daily, although patients are often started at 10 mg daily to minimize the initial worsening of disease that often occurs. Side effects and their management are as noted above.

- **Bexarotene (Targretin)** at initial doses of 150 mg/m² titrated to 300 mg/m² daily is FDA approved for the treatment of CTCL, but doses as low as 75 mg can be effective. Additional side effects not previously noted above include hypothyroidism, leukopenia, and agranulocytosis. Patients on therapy require thyroid hormone replacement and lipid-lowering treatment.

4. PHOTOTHERAPY

A number of dermatologic disorders have been known for years to respond to ultraviolet (UV) radiation. More recent advances have moved from using broad-spectrum light to highly specific wavelengths of the UV spectrum. The UV spectrum is between 200 and 400 nm and can be divided, from shortest to longest wavelength, into UVC (200 to 290 nm), UVB (290 to 320 nm), UVA2 (320 to 340 nm), and UVA1 (340 to 400 nm). Two common and important types of light-based therapies in dermatology are narrow band UVB (NBUVB), which uses high-intensity UV radiation limited to 311 to 313 nm, and photochemotherapy with psoralens plus UVA (PUVA).

4.1. Determining Response to UV Radiation

In the phototherapy setting and general clinical practice, dermatologists often determine a given patient's intrinsic photosensitivity, reflecting not only pigmentation levels but also other genetic factors. This can be done with Fitzpatrick skin phototyping, which utilizes a clinical scale based on pigmentation and response to sunlight ranging from one to six (Table 15-3). A more objective assessment can be obtained with phototesting, where small areas of normally covered skin are exposed to a range of UV doses to determine a minimal erythema dose (MED). Erythema is assessed at its peak, 24 hours after UVB exposure. In general, light-based dermatologic therapies are contraindicated in patients with known history of a photosensitizing disorder or genetic susceptibility to UV-induced carcinogenesis.

4.2. NBUVB

- **Mechanism of action.** UV light is absorbed by DNA, forming DNA photoproducts (primarily pyrimidine dimers). This induces p53 and causes cell cycle arrest or apoptosis, thus decreasing epidermal or immune cell proliferation. UVB also alters cytokine expression patterns (in both DNA damage–dependent and DNA

Table 15-3	Skin Phototypes (Fitzpatrick Scale)			
Skin type	Unexposed skin color	Burn	Tan	Associated features
I	White	Always	Never	Blue or green eyes, red or blond hair, freckles
II	White	Easily/ usually	Minimal/ difficult	Variable
III	White to beige	Sometimes/ mild	Average/ gradually	Variable
IV	Beige to light brown	Rarely	Easily	Variable
V	Dark brown	Extremely rare	Very easy/ dark	Variable
VI	Black	Never	Very easy/ dark	Dark brown eyes, dark brown or black hair

From Fitzpatrick TB. The validity and practicality of sun-reactive skin types I through VI. *Arch Dermatol* 1988;124(6):869–871.

damage–independent mechanisms) and causes associated immunosuppressive and anti-inflammatory effects.

- **Indications/use.** NBUVB is used to treat psoriasis, atopic dermatitis (Chapter 3), pruritus, vitiligo (Chapter 6), and CTCL (Chapter 8).
- **Dosing.** Patients are typically treated three times per week initially until remission or maximal improvement is achieved. Dose (ranging from 200 to 1,200 mJ/cm^2) is initially determined based on phototesting or phototyping and then increased in standard increments until persistent asymptomatic erythema is obtained. Treatment is paused and resumed at lower doses if painful erythema develops. After maximal response is achieved, maintenance therapy of twice and then once weekly treatments is continued for several months.
- **Therapeutic considerations.** Maximal response may not be evident until after 6 to 8 weeks of therapy (18 to 24 treatments). The major adverse effect is phototoxicity. Treatment compliance and/or availability is primarily hampered by the need for frequent office visits. UV carcinogenesis (Chapters 8 and 14) is a concern, but the risk appears to be quite low for NBUVB as opposed to sunlight exposure, tanning beds, broadband UVB, or PUVA.[10]

4.3. PUVA

In this treatment, patients are given a photosensitizing agent (psoralens), which absorbs light at 330 to 335 nm. The skin is then exposed to UVA radiation with peak emission at 352 nm. This combination produces a therapeutically beneficial phototoxic effect. Psoralens are a family of plant-derived compounds, several of which have been used for PUVA therapy.

- **Mechanism of action.** When activated by UV radiation, psoralens cross-link DNA, leading to cell cycle arrest and decreased cellular proliferation. It also forms

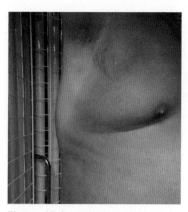

Figure 15-3. PUVA-induced hyperpigmentation. A patient on chronic therapy for CTCL demonstrates the characteristic dark, orange-hued pigmentation of a "PUVA tan." Once the pigmentation develops, the skin disease becomes less responsive (hardened) to equivalent doses of light. (Caroline Mann, MD and Pat Cashel-Lee, LPN.)

reactive oxygen species. Via these and other as yet undetermined pathways, keratinocyte and lymphocyte apoptosis occurs with resulting normalization of keratinocyte differentiation and decreased inflammation.

- **Indications/use.** Psoriasis (Chapter 3) and CTCL (Chapter 8). With the advent of new systemic therapies, the use of PUVA in psoriasis has greatly decreased because of equivalent efficacy and a better side effect profile.
- **Dosing.** 8-methoxypsoralens (8-MOP) 0.6 to 0.8 mg/kg is administered 1 to 3 hours prior to UVA exposure ranging from 0.5 to 5 J/cm² as determined by phototyping. Psoralens are also available via bath or topical applications. Treatments are 2 to 4 times per week during the initial clearing phase followed by maintenance treatments at decreased frequency. In contrast to NBUVB, erythema from PUVA peaks at 72 hours after treatment. Thus, dose increases are never more frequent than every 3 days.
- **Therapeutic considerations.** PUVA is carcinogenic, and patients are at an increased risk of cutaneous squamous cell carcinoma. Otherwise, the major side effects are nausea with oral psoralens, phototoxicity during treatment, and cumulative photodamage. PUVA induces melanogenesis and a distinctive increase in skin pigmentation (Fig. 15-3) to a greater degree than do other sources of UV light.

5. SELECTED ANTIMICROBIALS

The skin is a common site of a wide variety of infections and infestations (Chapter 4). The reader is referred to more detailed dermatologic or infectious disease texts for details of treatment,[1,4] although general principles of treatment should be already familiar to most generalist practitioners. However, several unique situations where antimicrobials are utilized in dermatology merit comment here.

5.1. Superficial Skin Infections

Folliculitis, minor wounds, paronychia, and impetigo (Chapter 4) may be amenable to topical treatment only. Clindamycin, erythromycin, gentamicin, mupirocin, and polymyxin B/neomycin/bacitracin are readily available in topical formulations. They can be applied to the affected areas of skin 2 to 4 times per day and are generally well tolerated without side effects. Gentamicin has activity where pseudomonal or other Gram-negative species may be a concern. Mupirocin has good activity against methicillin-resistant *Staphylococcus aureus* (MRSA).

5.2. Acne

The pathogenesis of acne (Chapter 3) is complex, with aseptic inflammation, sebum production, hormonal influences, and *Propionibacterium acnes* and other commensal bacteria all playing a role.

- Several topical and oral antibiotics are efficacious in the treatment of both acne vulgaris and acne rosacea because of their anti-inflammatory and antibacterial properties.
- Topical formulations of azelaic acid, benzoyl peroxide, clindamycin, and dapsone are effective in treating mild to moderate inflammatory acne. Of note, benzoyl peroxide–containing washes and gels do not require a prescription and have at least partial efficacy for most types and severity of acne. The major limitation to use of benzoyl peroxide is irritation and the fact that the compound will bleach clothing.
- Topical metronidazole and sodium sulfacetamide are first-line treatments for acne rosacea.
- For more severe inflammatory acne, oral tetracycline antibiotics are used. Doxycycline and minocycline at doses from 50 to 200 mg/d are both very effective at controlling acne. In contrast to isotretinoin, they unfortunately do not alter the natural history of the disease.
- Despite causing more gastrointestinal upset, doxycycline is preferred in most cases because of the risk of cutaneous hyperpigmentation and rare reports of severe drug reactions with minocycline therapy.

5.3. Atopic Dermatitis

Some dermatologic disorders are characterized by the propensity for chronic or periodic superinfection or overgrowth with *S. aureus* bacteria naturally present on the skin.

- Atopic dermatitis (Chapter 3) is the prototype for this phenomenon, but any clinical state with altered epidermal barrier function is susceptible. A more novel but growing population of these susceptible patients are those treated with targeted EGFRi (epidermal growth factor receptor inhibitor) chemotherapy for epithelial-derived malignancies.
- *S. aureus* overgrowth contributes to worsening of atopic dermatitis, and often, patients will require prolonged (1 month or more), repeated, or chronic antistaphylococcal antibiotic therapy. Skin swab culture to confirm infection and facilitate identification of susceptibility profile should always be performed prior to initiating therapy.

- Cephalosporins such as cephalexin 500 mg 2 to 3 times per day are used for methicillin-sensitive strains, while resistant strains are typically treated with trimethoprim/sulfamethoxazole 800/160 mg once or twice daily. Clindamycins and tetracyclins are other orally available anti-staphylococcal antibiotics.
- In this patient population, decontamination methods such as dilute bleach baths, mupirocin to nares and fingernails, or antibiotic washes such as chlorhexidine can also be helpful.

6. TOPICAL IMMUNOMODULATORS AND CHEMOTHERAPEUTICS

6.1. Topical Calcineurin Inhibitors (TCIs)

These drugs are nonsteroidal anti-inflammatory agents. They are a "steroid-sparing" option for treating steroid-responsive dermatoses such as atopic dermatitis and other inflammatory skin disorders. Calcineurin inhibitors avoid the main side effect of TCS, cutaneous atrophy. Thus, they are particularly useful around the eyes, on the face, or on the genital and intertriginous areas.

- **Mechanism of action.** These drugs bind to FK506 binding protein, interacting with calcineurin and preventing the dephosphorylation of the transcription factor NFAT and transcription of inflammatory cytokines.
- **Indications/use.** Atopic dermatitis, eyelid dermatitis, seborrheic dermatitis, perioral dermatitis, psoriasis, vitiligo (Chapters 3 and 6).
- **Dosing. Pimecrolimus (Elidel)** is supplied as a 1% cream, and **tacrolimus (Protopic)** is available as a 0.1% or 0.03% ointment. Both can be applied 1 to 2 times per day.
- **Therapeutic considerations.** The most common side effect that leads some patients to discontinue use is burning and stinging at the application site. Caution is advised in the setting of herpes virus (HSV or VZV) infection.

6.2. Imiquimod (Aldara)

This drug is a topical immune activating agent used in the treatment of viral (Chapter 4) or neoplastic (Chapter 8) lesions.

- **Mechanism of action.** Imiquimod stimulates antiviral and antitumor immune responses via activation of toll-like receptor 7 (TLR7), resulting in increased cytokines and cell-mediated immunity.
- **Indications/use.** It is first-line therapy for anogenital HPV infection (genital warts). It is also an effective option for treating superficial cutaneous malignancies, namely, actinic keratosis (AK), superficial basal cell carcinoma (sBCC), and squamous cell carcinoma in situ (SCCIS), should these lesions not be good candidates for destructive or excisional therapies (Chapters 8 and 11).
- **Dosing.** Imiquimod is supplied as a 5% or 3.75% cream. Warts and AK are treated with thrice weekly application for up to 16 weeks, while malignancies (sBCC or SCCIS) are treated five times per week for 6 weeks or more as tolerated.
- **Therapeutic considerations.** Patients should be counseled that irritation and inflammation is expected and desired at the treatment site (Fig. 15-4). Therapy can be discontinued or interrupted prior to the prescribed time period if excessive inflammation develops. In these cases, it is likely that the tumor or infection has

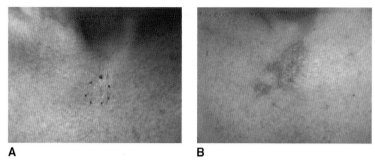

A   **B**

Figure 15-4. Inflammatory response in an sBCC treated with imiquimod. Before (**A**) and after (**B**) 7 weeks of treatment. (Courtesy Milan J. Anadkat, MD.)

cleared and the patient only needs to be observed at regular intervals for any sign of clinical persistence or recurrence after the inflammation has subsided.

6.3. 5-Fluorouracil (5-FU, Efudex)

This drug is a topical chemotherapeutic agent useful in the treatment of viral, premalignant, or malignant skin lesions (Fig. 15-5).

- **Mechanism of action.** 5-FU is a pyrimidine analog that blocks DNA synthesis and causes DNA breakage, leading to selective apoptosis of rapidly dividing and/ or malignant cells.
- **Indications/use.** This therapy is extremely useful for "field treatment" of patients with numerous actinic keratoses and areas of extensively UV-damaged skin where actinic keratoses are likely to arise but are not yet clinically evident. It is an alternative to the destructive or physical methods (cryotherapy or photodynamic therapy) discussed in Chapter 11. Similar to imiquimod, 5-FU is a topical treatment option for cutaneous or genital warts, superficial BCC, and SCCIS as well (Chapters 4 and 8).
- **Dosing.** The drug is supplied in a cream or solution at several concentrations. We typically use the 5% cream applied twice daily for 2 weeks for treatment of AK and up to 6 weeks for treatment of BCC or SCCIS.

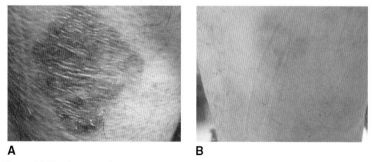

A   **B**

Figure 15-5. Clearance of SCCIS after treatment with 5-fluorouracil. Before (**A**) and after (**B**) 6 weeks of treatment. (Courtesy Milan J. Anadkat, MD.)

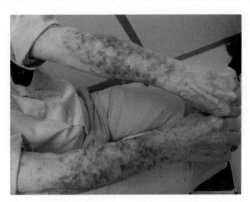

Figure 15-6. Inflammatory response to 2 weeks of 5-fluorouracil treatment of actinic keratosis of the arms.

- **Therapeutic considerations.** Again similar to imiquimod, 5-FU typically induces a marked inflammatory response characterized by variable degrees of erythema, pain, swelling, and crusting followed by eventual re-epithelialization (Fig. 15-6). The inflammation is related to the degree of actinic damage and underlying keratinocyte dysplasia and is a marker of therapeutic efficacy. Early cessation of therapy because of pronounced inflammation is acceptable and likely still results in significantly effective treatment. Patients should be assessed for persistent or recurrent lesions once the treated area has normalized. Topical 5-FU is pregnancy category X.

7. SYSTEMIC IMMUNOSUPPRESSIVE AND IMMUNOMODULATORY AGENTS

Many inflammatory and/or autoimmune skin disorders require systemic treatments. Prototypical examples include psoriasis (Chapter 3) and lupus (Chapter 10), respectively, but there are a great many additional diseases and therapies of interest to the dermatologic specialist that are beyond the scope of this manual. Commonly used therapies for this broad group of disorders include hydroxychloroquine, cyclosporine, azathioprine, mycophenolate mofetil, dapsone, methotrexate, and biologics. This last category refers to a wide variety of biomolecules including proteins, receptors, or antibodies that specifically target specific immune and/or cell signaling pathways. The development of biologics has only been possible because of recent technologic advances in molecular biology. These agents represent a profound leap forward in therapy for a wide variety of dermatologic and nondermatologic systemic autoimmune, inflammatory, and neoplastic diseases. Drugs in common use in dermatology and their targets include rituximab (Rituxan, CD20, B cells), ustekinumab (Stelara, IL-12/IL-23, T cells), omalizumab (Xolair, IgE, mast cells), anakinra (Kineret, IL-1) and the antitumor necrosis factor α (anti-TNF) agents etanercept, adalimumab, and infliximab that target dendritic cells, neutrophils, and IL-17–secreting T cells. Common first-line systemic treatments for plaque psoriasis will be discussed here; the reader is referred to additional resources for complete information.[1,2]

7.1. Methotrexate

- **Mechanism of action.** The drug exerts its anti-inflammatory effect by decreasing immune cell proliferation. It blocks key enzymes required for nucleotide synthesis and thus inhibits DNA replication and cell division.
- **Indications/use.** Methotrexate is a steroid-sparing immunosuppressive agent FDA approved for treatment of severe, debilitating, or recalcitrant psoriasis (Chapter 3). Additional indications include CTCL (Chapter 8), dermatomyositis, systemic sclerosis, and other glucocorticoid-responsive dermatoses (Chapter 10).
- **Dosing.** Supplied in 2.5-mg tablets, methotrexate is given orally once weekly and titrated to clinical response. Standard doses are between 10 and 25 mg. To decrease toxicity, we generally prescribe all patients 1-mg folic acid tablets to be taken daily except on the day of methotrexate administration. It is also available in parenteral (intramuscular or intravenous) formulations.
- **Therapeutic considerations.** A number of adverse effects are possible with methotrexate therapy; thus, patients should be selected, counseled, and monitored appropriately.
    - GI toxicity (oral ulcers, nausea, vomiting) is common and reduced with folate supplementation and/or parenteral administration.
    - Serious hematologic toxicity in the form of pancytopenia can occur even early in the course of therapy and at low doses. This can be potentiated by other drugs that inhibit folate metabolism; common examples are dapsone or trimethoprim/sulfamethoxazole.
    - There is a risk of hepatotoxicity in the form of cirrhosis and fibrosis; it is increased with cumulative dose and duration of therapy and/or additional hepatic insults such as chronic hepatitis, current or former alcohol use, or other pre-existing liver disease. Patients should be tested for hepatitis virus infection prior to initiating therapy.
    - The need for screening liver biopsy is no longer absolutely recommended; it can be determined by patient risk factors and consultation with a hepatologist.
    - Methotrexate is renally cleared, and drug levels may be elevated in patients with chronic kidney disease.
    - Complete blood count (CBC) and assessment of hepatic and renal function (CMP) should be performed at regular intervals (no less frequent that monthly with changes in dose and every 3 to 4 months when on a stable dose).
    - Methotrexate is an abortifacient and teratogen. Its use is contraindicated in pregnant or lactating patients. Reliable contraception and serum pregnancy testing are required.
    - The risk of infection is increased with therapy, and caution should be exercised in patients with active infection or additional underlying immunosuppressive conditions. Consideration should be given to HIV testing prior to initiating therapy.

7.2. Anti-TNF Agents

- **Mechanism of action.** These drugs bind to soluble or membrane bound TNF-α, thus blocking signaling and inducing apoptosis with resulting decrease in downstream inflammatory cytokines (IL-17, IL-22, IL-23) and cell types (dendritic cells, macrophages, neutrophils, Th17, and Th22 T cells).[11]
- **Indications/use.** Severe psoriasis or psoriatic arthritis (Chapter 3). Also approved for rheumatoid arthritis, juvenile idiopathic arthritis, and inflammatory bowel

disease (adalimumab and infliximab). A number of off-label dermatologic uses have been reported, including cutaneous lupus, dermatomyositis, and sarcoidosis (Chapter 10).

- **Dosing. Etanercept (Enbrel)** is a fusion protein of the TNF receptor and IgG. It is available in 25-mg or 50-mg syringes for subcutaneous administration. Standard dosing is 50 mg twice weekly for the first 3 months and then once weekly thereafter, but 25 mg twice weekly or an initial dose of only 50 mg weekly can also be used. **Adalimumab (Humira)** is a fully human monoclonal antibody directed against TNF. Standard maintenance dosing is 40 mg subcutaneous every 2 weeks. Frequency can be increased to weekly for recalcitrant disease, and at the initiation of therapy, higher and more frequent doses are given (i.e., first dose of 80 mg followed by 40 mg 1 week later). **Infliximab (Remicade)** is a mouse-human chimeric anti-TNF antibody. It is administered intravenously at 5 mg/kg, initially at weeks 0, 2, and 6 and then every 8 weeks, although the dose frequency and level can be adjusted up to 10 mg/kg to achieve a satisfactory response.
- **Therapeutic considerations.** Given their efficacy, TNF inhibitors have a favorable side effect profile compared to traditional, nonbiologic immunosuppressives. Serious infections are the most important adverse effect.
  - Patients are particularly susceptible to tuberculosis (TB) infection. Therefore, baseline and annual monitoring of TB infection status is required for all patients on therapy and can be accomplished via testing of the skin (PPD test), serum (Quantiferon or T-SPOT interferon-γ release assays), or lungs (chest x-ray).
  - Other reported adverse effects are the development of malignancy including melanoma and other skin cancers or lymphoma, heart failure, multiple sclerosis, or lupus-like autoimmune disease.
  - Hepatitis B reactivation has occurred, but patients with hepatitis C can often be successfully treated.
  - Infusion reactions and/or hypersensitivity can occur. In the case of infliximab, these can be managed with slow infusion rates and premedication.
  - Development of antidrug antibodies with concomitant loss of efficacy, particularly with infliximab, can be managed with concurrent low-dose immunosuppression with corticosteroids, azathioprine, or methotrexate.
  - Anti-TNF agents are category B, so they can be used if necessary in pregnant patients.
  - Baseline assessment of blood counts, electrolytes, kidney function, liver function, hepatitis serology, and TB status should be obtained prior to starting therapy. HIV status should also be assessed in at-risk individuals.

7.3. Vaccination

If feasible, clinicians should attempt to have patients up-to-date on vaccinations prior to initiating immunosuppressive therapy.[12] Live vaccines should be given at least 6 weeks prior to therapy, while inactivated vaccines are given up to 2 weeks prior to treatment. Inactivated vaccines can be given while on therapy, but the immunologic response and resulting immunity may be suboptimal. Live vaccines are contraindicated in immunosuppressed patients including those on TNF inhibitors. Common live vaccines to avoid include varicella, herpes zoster, intranasal flu, and MMR. Other live vaccines sometimes given to select populations include BCG, smallpox, and yellow fever.

REFERENCES

1. Bolognia J, Jorizzo J, Schaffer JV, eds. *Dermatology*. 3rd ed. Philadelphia, PA: Elsevier/Saunders; 2012.
2. Wolverton SE, ed. *Comprehensive dermatologic drug therapy*. 3rd ed. Edinburgh, UK: Saunders/Elsevier; 2013.
3. Mann MW, Berk DR, Popkin DL, et al. *Handbook of dermatology: a practical manual*. Chichester, UK: Wiley; 2009.
4. Saag MS, Eliopoulos GM, Chambers HF, et al., eds. *Sanford Guide to Antimicrobial Therapy 2014*. 44th ed. Sperryville, VA: Antimicrobial Therapy; 2014.
5. Jacob SE, Steele T. Corticosteroid classes: a quick reference guide including patch test substances and cross-reactivity. *J Am Acad Dermatol* 2006;54(4):723–727.
6. Tadicherla S, Ross K, Shenefelt PD, et al. Topical corticosteroids in dermatology. *J Drugs Dermatol* 2009;8(12):1093–1105.
7. Long CC, Finlay AY. The finger-tip unit—a new practical measure. *Clin Exp Dermatol* 1991;16(6):444–447.
8. Long CC, Mills CM, Finlay AY. A practical guide to topical therapy in children. *Br J Dermatol* 1998;138(2):293–296.
9. Drake LA, Dinehart SM, Farmer ER, et al. Guidelines of care for the use of topical glucocorticosteroids. American Academy of Dermatology. *J Am Acad Dermatol* 1996;35(4):615–619.
10. Hearn RMR, Kerr AC, Rahim KF, et al. Incidence of skin cancers in 3867 patients treated with narrow-band ultraviolet B phototherapy. *Br J Dermatol* 2008;159(4):931–935.
11. Lynde CW, Poulin Y, Vender R, et al. Interleukin 17A: toward a new understanding of psoriasis pathogenesis. *J Am Acad Dermatol* 2014;71(1):141–150.
12. Chirch LM, Cataline PR, Dieckhaus KD, et al. Proactive infectious disease approach to dermatologic patients who are taking tumor necrosis factor-alfa antagonists: Part II. Screening for patients on tumor necrosis factor-alfa antagonists. *J Am Acad Dermatol* 2014;71(1):11.e1–e7; quiz 18–20.

16 Differential Diagnoses Tables

Jamie L. Mull, MD and M. Laurin Council, MD

Table 16-1	Differential Diagnosis by Primary Lesion

Macules and Patches

Macular hyperpigmentation

Acanthosis nigricans	Associated with insulin resistance and obesity
Café au lait spots	Multiple seen in neurofibromatosis
Drug-induced hyperpigmentation	May be seen with minocycline, clofazimine, amiodarone
Ephelides (freckles)	Become more pronounced with UV exposure
Fixed drug eruption	Recurs at same location upon drug rechallenge
Hemochromatosis	"Bronze diabetes" secondary to iron deposition
Junctional melanocytic nevus	Flat, generally darker in color compared to intradermal nevi
Lentigines	Multiple perioral seen in Peutz-Jeghers syndrome
Melanoma in situ	Early melanoma, a subtype is known as lentigo maligna
Melasma	F > M; associated with pregnancy, OCPs, UV exposure
Mongolian spot	Congenital blue/gray patch on lumbar region
Postinflammatory hyperpigmentation	More common in darker skin types
Stasis dermatitis	Common on lower legs; may cause pruritus

Macular hypopigmentation/depigmentation

Albinism	Associated with ocular abnormalities
Lichen sclerosus et atrophicus	Affects genitalia causing dyspareunia, scarring, and SCC
Postinflammatory hypopigmentation	Seen with seborrheic dermatitis, atopic dermatitis
Tuberous sclerosis (ash leaf macule)	Other findings: mental retardation, seizures, shagreen patch, ungual fibromas, and facial angiofibromas
Vitiligo	Autoimmune; often periorificial

Papules and Plaques

Inflammatory

Acne rosacea	Erythematous papules and pustules with facial erythema
Acne vulgaris	Multifactorial; more severe in males
Arthropod bites	Pruritic, often clustered

Contact dermatitis	Itching or burning rash in distribution of exposure to allergen
Discoid lupus	"Carpet-tack" scale
Drug eruption	May occur weeks to months after starting offending agent
Erythema multiforme	"Target lesions" with three zones
Folliculitis	Red follicular-based pustules
Granuloma annulare	Annular papules and plaques
Keratosis pilaris	Commonly located on extensor surface of upper arms
Lichen planus	Polygonal pruritic papules
Morphea	Sclerotic plaques; may cause significant disability
Mycosis fungoides	May present as chronic dermatitis
Necrobiosis lipoidica diabeticorum	Associated with diabetes mellitus
Pityriasis rosea	"Christmas tree" distribution following skin cleavage lines
Psoriasis	Auspitz sign—pinpoint bleeding with removal of scale
Sarcoidosis	Noncaseating granulomas on histology
Seborrheic dermatitis	Hypersensitivity to Malassezia species
Urticaria (hives)	No single lesion lasts >24 h.
Vasculitis	Etiologies include drug-induced, autoimmune, infectious

Infectious

Deep fungal infection	More common in immunocompromised
Folliculitis	Commonly caused by *Staphylococcus aureus*
Molluscum contagiosum	Poxvirus infection, common in children
Necrotizing fasciitis	STAT surgical consult
Scabies	Burrows in the interdigital web spaces
Tinea	"If it's scaly, scrape it"
Verruca vulgaris	Caused by human papillomavirus
Viral exanthema	Often nonspecific

Growths and neoplasms

Acrochordons	"Skin tags" often on neck, axilla
Actinic keratosis	May progress to SCC
Basal cell carcinoma	Most common primary skin cancer
Dermal melanocytic nevus	Monitor for atypical nevi with "ABCDEs"—asymmetry, border irregularity, color irregularity, diameter >6 mm, and evolving
Dermatofibroma	Dimple sign with lateral opposing pressure
Kaposi sarcoma	Associated with HHV-8; classic and AIDS-related types
Malignant melanoma	Familial forms associated with pancreatic cancer
Neurofibroma	Multiple seen in neurofibromatosis; buttonhole sign
Pyogenic granuloma	Common in children and pregnant women

continued on following page

Sebaceous hyperplasia	Yellow papule with central dell
Seborrheic keratosis	"Stuck-on" appearing
Squamous cell carcinoma	Marjolin ulcer in sites of chronic inflammation or scarring

Nodules and Tumors

Malignant

Basal cell carcinoma	Pearly papule with telangiectasia; "rodent ulcer"
Cutaneous metastasis	Breast cancer and melanoma are most common causes.
Kaposi sarcoma	Classic form seen in elderly men of Ashkenazi Jewish or Mediterranean origin
Leukemia cutis	Most commonly AML
Malignant melanoma	Prognosis related to tumor depth
Mycosis fungoides	Patch, plaque, and tumor stages
Sarcoma	Primary cutaneous or metastatic; examples include leiomyosarcoma, dermatofibrosarcoma protuberans
Squamous cell carcinoma	Increased risk in immunosuppressed, that is, transplant patients

Benign

Abscess	Recurrent in chronic granulomatous disease
Deep fungal infection	Opportunistic infections include aspergillosis and Cryptococcosis
Epidermal inclusion cyst	Overlying central punctum
Erythema nodosum	Associated with sarcoid, infection, inflammatory bowel disease
Furuncle	Deeper form of folliculitis
Gouty tophus	Uric acid crystals are negatively birefringent under polarized light microscopy.
Keloid	May be seen on earlobe after piercing
Lipoma	Soft mobile subcutaneous mass
Polyarteritis nodosa	Cutaneous and systemic forms; associated with hepatitis B
Rheumatoid nodule	Overlying bony prominences, especially the elbows
Sarcoidosis	Associated with bilateral pulmonary lymphadenopathy
Tuberculosis	Primary inoculation may lead to painless TB chancre.

Vesicles and Bullae

Arthropod bites	Exuberant reactions seen in adults with hematologic malignancy
Behçet disease	"Ocular-oral-genital" syndrome with oral and genital ulcerations, posterior uveitis
Bullous pemphigoid	Subepidermal autoimmune blistering disorder; antibodies to the hemidesmosome

Burn	*Pseudomonas* is the most common cause of secondary infection
Contact dermatitis	Vesicular in acute stage
Dermatitis herpetiformis	Associated with celiac disease/gluten sensitivity
Herpes simplex	Grouped, on an erythematous base
Pemphigus vulgaris	Intraepidermal flaccid bullae; severe mucosal involvement
Porphyria cutanea tarda	Hypertrichosis, milia, and scarring in sun-exposed areas
Stevens-Johnson syndrome/toxic epidermal necrolysis	SJS <10% BSA, TEN >30% BSA
Varicella/zoster	"Dew drop on a rose petal" appearance

Pustules

Acne rosacea	Commonly affects fair-skinned adults; no comedones
Acne vulgaris	1st-line treatments: topical and oral antibiotics and retinoids
Candidiasis	Yeast and pseudohyphae on microscopy
Cellulitis	Risk factor includes tinea pedis, providing portal of entry
Folliculitis	Infectious, drug induced, or idiopathic
Gonococcemia	Disseminated infection more common in menstruating women and patients with complement deficiency
Impetigo	"Honey-colored" crust
Pustular psoriasis	May be triggered by rapid tapering of corticosteroids
Tinea	Confirm diagnosis with KOH preparation of skin scraping

Ulcers

Arterial insufficiency	Preceding claudication, diminished peripheral pulses, hair loss of the extremity
Bacterial infection	Syphilis, anthrax, etc.
Cutaneous malignancy	For example, "rodent ulcer" of BCC
Deep fungal infection	Causes include histoplasmosis, coccidioidomycosis, and blastomycosis
Factitial	Look for bizarrely shaped lesions
Pyoderma gangrenosum	Raised undermined border; cribriform scarring
Venous insufficiency	"Stasis ulcer"; common near medial malleolus

Purpura

Actinic purpura	Blood vessel fragility
Coagulopathies	Rule out protein C or S deficiency, antiphospholipid antibody syndrome
Livedo reticularis	Reticular or "net-like" pattern; possible underlying coagulopathy
Thrombocytopenia	Macular petechial eruption
Vasculitis	"Palpable purpura" in leukocytoclastic vasculitis, that is, HSP

OCPs, oral contraceptive pills; SCC, squamous cell carcinoma.

Table 16-2	Differential Diagnosis by Morphologic Groups

Annular

Discoid lupus	Heals with atrophic scarring and dyspigmentation
Granuloma annulare	Unknown etiology; commonly located on extremities
Necrobiosis lipoidica diabeticorum	Often located pretibial region
Nummular eczema	"Coin shaped"; often on lower legs
Tinea	"Leading scale"

Atrophic

Lichen sclerosus et atrophicus	Idiopathic, autoimmune; more common in women
Morphea	En coup de sabre—linear form involving forehead of children
Scleroderma	Systemic findings: lung, renal, gastrointestinal, cardiac
Striae	"Stretch marks"

Papulosquamous

Atopic dermatitis	Severely pruritic; lichenification (accentuation of skin lines)
Contact dermatitis	Confirm diagnosis with patch testing
Pityriasis rosea	Suspected viral etiology; self-resolving
Psoriasis	Genetic predisposition; association with arthritis
Seborrheic dermatitis	Affects scalp, glabella, nasolabial folds, chest
Subacute lupus erythematosus	Photodistributed, scaly polycyclic plaques
Syphilis	May resemble pityriasis rosea
Tinea corporis	Most common cause: *Trichophyton rubrum*

Morbilliform

Acute hepatitis	Also associated with vasculitides, lichen planus, porphyria cutanea tarda
Acute HIV (acute retroviral infection)	Associated flu-like symptoms
Drug eruption	Occurs in EBV mononucleosis treated with ampicillin
Kawasaki disease	Fever, conjunctivitis, "strawberry tongue," LAD, desquamation
Measles	Cephalocaudal progression
Other viral infections	May have associated fever and upper respiratory or gastrointestinal symptoms
Secondary syphilis	Involvement of the palms and soles

Alopecia

  Scarring

Discoid lupus	5% to 15% risk of developing systemic lupus erythematosus
Malignancy	Secondary to cutaneous metastases, CTCL

Nonscarring

Alopecia areata	Autoimmune; "exclamation-point hairs"
Anagen effluvium	Triggered by chemotherapy
Androgenic alopecia	Common in men and women
Malnutrition	Flag sign—alternating bands of pigment along hair shaft
Secondary syphilis	"Moth-eaten" appearance
Telogen effluvium	Begins months after a physiologic or emotional stressor
Thyroid disorders	Hypothyroidism also associated with dry, brittle hair
Tinea capitis	Most common cause in United States: *Trichophyton tonsurans*
Trichotillomania	Bizarre, often geometric-shaped patterns of hair loss

Vascular

Angioma	"Cherry angiomas" common finding in adults
Vasculitis	Rule out systemic disease
Telangiectasia	Multiple seen in hereditary hemorrhagic telangiectasia (Osler-Weber-Rendu)

Erythema

Localized erythema

Acral erythema of chemotherapy	Painful; "hand-foot syndrome"
Acute lupus erythematosus	Malar rash sparing the nasolabial folds
Cellulitis	Most commonly caused by *Streptococcus pyogenes* or *S. aureus*
Dermatomyositis	"Heliotrope" eyelid eruption, shawl sign
Erythema chronicum migrans	Lyme disease; "bulls-eye" expanding lesion
Erythema multiforme	Often recurrent, triggered by infection (HSV) or drug
Urticaria (hives)	Pruritic; wheel and flare

Diffuse erythema

Carcinoid syndrome	Flushing, diarrhea, and bronchospasm; workup for malignancy
Contact dermatitis	Causes include poison ivy and nickel
Drug rash with eosinophilia and systemic symptoms (DRESS)	Associated with facial edema, elevated liver enzymes; Common causes: anticonvulsants, sulfa
Graft versus host disease	Acute and chronic presentations; follows bone marrow transplant
Necrolytic migratory erythema	Glucagonoma

continued on following page

Photosensitivity/photo-toxic drug eruption	Causes include doxycycline, sulfa, diuretics
Psoriasis	May occur in setting of previous plaque psoriasis
"Red man" syndrome	From vancomycin infusion
Scarlet fever	Group A Strep infection; "strawberry tongue"
Sézary syndrome	Erythroderma, circulating Sézary cells, lymphadenopathy
Staph scalded skin syndrome (SSSS)	Toxin mediated; noncutaneous primary focus of infection
Stevens-Johnson syndrome/ toxic epidermal necrolysis	Causative drugs include sulfa, anticonvulsants, allopurinol.
Toxic shock syndrome	Due to Staph or Strep; also see mucosal hyperemia

EBV, Epstein-Barr virus; LAD, lymphadenopathy; CTCL, cutaneous T-cell lymphoma; HSV, herpes simplex virus.

Table 16-3   **Differential Diagnosis by Anatomical Region**

Oral Mucosa

Amyloidosis	Macroglossia; apple green birefringence with Congo red stain under polarized light microscopy
Aphthous ulcers	May be recurrent; etiology unknown
Behçet disease	Recurrent oral and genital ulcerations; ocular findings
Cicatricial pemphigoid	Subepidermal autoimmune bullous disorder; also ocular involvement
Candidiasis	"Thrush"; mucosal plaques are easily scraped away.
Crohn disease	May also see fissures of the perianal skin
Drug-induced stomatitis	Especially chemotherapeutics, for example, methotrexate
Erythema multiforme	Mucosal involvement in EM major; no progression to TEN
Hand-foot-and-mouth disease	Oral ulcerations in addition to palm/sole involvement
Herpes simplex	Recurrences usually localized to vermilion border
Leukoplakia	May progress to SCC
Lichen planus	Reticular, lacy white plaques
Mucocele	Secondary to salivary gland rupture
Oral hairy leukoplakia	Lateral tongue; associated with EBV in HIV+
Pemphigus vulgaris	Oral ulcerations; autoantibodies to desmosomal (intercellular) proteins
Syphilis	Syphilitic chancre in primary disease; mucous patches in secondary disease
Squamous cell carcinoma	Risk factors include smoking, HPV infection

| Stevens-Johnson syndrome | Mucosal involvement is a hallmark feature |
| Systemic lupus erythematosus | Oral ulceration is a diagnostic criterion for SLE |

Palms and Soles

Dyshidrotic eczema	Pruritic; commonly affects hands of adults
Erythema multiforme	May prevent recurrence with prophylactic HSV therapy
Hand, foot, and mouth disease	Vesicular eruption, nail changes
Keratoderma blenorrhagicum of reactive arthritis	May see uveitis, urethritis, arthritis—"Can't see, can't pee, can't climb a tree"
Palmoplantar psoriasis	Pustular or scaly erythematous plaques
Raynaud phenomenon	"White, blue, then red" color change; digital ulceration
Rocky mountain spotted fever	Petechiae begin on wrists and ankles
Secondary syphilis	Copper-colored papules and plaques
Tinea manuum and pedis	Most commonly affects interdigital web spaces of toes
Verrucae	Cause interruption of skin lines

Scalp

Acne keloidalis nuchae	More common in African American men
Alopecia	Scarring forms are permanent, resulting in loss of follicular ostia
Cyst	May become inflamed, painful, and enlarged
Discoid lupus	Scarring alopecia
Folliculitis	Often pruritic
Metastases	Often associated with alopecia
Psoriasis	Commonly located on the scalp, elbows, and knees
Seborrheic dermatitis	Severe in patients with HIV and Parkinson disease
Tinea capitis	Scaly patches of hair loss

Nails

Lichen planus	Other commonly affected locations include the volar wrists, oral mucosa, and genitalia
Onychomycosis	Most common cause: *T. rubrum*
Paronychia	Acute often due to Staph or Strep; chronic due to *Candida*
Pseudomonas infection	Green discoloration of the nail plate
Psoriasis	Nail pitting, onycholysis (lifting of the nail plate)
Trauma	May result from cuticle destruction

Intertriginous

Acanthosis nigricans	Velvety hyperpigmentation of the skin folds
Hidradenitis suppurativa	Exacerbated by obesity, smoking
Intertrigo	Commonly exacerbated by *Candida*

continued on following page

Groin/Genitalia

Sexually transmitted infections

Chancroid	Painful genital ulcer; due to *Haemophilus ducreyi*
Granuloma inguinale	Vegetative ulcerations; due to *Klebsiella granulomatis*
Herpes simplex	More commonly HSV-2; risk of CNS involvement
Lymphogranuloma venereum	Painful draining lymph nodes; due to *Chlamydia trachomatis*
Molluscum contagiosum	More severe in AIDS
Syphilis	Painless chancre (primary); condyloma lata (secondary)

Others

Balanitis circinata of reactive arthritis	HLA-B27 haplotype
Behçet disease	May also see arthritis, erythema nodosum
Condyloma acuminata	HPV infection; verrucous moist plaques
Extramammary Paget's disease	"Strawberries and cream" appearance
Hidradenitis suppurativa	Chronic abscesses and draining sinus tracts
Intertrigo	Multifactorial; also seen under breasts, pannus, and other skin folds
Lichen planus	Association with hepatitis C
Lichen sclerosus et atrophicus	Monitor for development of SCC
Psoriasis	May involve the penis and scrotum
Scabies	Penile and scrotal involvement is common
Squamous cell carcinoma	Risk factors include HPV infection, lichen sclerosus
Tinea cruris	Involvement of crural folds; generally spares scrotum

EM, erythema multiforme; SCC, squamous cell carcinoma; EBV, Epstein-Barr virus; SLE, systemic lupus erythematosus; HSV, herpes simplex virus.

Table 16-4	Pediatric Differential Diagnosis

Growths and Neoplasms

Capillary malformation (port wine stain)	Often segmental; seen in Sturge-Weber syndrome
Congenital melanocytic nevus	Except for "bathing trunk nevi," low risk of melanoma
Infantile hemangioma	Spontaneously involute; rule out visual or laryngeal obstruction, systemic involvement
Pyogenic granuloma	Rapidly growing, bleeds easily
Spider angioma	Telangiectasia, common on face
Spitz nevus	Despite generally benign clinical course in children, complete excision recommended

Inflamatory

Atopic dermatitis	Associated with asthma, allergic rhinitis
Dermatomyositis	"Gottron's papules," "mechanic's hands"
Diaper dermatitis	Irritant dermatitis spares the folds.
Erythema toxicum neonatorum	Common finding in neonates; spontaneous resolution
Henoch-Schönlein purpura	"Palpable purpura," renal disease, intussusception
Kawasaki disease	Treat with aspirin to prevent coronary artery aneurysms
Neonatal lupus	Associated with maternal anti-Ro antibodies
Psoriasis	May be triggered by Group A Strep infection
Seborrheic dermatitis	"Cradle cap" in infantile form
Transient neonatal pustular melanosis	More common in darker skin types; resolves with hyperpigmentation

Infectious

Candida diaper dermatitis	Surrounding satellite lesions
Erysipelas	Group A Strep; raised, sharply demarcated border
Erythema infectiosum	Fifth disease; parvovirus B19
Erythema marginatum	Rheumatic fever; Diagnosis made with Jones Criteria
Extramedullary hematopoiesis	"Blueberry muffin baby"; congenital TORCH infections
Hand, foot, and mouth disease	Most commonly caused by coxsackievirus A16
Herpes simplex	Primary infections generally more severe
Impetigo	Most commonly caused by *S. aureus*
Lice (pediculosis)	Nits firmly attached to hair shaft
Measles	Cough, coryza, conjunctivitis, Koplik spots
Molluscum contagiosum	Dome-shaped umbilicated papules
Rubella	"German measles"; "blueberry muffin baby" in congenital rubella syndrome
Scabies	Diffuse crusted scabies in immunocompromised
Scarlet fever	Sandpaper-like texture; resolves with desquamation
Staph scalded skin syndrome (SSSS)	Flaccid bullae, positive Nikolsky sign
Tinea	Human-to-human and animal-to-human transmission
Varicella/zoster	"Chickenpox" as primary infection, "shingles" as recurrence
Verruca vulgaris	May spontaneously remit over months to years

Genodermatoses

Marfan syndrome	Upward lens dislocation, risk of aortic dissection
Neurofibromatosis	Neurofibromas, café au lait spots, optic gliomas, Lisch nodules, CNS tumors
Sturge-Weber syndrome	Tram-track sign on imaging suggestive of leptomeningeal involvement
Tuberous sclerosis	Autosomal dominant; mutation in tuberin and hamartin

Index

Note: Italicized *f* and *t* refer to figures and tables